Improving Health Service Delivery in Developing Countries

Improving Health Service Delivery in Developing Countries

From Evidence to Action

Editors
David H. Peters
Sameh El-Saharty
Banafsheh Siadat
Katja Janovsky
Marko Vujicic

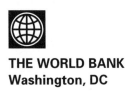

THE WORLD BANK
Washington, DC

1818 H Street NW
Washington DC 20433
Telephone: 202-473-1000
Internet: www.worldbank.org
E-mail: feedback@worldbank.org

ISBN: 978-0-8213-7888-5
eISBN: 978-0-8213-7943-1
DOI: 10.1596/978-0-8213-7888-5

Cover photo: © World Bank/Tran Thi Hoa

Library of Congress Cataloging-in-Publication Data

Improving health service delivery in developing countries : from evidence to action / edited by David H. Peters ... [et al.].
    p. ; cm. — (Directions in development)
    Includes bibliographical references and index.
    ISBN 978-0-8213-7888-5 (alk. paper)
    1. Medical care—Developing countries. 2. Public health—Developing countries. 3. Health services accessibility—Developing countries. I. Peters, David H., 1962- II. World Bank III. Series: Directions in development (Washington, D.C.)
    [DNLM: 1. Delivery of Health Care. 2. Developing Countries. 3. Evaluation Studies as Topic. 4. Health Services. 5. Outcome and Process Assessment (Health Care) WA 395 I343 2009]

    RA441.5.I47 2009
    362.109172'4—dc22

                                                                    2009008335

Contents

John Ovretveit, Banafsheh Siadat, David H. Peters,
Anil Thota, and Sameh El-Saharty

**Chapter 2   Review of Strategies to Strengthen the
Performance of Health Organizations   69**
*Anbrasi Edward, David H. Peters, Amy Daniels,
Yong Rang, and Toru Matsubayashi*

**Chapter 3   Review of Strategies to Improve Health Care
Provider Performance   101**
*Alexander K. Rowe, Samantha Y. Rowe,
Marko Vujicic, Dennis Ross-Degnan, John Chalker,
Kathleen A. Holloway, and David H. Peters*

Boxes

Figures

Tables

setting international targets for health services and offers an alternative based on each country's experience.

This book helps us think beyond what can be learned from the simpler, reproducible, and controlled interventions that are commonly described in research but are less applicable in practice. It demonstrates how a better understanding of implementation processes—the "how to"—is a crucial complement to the evidence addressing which health intervention should be selected. By better recognizing how context matters—how enabling and inhibiting factors influence even the most standardized or well-intentioned health strategy—the book points a way for managers and decision makers to deal with the complexities they regularly face. Chapter 6 outlines a way of thinking of the institutional factors that influence the delivery of health services, which should be helpful for analysts, managers, and policy makers. In chapter 8, the book describes how strategies were developed and implemented in the context of seven country case studies.

The World Bank does not emerge untouched in this analysis. Chapter 7 highlights how little attention has been paid, in the evaluation of World Bank–assisted projects, to measuring changes in health services, health financing, or health outcomes, even though such measuring pinpoints important markers of a project's success. A recent 10-year review of the Health, Nutrition, and Population operations and analytical work within the World Bank clearly recommends that much more emphasis and resources need to be focused on monitoring and evaluation. With the recent launch of such initiatives as the International Health Partnership, the High Level Taskforce on Innovative International Finance for Health Systems, and Health Results Based Financing for Millennium Development Goals Four and Five, the World Bank is committed to supporting results and the necessary monitoring capacity in countries.

The messages emerging from this book are clear and hopeful: there are many ways to improve health services. Measuring change and using information to guide decisions and inform stakeholders are critically important factors for successful implementation. The consistent lack of information on how the poor are affected by health strategies is disturbing, yet remediable. It is a call to continually focus on how strategies affect poor and vulnerable populations and to measure their results. It is also important to involve key stakeholders and institutions in seeking ways to improve health services, since it is not sufficient for governments, researchers, or professionals to work on their own or to ignore the important roles played by households and civil society organizations. A brighter future involves learning and doing through a collaborative and informed approach to implementing strategies for improving health services.

Acknowledgments

This book was prepared by a core team consisting of David Peters, Sameh El-Saharty, Banafsheh Siadat, Katja Janovsky, and Marko Vujicic. We are grateful for the generous funding support of the Netherlands government through the World Bank–Netherlands Partnership Program.

Background papers were prepared for this book by John Ovretveit, David Peters, Banafsheh Siadat, and Anil Thota (*Strengthening Health Services in Low Income Countries: Lessons from a Review of Research*); Gerry Bloom, Hilary Standing, and Anu Joshi (*Institutional Arrangements and Health Service Delivery in Low Income Countries*); Laura Morlock (*Issues in the Design and Conduct of Country Case Studies: Toward an Analytic Approach*); Savitha Subramanian, David Peters, and Jeffrey Willis (*How Are Health Services, Financing and Status Evaluated?*); Toshihiko Hasegawa, Leizel Lagrada, Atsushi Koshio, Tomoko Kodama, Yashushi Shimada, and Norio Yamada (*Evaluation of Health Services Delivery Based on Millennium Development Goals*); Toru Matsubayashi, Toshihiko Hasegawa, David Peters, Koshio Atsuchi, and Leizel Lagrada (*A Longitudinal Analysis of Trends in Health Services in Low and Middle Income Countries*); Alex Rowe, Samantha Rowe, John Chalker, Kathy Holloway, David Peters, Dennis Ross-Degnan, and Marko Vujicic (*Preliminary Results of a Systematic Review of the Effectiveness and Costs of Strategies to Improve Health Care Provider Performance and Related Health*

Outcomes in Low- and Middle-Income Countries); Bahie Rassekh and Nathanial Segaren (*A Systematic Review of Community Empowerment Strategies in Low and Middle Income Countries Globally*); and Anbrasi Edward, David Peters, Rong Yang, Amie Daniels, and Toru Matsubayashi (*A Systematic Review of Health Organization Performance in Low and Middle Income Countries*). Country case studies were prepared by Stephanie Simmonds, Ferozuddin Feroz, and Banafsheh Siadat (Afghanistan); Sameh El-Saharty, Sosena Kebede, and Petros Olango (Ethiopia); David Peters and Jessica St. John (Ghana); Laurence Lannes, Banafsheh Siadat, Miche Kibera, Jacky Mathonnat, and Agnes Soucat (Rwanda); Katja Janovsky, Phyllida Travis, and Banafsheh Siadat (Uganda); Joseph Capun and Kelechi Ohiri (Vietnam); and John Ovretveit and Nathaniel Segaran (Zambia). Advice and support for the country cases were provided by numerous World Bank staff, including Benjamin Loevinsohn (Afghanistan); Mukesh Chawla (Ethiopia); Laura Rose (Ghana); Agnes Soucat (Rwanda); Peter Okwero and Julie McLaughlin (Uganda); Sandy Lieberman (Vietnam); Rosemary Sunkutu and Monique Vledder (Zambia); and Christopher Walker.

Many people participated in the systematic reviews, including many who tirelessly assessed research papers and abstracted data: Charity Akpala, Aneesa Arur, Adrijana Corluka, Amy Daniels, Onnalee Gomez, Karen Herman, Quin Li, Constance Liu, Toru Matsubayashi, Dawn Osterholt, Bahie Rassekh, Alex Rowe, Samantha Rowe, Nathaniel Segaren, Nirali Shah, Jeffrey Willis, Karen Wosje, and Rong Yang.

The team was guided by many people along the way, including a core set of advisors including Tonia Marek, Joseph Naimoli, John Ovretveit (Karolinska Institute), Finn Schleimann, and Agnes Soucat. The work was initiated with guidance on study selection and design by Cristian Baeza, Paolo Belli, Peter Berman, Jonathan Brown, Jan Bultman, Karen Cavenaugh (USAID), Shiyan Chao, Dominique Egger (WHO), Jean Jacques Frere, Paul Gertler, Dave Gwatkin, Eva Jarawan, Kei Kawabata, Kees Kostermans, Magnus Lindelow, Katherine Marshall, Tawhid Nawaz, Ok Pannenborg, Khama Rogo, Jean-Jacques de St. Antoine, George Schieber, Finn Schleimann (then DANIDA), Agnes Soucat, Phyllida Travis (WHO), Abdo Yazbeck, and Feng Zhao. Helpful comments on drafts of the book were received from Mukesh Chawla, Aissatou Diack, Ariel Fiszbein, Pablo Gottret, Kathy Holloway (WHO), Jack Langenbrunner, Benjamin Loevinsohn, Julie McLaughlin, Sebastian Martinez, George Schieber, Agnes Soucat, Phyllida Travis (WHO), and Feng Zhao. Superb editing support was provided by Jonathan Aspin.

About the Editors

David H. Peters has worked in health systems as a researcher, policy advisor, educator, bureaucrat, manager, and clinician in more than 20 developing countries over the last two decades. His work concerns the performance of health systems and how they affect disadvantaged populations. It has also involved examining such issues as innovations in organization, technology, and financing, as well as the role of health-related markets. While at the World Bank, he worked in the Africa and South Asia Regions, as well as the network hub for health, nutrition, and population, helping to develop Sector Wide Approaches (SWAps) in health, and leading policy dialogue, sector operations, and analytical work in health systems across numerous low- and middle-income countries. Throughout his career, he has sought ways to use evidence and development assistance to improve decision making and strengthen local capacity in low-income countries. He is an associate professor in international health at Johns Hopkins University, where he is also deputy director of the health systems program, and director of the future Health Systems Research Consortium. He has a medical degree from the University of Manitoba and master of public health and doctor of public health degrees from Johns Hopkins University.

Dr. Sameh El-Saharty is senior health policy specialist in the Middle East and North Africa (MENA) Region at the World Bank. He is a medical doctor and holds a master of public health (MPH) degree from the Harvard School of Public Health in International Health Policy and Management. Before joining the World Bank, he held several positions with international donors, academic institutions, and consulting firms, such as USAID, UNFPA, Harvard University, the American University in Cairo, and Pathfinder International. He has had extensive experience for more than 25 years working as a researcher, technical advisor, and international consultant on child survival, reproductive health, public health, health management, and health sector reform programs in more than 15 countries in the MENA region, Africa, and the U.S. His recent work has focused on health systems, with particular interest in health service delivery and improving the performance of health sector organizations. He authored and contributed to many studies and articles on these subjects, including *Public Health Challenges in the MENA region* (The Lancet), *The Millennium Development Goals: Challenges and Opportunities, Tunisia: Health Sector Strategy, Egypt: Health Policy Note, Yemen: Health Sector Strategy, Oman: Cost Effectiveness of Health Programs,* and *Egypt's Health Sector Reform Strategy.*

Banafsheh Siadat is a doctoral student in the Global Health and Population department, with a concentration in health financing and health systems. Siadat previously worked in the Health, Nutrition, and Population department of the World Bank during research for this volume. While at the World Bank, Siadat also worked on issues related to aid effectiveness and health systems governance indicators, national health accounts, fragile states, and health finance in East Asia. She has also worked outside the World Bank as a management consultant on U.S. health systems. Siadat holds a master's degree in international development from the the Fletcher School at Tufts University and a BA from the University of California at Berkeley.

Marko Vujicic is an economist specializing in issues related to the health care sector. He is currently working in the Health, Nutrition and Population unit of the World Bank. His main area of expertise is health labor market policy in developing countries, including such topics as health worker productivity, labor force participation, rural retention and the migration of health workers. He is lead author of the book *Working in Health,* which examines public sector wage bill and management policies and their impact on health workforce performance. He has also worked in the area of health service delivery and health financing in several countries in Africa, eastern Asia, the Caribbean, eastern Europe, and central Asia. Mr. Vujicic has lectured at Harvard University, George Washington University, University of Pennsylvania, and New York University. He completed his PhD in economics at the University of British Columbia in Canada and has an undergraduate degree in business from McGill University. He has worked as a consultant with PricewaterhouseCoopers Consulting and worked at the World Health Organization prior to joining the World Bank. He is a Canadian national.

Katja Janovsky is a health policy and systems consultant, predominately at the World Bank and the World Health Organization (WHO). From 1988 to 2004 she held various positions at WHO, including director for strategy, cooperation and partnership in the director general's office in Geneva and director for liaison with the World Bank and IMF in Washington. Between 1978 and 1986 she lived and worked in eastern Africa, one year with the Kenya Ministry of Health as health planner and six years with the African Medical and Research Foundation (AMREF) as director for planning and evaluation. Prior to this, she worked as a program associate at Harvard University, the Harvard Institute for International Development (HIID), and the Office of International Health Programmes at the Harvard School of Public Health. Ms. Janovsky holds an MA in education and a doctoral degree in planning and social policy from Harvard University (joint committee, School of Education, School of Public Health, and School of Business Administration). She is an Austrian national.

Abbreviations

BAT	before-after trial (uncontrolled)
CHPS	Community-Based Health Planning and Services (Ghana)
CHW	community health worker
CI	confidence interval
DPT3	diphtheria, pertussis, and tetanus vaccine
EPI	Expanded Programme on Immunization
GHS	Ghana Health Service
GNI	gross national income
HCP	health care provider
HSSP	Health Sector Strategic Plan (Uganda)
LMIC	low- and middle-income country
MOPH	Ministry of Public Health (Afghanistan)
MOPH-SM	Ministry of Public Health Strengthening Mechanism (Afghanistan)
NGO	nongovernmental organization
NHIS	National Health Insurance Scheme (Ghana)
NRCT	nonrandomized controlled trial
ODA	official development assistance
OECD	Organisation for Economic Co-operation and Development

OR	odds ratio
PAR	public administration reform (Afghanistan)
PBF	performance-based financing
PNFP	private not-for-profit
RCT	randomized controlled trial
SNNPR	Southern Nations, Nationalities, and People's Region (Ethiopia)
STI	sexually transmitted infection
SWAp	sectorwide approach
TA	technical assistance
TB	tuberculosis
UN	United Nations
USAID	United States Agency for International Development
WHO	World Health Organization

All dollar amounts are U.S. dollars unless otherwise indicated.

Overview

Summary

Decision makers and the public are in need of information to guide their decisions about how to strengthen health services. This book pulls together available evidence concerning strategies to improve health services delivery in low- and middle-income countries (LMICs), using current methods to assemble a knowledge base and analyze the findings. It describes the results of reviews of such strategies, and how such strategies can produce gains for the poor. This type of information is intended to help decision makers in LMICs learn from others and from their own experiences, so that they may develop and implement strategies that will improve health services in their own setting.

Local solutions on their own are unlikely to be easily scaled up. The institutional arrangements within which local service providers operate strongly influence their performance. These arrangements include the ways in which governments use their financial resources and regulatory powers and the roles of a variety of organizations

(continued)

that may include civil society organizations, nongovernmental organizations, as well as associations of professionals and other service providers and private companies. The arrangements also include the degree to which the health facilities are competitive or cooperative in their relationships with each other.

The book provides some suggestions for what works and how to improve implementation, as the evidence does not hold up for "blueprint" planning. It finds that there are many ways that can succeed in improving health services. But not nearly enough attention has been paid to demonstrating how to improve services for the poor. Approaches that ask difficult questions, use information intelligently, and involve key stakeholders and institutions are critical to "learning and doing" practices that underlie successful implementation of health services.

Health Services and the Challenge of Implementation

In recent years, as decision makers[1] have become more aware of their health sector problems and the interdependence of health and development, higher priority has been given to delivering health services and meeting the health needs of the poor. Strengthening health services is recognized as a priority for countries to be able to meet the basic health needs of their people, especially for poor and vulnerable populations. A challenge in most low- and middle-income countries (LMICs) remains finding ways to enable the many actors in the health sector to address these basic health needs more effectively. Progress on the Millennium Development Goals (MDGs) and on disease-specific programs depends on the ability of health systems to provide services (Jha et al. 2002; World Bank 2007; WHO 2007; GAVI Alliance 2007). Yet decision makers have little evidence to guide their decisions about how to most effectively, equitably, and affordably provide health services.

The aim of this book is to bring together a wide range of evidence that is not restricted to a particular outcome measure or single set of methodologies. The various chapters examine—by means of systematic reviews; quantitative and qualitative analyses of existing data; and country studies—the evidence on what strategies work to strengthen health services, and how they have been implemented in real situations.

In the last decades, a considerable amount of evidence has been amassed about how well particular health interventions can improve specific health conditions. Much of the discussion focuses on selecting priority interventions among those affordable in LMICs. Analyses such as the *World Development Report 1993* (World Bank 1993), the Disease Control Priorities Project 2 (Jamison et al. 2006),[2] and several *Lancet* series[3] carefully catalogue the research evidence around the costs and effectiveness of specific health interventions. A common and compelling argument is that the technical interventions are available to save millions of lives in LMICs, but that they need health systems and financial support to increase coverage to those in need (Jha et al. 2002; Victora et al. 2004a). Some papers have estimated the global cost of scaling up packages of interventions for priority diseases, using assumptions that the costs and effectiveness of interventions based on small-scale and public sector delivery can be reproduced and enlarged to cover entire countries. (Johns and Torres 2005, for example, review other papers and interventions.)

Yet these analyses and the debates on prioritization fall short of the evidence needed by decision makers on how to deliver effective health services in their own country in a coherent way and—where they are not already—on a large scale. In addition to the complexity of the number and types of proposed interventions, each country has its own set of conditions and stakeholders that make it unrealistic to simply copy prescriptions on providing and financing a wide variety of health services to very different populations. Even if packages of these interventions are adopted as priorities for a country, is it reasonable to expect that any country can obtain results like those achieved elsewhere in research environments where only a limited set of interventions and outcomes are considered at a time?

Strengthening health services is concerned with the challenge of implementation. To answer questions about implementation, decision makers and the public need to go beyond the question of which intervention has been able to produce a cost-effective result when examined on its own. Improving implementation does not ignore the question of *what* should be done, but places greater emphasis on *how* to do it. Which strategies can be used to best improve the delivery of a range of health services in a given context? What are the factors that help or hinder implementation of these strategies, and how should they be addressed? Which approaches will be quicker, or more sustainable? Which strategies will ensure that the poor and disadvantaged benefit?

Decision makers and the public are in need of information to guide their decisions on how to strengthen health services—how to identify strategies and implement them effectively within their own environ-ments. This book pulls together available evidence concerning strategies to improve health services delivery in LMICs, using current methods to assemble a knowledge base and analyze the findings. It describes the results of reviews of strategies that aim to improve the delivery of health services in LMICs, and how such strategies can produce gains for the poor. This type of information is intended to help decision makers in LMICs learn from others and from their own experiences, so that they may develop and implement strategies that will improve health services in their own setting.

Common Strategies to Strengthen Health Services

In addition to the many types of specific health interventions that have been tested on their own or as packages of services in LMICs, there have also been many strategies to strengthen health services. Some of these strategies are designed specifically to implement a set of techni-cal interventions in a fairly reproducible way, such as the strategy for integrated management of childhood illness (IMCI). Others have been developed as part of broader health sector reform programs.

International agencies and other funding bodies have encouraged devel-oping countries to initiate a bewildering range of health strategies in the last decades. Some of the more common strategies have been associated with major international initiatives. These include the expansion of community-based health workers and community participation strategies and the Health for All movement; the establishment of user fees and community management and The Bamako Initiative; and immunization campaign days and the Polio Eradication Initiative. A 2006 study of 12 LMICs examined eight strategies to improve coverage, quality, or access to health services—community engagement, contracting, decentralization, performance incen-tives, reorganizing outreach workers, social marketing, subsidies for the poor, and user fee exemptions—and found that most countries had adopted and tested several of these strategies in the last 10 years. With a few exceptions, such as for social marketing and user fee exemptions, most of these strategies were implemented only as pilot projects, and rarely did these strategies include strong evaluations (Janovsky and Peters 2006).

In assembling evidence on health strategies, it is useful to identify the types of strategies that can be chosen by decision makers. The annex to this overview lists strategies under four main descriptive categories; it is also clear that strategies may well fit into more than one category. Partly for this reason, the structure of this book does not mirror exactly these four main categories:

- public oversight strategies, usually led by governments or agencies representing governments
- provider-based strategies led by provider organizations, whether public or private
- household and community empowerment strategies
- financing strategies.

Framework

There are many frameworks that can be used in an examination of health services strengthening strategies. Figure 1 depicts the framework used in this book. This framework attempts to show how such strategies relate to, and are affected by, their environments. It schematizes the relationships between the three key players and the related health systems (three dark shaded boxes) within a country's health sector "micro environment" in which a strategy (the central light shaded area) is implemented, which in turn must be viewed within the country context of a wider "macro" environment (the whole figure): the net effect of both environments is seen distilled in the enabling and inhibiting factors that influence *how* the strategy is implemented.

In figure 1, the overall *purpose* of health systems including health services is shown in the small, top right rectangle, namely to improve *health status*, ensure *financial protection* from impoverishment due to ill health, and enhance *trust* of the population in the health system. Other authors have focused on "consumer satisfaction" (Roberts et al. 2008) or "responsiveness" (WHO 2007) as describing the third main purpose of a health system, which we consider as contributing to people's trust in the health system, and critical to its sustained integrity. These three goals—health status, financial protection, and trust—describe the main measures of impact, and are affected by health services delivery and other factors outside the health system, such as demographic conditions (aging, youth bulge) and epidemiologic conditions (prevalence of malaria, HIV/AIDS, or chronic diseases) of a population, as well as economic development and macroeconomic stability.

The right *health services* rectangle characterizes the intermediate results or outcomes of health services delivery and financing, which are sometimes called performance measures and which, too, contribute to the

Figure 1 Descriptive Health Services Framework

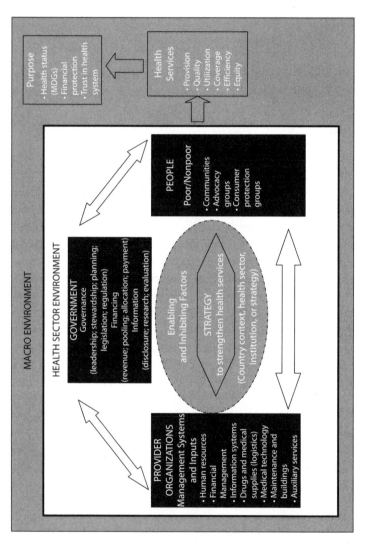

Source: Authors.

overall purpose. Strategies to strengthen health services are aimed at improving the provision, quality, utilization, coverage, efficiency, and equity of health services, usually with an implicit intent to improve effectiveness in terms of achieving the intended health outcomes. Such strategies are discussed in chapter 1. Most of the studies in this book examine health services utilization, but also assess the quality, costs, and efficiency of services. How these results are distributed between poor and other disadvantaged groups on the one hand, and the nonpoor on the other, is of particular interest (also see box 1).

The twin-headed arrows represent some key accountability relationships between actors in the health sector. For example, *people* can influence their *provider organizations* through direct consumer redress, or by direct payments from clients to providers. A *government* can hold *provider organizations* accountable through its governance system, including policies, regulation, and performance contracts. Chapter 2 reviews strategies to strengthen the performance of health organizations in general, while chapter 3 reviews strategies to improve the performance of health workers. In addition, *people* may hold a *government* accountable, often through voting, or *government* may give more authority to *people* through decentralization. Chapter 4 reviews the success of strategies empowering households and communities to improve their health.

To examine how strategies are implemented to improve health services, it was also important to assess the *implementation process* over time.

Box 1

Innovations and the Poor

In pluralistic health systems, markets on their own do not provide cost-effective services, and they tend to exclude the poor. Many of the innovations in service delivery strategies have developed in the context of the reality of high degrees of marketization in developing countries and poor public sector performance. These innovations include using market-based mechanisms to improve access and quality, new kinds of governance and accountability arrangements for local service providers, new ways to contract and pay health workers, community organization to provide support to households coping with sick family members, and ways of using new channels of information to enable people to cope more effectively with health problems or to make better-informed choices.

Source: Bloom et al. 2008.

Chapter 5 analyzes whether utilization of certain *health services* related to the MDG targets can change as rapidly as expected by international agencies and governments, how some country characteristics (*enabling and inhibiting factors*) influence these changes at a national level, and whether changes in *coverage* of different types of health services can affect each other positively or negatively.

The set of *enabling and inhibiting factors* (the oval shape in the framework) influences how strategies are adopted and implemented. Some factors are specific to the strategy pursued, while others are more general both to the health sector and to the wider macro context (hence the dashed outline of the oval as these factors permeate the different levels). Chapter 6 reviews governance issues and the institutional context in which health services operate in relation to two dimensions: the degree of institutionalization, associated with government effectiveness, voice and accountability, and corruption control; and the degree of statehood, linked to political stability, rule of law, and regulatory quality.

Cross-country improvements to *health services*, their *financing*, and the *health status* of the population—underlying features of the whole framework—are reviewed in chapter 7, on the basis of data from the World Bank, which financed large-scale programs intended to support LMICs to achieve these outcomes.

The above is the analytical framework: chapter 8 reviews, in a real-life context, seven low-income country case studies in which different health services strengthening strategies were implemented.

How to Gain Knowledge on Strengthening Health Services

Knowing *how* to strengthen health services is different from knowing *what* to strengthen; and the type of scientific evidence needed to answer *how* questions is different from evidence used to answer the *what* questions. Both types of knowledge are important for decision makers. To provide a useful knowledge base to inform decision makers on strategies to strengthen health services, multiple approaches to obtaining knowledge are needed. Each approach is grounded in different disciplines, and carries different values, purposes, and philosophies of knowledge (epistemologies). Much of the existing research methodology for health services is concerned with propositional knowledge, the purpose of which is to "know that" something is true, and that there is justification for that belief. The challenge of implementation is concerned more with the question of "knowing how" something can work. This type of practical knowledge can be built up from more in-depth inquiry of determinants of improved health services. For example, for any specific intervention involving health workers to succeed, it is likely that health workers will need to be trained to provide the specific intervention. The larger challenges lie in how to provide effective training, supportive supervision, ensuring that materials are available to do the job, and that the right incentives and accountabilities for health workers to perform well are in place. A more complete strategy would also need to know how to build up appropriate demand for the intervention, which may be even more challenging.

When assessing information used to influence decision making, it is useful to understand who the decision maker is and what types of decisions are being made, and what type of judgment is being made about a strategy. A basic set of questions for national decision makers is whether to initiate, continue, change, or expand a strategy. For strategies that have already been initiated in some way, decision makers ought to make judgments about the results in order to inform a decision (table 1). Many managers will be primarily interested in whether a strategy has resulted in a certain level of coverage in a population (overall or for a target group), or whether the quality of services meets certain standards. In the language of Habicht et al. (1999), this type of inference is known as an *adequacy* statement, which answers the question of whether an expected change occurred. The level of confidence that decision makers need to attribute an observed change (or lack of change) to the strategy is usually relatively low. The design of an evaluation that can provide this type of information is a before-after trial or time-series study (both uncontrolled interventions), which examines changes within the beneficiaries of a strategy or program.

If decision makers need greater confidence that an observed change is due to the strategy rather than to other external factors that may have caused the changes, the type of inference is called a *plausibility* statement (Habicht et al. 1999; Victora et al. 2004b). Unlike assessments of adequacy, evaluation designs that support plausibility assessments need to control for the influence of external factors by choosing comparison groups before a strategy is implemented and evaluated, or is otherwise addressed during the analysis.

Research organizations and donor organizations often want to know whether a strategy (or program) results in statistically significant improvements in health outcomes. These statements of *probability* try to show that there is only a small but known probability that the difference between where a strategy was implemented and where it was not is due to chance

Table 1   Judgments about Health Strategies and Their Implications for Evaluation and Research Design

Type of judgment	Primary question to be answered	Type of inference	Research design implications
Demonstration of expected changes in behaviors, health services, or health status	Are behavioral, health services or health indicators changing among beneficiaries of a strategy?	Adequacy	Before-after or time-series study in program recipients only
Demonstration that the strategy is likely effective	Is any measured effect on health services or health status likely due to the strategy rather than other influences?	Plausibility	Concurrent, nonrandomized clusters where strategy is implemented compared to where it is not; before-after or cross-sectional study in program recipients and nonrecipients
Proof that the strategy is efficacious or effective	Is any measured effect on health services or health status due to the implemented strategy?	Probability	Controlled trials, usually randomizing clusters rather than individuals; health strategy implemented in some areas and not in others
Explanation of how or why a strategy works	How did implementation of the strategy lead to measured effects on health services or health status?	Explanatory	Mixed methods: Designs above, including repeated measurement of many variables on context, actors, depth, and breadth of implementation across subunits; and qualitative methods, including key informant interviews, focus groups, historical reviews, and triangulation of data sources

Source: Adapted from Habicht et al. 1999.

alone rather than the strategy itself.[4] Probability assessments require randomization of "treatment" and "control" activities. These evaluation designs are called randomized controlled trials (RCTs), which usually involve the random allocation of a strategy (or program) to clusters (geographic areas or populations) in comparison with a control. The main advantages of randomization are that it minimizes selection bias (where the results can be explained because of the characteristics of who is selected for "treatment" and who is not); it allows for the quantification of differences between "treatment" and "control" groups; controls for both observable and unobservable factors that can explain the differences; and generally provides greater confidence in the causal role of the "treatment" on the outcome (Deaton 2005). There are many difficulties in conducting a good RCT for health services strategies (including lack of feasibility, inability to "control" the allocation of a strategy to particular recipients or to hide the allocation status from recipients or implementers, and bias due to participation dropout because of randomization). Nonetheless, RCTs have become the "gold standard" in academic literature for assessing the efficacy of an intervention.

The applicability of RCTs to "treatments" that involve complex strategies, including most approaches to strengthening health services, is limited. A major concern is related to their "generalizability"—the fact that the study population, the sets of actors and factors that influence a strategy, and the strategy itself, are rarely comparable to other locations, even in the same country (Eldridge et al. 2008). This limits the ability to apply the evidence from these studies to situations and populations other than those in which they were tested (Victora et al. 2004b; Green and Glasgow 2006). As will be seen in later chapters, many health strategies are complex and not simply replicable, even if the specific interventions they involve at the individual level are more replicable. Another concern is that RCTs typically provide information on the average effect of a strategy and not on the distribution of effects across a population (Heckman and Smith 1995), even though that distribution is particularly important when there is a concern to ensure that health services reach the poor. Finally, many RCTs are "black box" experiments that will usually be able to assess whether a strategy succeeded or failed, but that will provide little explanation about how or why a strategy may have worked, or for whom. If decision makers are concerned with *explanatory* inferences about how or why a strategy works or fails, nonexperimental methods are more likely to provide this type of information, often supplementary to other research methods (Victora et al. 2004b). The findings and implications for decision makers draw on all four types of inferences (table 1, and table 2 below).

In practice, both clinical and policy decisions cannot depend entirely on the conduct of RCTs as the source of "evidence" (Grahame-Smith 1995; Smith and Pell 2003; Smith et al. 2001; Victora et al. 2004b). In Victorian England, no controlled trial was available to demonstrate that sending children under nine years to work in the cotton mills or having them work more than 10 hours a day was bad for their health, and

Table 2   Summary of Health Services Reviews, Other Analyses, and Country Case Studies

Chapter	Main issues addressed	Methodology	Main limitations	Main lessons and implications
1. Review of strategies to strengthen health services	What is the evidence of the effect of different approaches to strategies to strengthen health services? What are the main enabling and inhibiting factors influencing their effect?	Modified systematic review of published literature	Weak ability to generalize findings because: • Many studies do not give sufficient details of the strategies or interventions that are being pursued or whether it was fully implemented. • Different strategies are often given the same label. • Strategies often involve multiple components that are not specified, nor studied in a way that would indicate which component is essential, or where there are synergies between components. • Few studies examine factors beyond the health system or the intervention itself.	• The evidence base is weak for claiming success of any particular health services strengthening strategy in one LMIC. • More and better research and evaluation of health services strategies in developing countries is greatly needed. • How a strategy is implemented is as important as the type of strategy implemented. • Strategies that are more effective in strengthening service delivery for the poor involve planning for benefits to reach the poor, ensuring regular measurement of impact on the poor, and providing oversight to ensure that the poor benefit.

- Stakeholder involvement and consultation are necessary for effective implementation.
- Successful implementation is linked to interventions to identify and minimize constraints.
- There was no evidence that certain strategies are less dependent on the local environment and work in more countries than other strategies.
- Mobilization of adequate resources is linked to successful strategy implementation.
- The initial and continuous adaptation of the strategy to the local context is associated with more complete strategy implementation, and adaptation is easier in small-scale interventions.

- It is unclear how much the studies' results can be attributed to the strengthening actions.
- Plausibility and limited probability inferences only can be made.
- There may be publication bias.

(continued)

Table 2 Summary of Health Services Reviews, Other Analyses, and Country Case Studies *(Continued)*

Chapter	Main issues addressed	Methodology	Main limitations	Main lessons and implications
				• Multiple strategies are more effective than single strategies, but risk of failure is greater. • Moderate evidence suggests that strategies to strengthen disease-specific programs that are effective in one area can be successfully scaled up nationally. • The evidence is inconclusive as to whether disease-specific programs are an effective way to strengthen health services.
2. Review of strategies to strengthen the performance of health organizations	What is the evidence of the effect of different strategies to improve the performance of health services organizations?	Systematic review of published and gray literature	Weak ability to generalize findings because: • It is impossible to tell which approaches were more successful or sustainable, given the small number of studies involved, and the fact that few organizational changes are really comparable to each other.	• The strategies for improving the performance of health organizations, including human resource strategies, are not likely reproducible across countries.

- It is unrealistic to claim probabilistic statements, although the conclusions are still plausible.
- The very high positive result rate raises suspicions of publication bias and limits the ability to test if some broad strategies are more successful than others.

- There are no blueprints for improving the performance of health organizations in LMICs; many methods seem to improve overall organizational performance.
- Strategies involving organizational change had widely variable results.
- Provider-based performance improvement strategies seemed to hold the most promise, with a large effect size.
- The types of strategies were usually not the same, even when carrying similar labels.
- Conclusions are plausible (strategies led to positive results), but it is unrealistic to claim probabilistic statements about the magnitude of change attributable to particular strategies.

(continued)

Table 2 Summary of Health Services Reviews, Other Analyses, and Country Case Studies (*Continued*)

Chapter	Main issues addressed	Methodology	Main limitations	Main lessons and implications
3. Review of strategies to improve health care provider performance	What is the evidence of the effect on the performance of health workers of different strategies to improve that performance?	Systematic review of published and gray literature	Weak ability to generalize findings because: • Methodological differences complicate comparisons across studies. • Few studies report costs or cost-effectiveness. • Plausibility and limited probability inferences only can be made.	• Most strategies, including the common ones such as training only, have small effect sizes (less than 10 percentage points). • Most strategies have multiple components, but there is no clear relationship between the number of components in a strategy and the strategy's effect size. • Strategies with the same label often have heterogeneous effects. • Effect size seems to vary by scale of implementation, with strategies implemented at state, province, or national level generally more successful than those at the district level or lower.

	Research question	Method	Weaknesses	Implications
4. Review of community empowerment strategies for health	What is the evidence of the effect on health services or outcomes of different strategies to empower communities?	Systematic review of published and gray literature	Weak ability to generalize findings because: • Data are pooled on widely different interventions (often with the same label or name) and on multiple outcomes. • Many very different and changing factors influence outcomes. • Many large-scale strategies are unsuitable for controlled designs, so were not included • How implementation occurs is not captured. • Plausibility and limited probability inferences only can be made. • There may be publication bias.	• Initial conditions are important, especially strong local leadership. • There is no clear pattern in the scale of the strategy and the likelihood of a positive outcome. • Planning for scaling up and using local adaptive learning processes should be considered in designing and implementing strategies. • More robust research on community empowerment strategies is needed, to facilitate learning and testing of approaches for scaling up strategies nationally.
5. Analysis of cross-country changes in health services	What are the trends over time of specific health service outputs across LMICs? How do changes in one priority health service affect changes in other health services?	Longitudinal statistical analysis of cross-country data on health services and contextual factors	• Few health services are recorded consistently across countries, with variable data quality. • The ability is limited to track relevant events	• Identifying negative or slow rates of change in a country is probably a more important strategy than setting universal targets for health attainment.

(continued)

17

Table 2 Summary of Health Services Reviews, Other Analyses, and Country Case Studies (*Continued*)

Chapter	Main issues addressed	Methodology	Main limitations	Main lessons and implications
	What are the contextual factors that most influence health service outputs at the national level?		(and timing) that are particular to individual countries. • Only national averages are included, so variability within a country is not captured. • Plausibility inferences only may be made. • Some important health services (such as for HIV/AIDS) do not have adequate data for these analyses.	• Individual country differences (in delivery of health services, health status, and macro context) may be more important than international averages imply, undermining the relevance of targets set without reference to country-specific experience. • Rather than showing a common pattern of progress for health services, countries tend to follow their own pathways. • Countries' very different starting points affect their prospects of achieving the targets and their rate of change.

6. Institutional context of health services	What are the main institutional factors influencing the delivery of health services in LMICs?	Literature review	• Specific institutional factors cannot be identified by country. • Comparable data are few, hence a weak ability to generalize the role of specific institutional factors. • Plausibility inferences only may be made.	• Improvements in health services are usually not associated with changes in other health services (with one or two exceptions). • Since changes in national governance are significantly associated with health status improvements, health programs should be planned within a broader framework. Implementation of health services is dependent on the following eight key dimensions: • Degree and breadth of commitment to the stated objectives of the strategy or intervention • Rules about how critical stakeholders are involved, and the incentives to make them work • Incentives and disincentives for health workers (and ultimately organizations) to perform well

(continued)

19

Table 2 Summary of Health Services Reviews, Other Analyses, and Country Case Studies *(Continued)*

Chapter	Main issues addressed	Methodology	Main limitations	Main lessons and implications
				• Capacity of government to be a regulator of the health system • Mechanisms for accountability in health systems • Co-accountability of national health systems to external bodies providing financial and technical support • Level of statehood • Institutional development
7. Evaluation of changes in health results in World Bank-assisted health projects	How well do World Bank-assisted project evaluations measure changes in health services, financing, and health status? What are the main factors associated with measuring changes?	Documentation analysis using standardized definitions and cross-sectional statistical analysis	• Conclusions are drawn only from health systems receiving World Bank assistance. • Information is limited by what is documented in World Bank implementation completion reports. • Retrospective approach only allows for analysis of associations, not causes.	• Sectorwide approaches may well improve health services or health status more than other programs. • Among project activities, contracting and logistics support are likely to show improvements in health services and status, respectively. • Projects organized around disease-control programs

			• promote improvements in health services and outcomes related to those specific programs. • No type of project input is associated with improvements in health services or status. • More consistent measurement of results is needed, to better assess whether individual country efforts produce the desired changes. • Adequacy inferences only may be made.
8. Seven country case studies	Describe the strategies of significant scale for strengthening health services delivery in the real-life context in which they occurred. What are the presumed causal links between the strategies and their effects? What are the lessons learned?	Mixed methods case studies (documentation review, key informant interviews, and quantitative analysis of health services data)	• Each country situation is virtually unique. Hence generalizations and comparisons across countries are limited. • Success in implementation of the selected health services delivery strategies is driven largely by several factors related to the country-specific macro environment and/or to the health sector micro environment. • Country cases may not represent experience of others, or provide complete picture. • What drives change is very context specific. • Plausibility inferences only may be made.

(continued)

Table 2   Summary of Health Services Reviews, Other Analyses, and Country Case Studies *(Continued)*

Chapter	Main issues addressed	Methodology	Main limitations	Main lessons and implications
				• As the country context changes, the health system components also evolve and adapt in response to the changing environment. • In virtually no country can overall health services improvements be linked to a particular strategy. • Political stability, security, and economic growth, as well as the legislation, regulation, and the capacity to monitor and enforce, are all macro-environment factors that influence how strategies are implemented. They are usually outside the control of the strategy implementers. • Leadership, status of NGOs and faith-based organizations, size of donor support, and aid approaches are not

		under the control of the strategy implementers, but they directly influence how the strategy is implemented. • Some "strategy-related" factors are critical. They are directly related to strategy design, adaptation, and implementation, and are usually under the control of strategy implementers. • See chapter 9
9. From evidence to learning and doing	What are the main lessons and implications for future work based on the body of evidence on strengthening health services in LMICs?	Synthesis of quantitative and qualitative work	• See chapter 9

Source: Authors.

Note: Systematic reviews (chapters 1–4) involve a standardized approach to gathering and interpreting the literature on the same research question (with regard to the effectiveness of a particular intervention or strategy), categorizing evidence by the quality of the study (largely determined by study design, with the strongest designs being randomized controlled trials, followed by nonrandomized controlled trials, time-series studies, before-after trials, and case-control designs), and pooling the size of the effects to determine the strength of the evidence for a given set of questions.

demanding such evidence would likely have delayed the implementation of the Factories Act (Bennett 1995). RCTs of smoking cessation programs have not demonstrated significant effects on health status outcomes in the United States, and until recently, have shown little effect on smoking rates. However, there have been impressive reductions in adult smoking over the last decades and declines in tobacco-related cancers and other tobacco-related health outcomes. A review of RCTs concerning the promotion of abstinence plus safe sex or use of condoms has shown unimpressive gains in preventing the transmission of HIV or other sexually transmitted infections (Underhill et al. 2007). Yet it would still make good public health policy to promote smoking reduction and safe sexual practices.

In summary, the type of inference (adequacy, plausibility, probability, and explanatory) and level of certainty needed by the decision maker should determine the type of research that will produce the evidence needed to support decisions. There are trade-offs in the types of research that can provide different types of evidence, and so usually more than one type of information and research design are needed. For example, research that produces a probability statement with a high level of certainty may involve a well-designed RCT, but unless the intervention is very simple and replicable, the study will have limited ability to provide much information about how to implement a more complicated strategy in conditions that were not set up in the trial.

Overview of the Studies

Summary of Methods Used

In chapters 1–4, we draw on the tradition of "evidence-based medicine" and "evidence-based policy" to pull together the information that can be gleaned from experimental, quasi-experimental, and observational research, as consolidated through systematic reviews of the literature. The methods rely on the disciplines of epidemiology, economics, and library and evaluation sciences, and tend to give greater weight to inferences of probability than of plausibility or adequacy. In chapter 5, we have collected the available national data on health services to assess how changes over time in different types of health service are related to each other, and to identify plausible factors that influence changes in health services delivery. Chapter 6 reviews the literature on institutional frameworks for providing health services in LMICs to identify key institutional factors. In chapter 7, we analyze the data used for all the evaluations of World Bank-supported health projects completed in the fiscal years 2003 to 2005 to provide insights on how the main channels of World Bank assistance have been used to demonstrate changes in health services, health financing, and health impact. The nature of the data limits the inferences to inferences of adequacy, but nonetheless the data show large gaps in the way that large-scale health projects can lead to improvements in the sector. Chapter 8 uses contextual (largely qualitative) methods to outline how strategies to develop and implement strategies to strengthen health services were developed in seven low-income countries over the last 10 years, while tracking trends in the delivery of health services. Both chapters are limited to inferences of plausibility. Chapter 9 is a summary of the studies, and points to possible future directions.

Table 2 outlines the main reviews of this book, noting their main questions, methods, and limitations.

Systematic review methods. In chapters 1–4, we begin with a series of systematic reviews of the literature as a means of using the best available approach to synthesizing quantitative research evidence on effectiveness of health strategies. We use this approach to evaluate the effectiveness of overall strategies to strengthen health services in LMICs (chapter 1), strategies to improve the performance of organizations that deliver health care (chapter 2), supply-side strategies to improve health worker performance (chapter 3), and demand-side approaches to empower households and communities in health (chapter 4). The results obtained through these approaches provide useful information about interventions and broad strategies that can work in various settings, as well as some of the main determinants of success.

The systematic reviews follow methods based on those used by Grimshaw et al. (2004), and involve the following steps.

Conducting comprehensive electronic and document searches. All literature searches were conducted in English, though this method still picked up the English abstracts of non-English articles, and a limited number of non-English articles. Such searches included:

- identification of key search terms for types of strategies, geographic areas, and types of outcome measurements;
- definition of inclusion and exclusion criteria of studies for review;
- screening the titles and abstracts of research results for relevant studies;
- review of full articles for final selection of studies for review;
- detailed abstraction of study information into standardized data entry formats by independent reviewers and reconciliation of differences.

A summary of the number of number of studies screened and finally included for review is shown below (table 3).

Evaluating the quality and strength of recommendations from each eligible study. During data abstraction, each study was assessed for relevance, scientific strength, outcome data, and quality of description, and classified accordingly. The studies were categorized based on the study quality criteria described in table 4. Studies were reviewed largely on the following criteria: quality of study methods (assignment to treatment and control group, blinding, degree of potential confounding, classification of outcomes and follow up, and appropriate analysis), magnitude of effect, consistency, and generalizability of findings to LMICs. The reviews concentrated on the strongest study types (D1 and D2 study designs), though they also looked at weaker study designs (D3 and D4).

Analysis of results. Studies were stratified according to the strength of the evidence largely on the basis of their design, as outlined in table 5. To use a single statistic on which to compare the articles, the effect size of each outcome was calculated for each of the studies reviewed. The effect size was calculated using four individual data points: post-intervention percentage for the intervention group; pre-intervention percentage for the intervention group; post-intervention percentage for the control group; and pre-intervention percentage for the control group using the following formula:

$$\text{Effect size} = (\%POST - \%PRE)_{intervention} - (\%POST - \%PRE)_{control}$$

Table 3   Number of Studies Screened and Included in Systematic Reviews

Systematic review	Number of studies screened	Number of studies with designs adequate for inclusion in final review
Chapter 1. Review of strategies to strengthen health services	208[a]	150
Chapter 2. Review of strategies to strengthen the performance of health organizations	127,000	88
Chapter 3. Review of strategies to improve health care provider performance	40,000[b]	127[b]
Chapter 4. Review of community empowerment strategies for health	27,000	282

Source: Authors.

a. Methods included screening of articles found in reviews and more specific search terms, supplemented by cascade sampling of articles identified from these papers (Ovretveit 2003).

b. Review is ongoing; results are as of February 2008.

Table 4 Categories of Study Designs Used for Inclusion and Exclusion in Systematic Reviews

Study type	Description	Study design
D1: Randomized controlled trials	Studies involving a random allocation of the intervention and comparison (such as "usual care") to different study groups, including measurement of the outcome before and after the intervention is made	Post-only randomized control design R E X O1 R C –X O1 Pre-post control design R E O1 X O2 R C O1 –X O2
D2: Nonrandomized controlled trials	Nonrandomized studies containing a before-and-after measurement that compare results in two or more groups. The comparison intervention may be "usual care" or another intervention. Those case-control studies where the assessment is made in a nested (that is, prospective) manner have a stronger design than those studies where the intervention or attributes occurred in the past	Pre-post or before-after with nonequivalent groups NR E O1 X O2 NR C O1 –X O2
D3: Uncontrolled interventions: before-after trials and time-series studies	Nonrandomized studies containing a before-and-after measurement, but without any comparison group for the intervention (such as a cohort study). Time-series studies, where data on the cohort involve more than three data points prior to an intervention and more than three points after an intervention, provide stronger evidence than those with only one baseline point	Group pre-post or before-after trials NR E O1 X O2 Time-series studies NR E O1 O2 O3 X O4 O5 O6 (at least three data points before and after; single or multiple groups)

(continued)

27

Table 4 Categories of Study Designs Used for Inclusion and Exclusion in Systematic Reviews (*Continued*)

Study type	Description	Study design
D4: Case-control studies (and cross-sectional studies with ≥2 comparison groups)	Case-control studies dividing groups based on different outcomes, and then assessing prior to "exposure" to an intervention. These studies are based on surveys conducted at one point in time. Nested case-control studies may be considered as having evidence comparable to D2 studies.	Post-only design with nonequivalent groups NR E X O1 NR C −X O1
D5: Cross-sectional studies	Measurement made at one point in time when an intervention has occurred without comparable control groups. Unless there are data to construct a time-series or case-control study, these studies are excluded from the systematic reviews.	Group post-only design (exploratory studies) NR E X O1
D6: Descriptive studies	Descriptive case studies and expert opinions, and reports lacking comparison groups or measurement of outcome variables. These studies are excluded from the systematic reviews.	No comparison and no measurements on outcomes

Source: Authors' adaptation of Grimshaw et al. 2004.
R = randomized, NR = nonrandomized, E = experimental, C = control, O = observation, X "treatment" or implementation of strategy, –X = no "treatment" or usual care or existing strategy such as continued training.

28

Table 5   Category of Strength of Evidence

Category	Strength of evidence
S1	Strong evidence of results: consistent findings of results in two or more D1 studies
S2	Moderate evidence: consistent findings of results in two or more scientific studies of acceptable quality (D2 and D3)
S3	Limited evidence: only one study giving results, or inconsistent findings of results of several studies. Studies of results showing perceptions are graded S3 if they were collected and analyzed according to accepted scientific methods using an appropriate design (for example, D2–D4)
S4	Evidence of implementation only: description of implementation collected and analyzed according to accepted methods using a reasonable design (for example, D4 or D5)
S5	Descriptive studies only: no studies demonstrating scientific evidence (D6 only)
S6	No evidence of any type

Source: Authors.

When outcomes were determined as percentages, the effect size was calculated as the net difference between percentage improvements in the intervention group and comparison group or the relative gain from the intervention (Ross-Degnan et al. 1997). If the outcome was not in the form of a percentage, then each value was first converted to a percentage and then the effect size was calculated. For example, if correct treatment rates in an intervention group increased from 25 percent to 55 percent (a 30 percentage point improvement), and correct treatment in the comparison group increased from 20 percent to 30 percent (a 10 percentage point improvement), the effect size for the strategy would be 20 percentage points (30 minus 10 percentage points). For each study, one effect size was used to measure the study's effectiveness, and that was the effect size of the primary outcome (or a median effect size for studies where there was more than one outcome). Each systematic review was then analyzed to identify which types of strategies and other determinants were related to whether there was a positive effect, or the size of the effect, through cross-tabulations and regression analyses where sample size was sufficient.

Other analytical methods. Chapter 5 involves the aggregation of national-level databases and applies new statistical methods (multilevel modeling) to assess how indicators of health services change over time across LMICs, in ways that account for each country's trends and critical enabling and inhibiting factors. The data sources and statistical methods are described in more detail in the chapter.

Chapter 6 offers a critical review of the literature on the influence of institutional arrangements on development to identify how they affect health services in LMICs.

Chapter 7 involves an analysis of all World Bank-assisted projects with a health component that were completed during 2003–2005. A standard checklist was used to systematically extract data on all the implementation completion reports by two independent analysts to document changes in health services, health financing, and health status, along with key features of the way projects were designed and implemented. Descriptive statistical analysis followed by cross-tabulations and multiple logistic regression analysis were then used to identify factors associated with positive changes in measures of health services, financing, and health status.

Case study methods. The quantitative methods used above point to what approaches have been shown to work, but are limited in their ability to provide the knowledge concerning how similar strategies can be implemented in other settings to achieve comparable results ("replicability").

Chapter 8 presents country case studies from seven low-income countries: Afghanistan, Ethiopia, Ghana, Rwanda, Uganda, Vietnam, and Zambia. The case studies use mixed methods to identify both how these low-income countries have adopted and implemented strategies to improve health services, and the factors that have enabled and inhibited their ability to make changes in their health services. These methods are grounded in political science, economics, public policy, management, and evaluation research, and are largely concerned with plausibility of findings: can specific factors affect how strategies are implemented and what effects do they have? These case studies are used to understand how policies and strategies are implemented in complex environments— where decision makers need to look for unintended consequences of these strategies—and to draw out principles for improving the prospects of successful implementation.

A standardized protocol was developed for use in each country to identify the key strategies to improve health services in the country, how these strategies were developed, and the critical stakeholders and factors affecting implementation.

Main Lessons and Implications

The research compiled in this book represents an attempt to bring together thinking about strategies to improve health services in LMICs, using the best currently available data and methodologies. Chapter 9 summarizes the book's findings and presents the main lessons and implications.

Although no "magic bullets" emerge, the reviews point to many ways that strategies have been successfully implemented, and identify some of the key factors that influence success. It is clear that many types of strategies can work in many settings. Some of the success factors, such as strong leadership, good management systems, clear accountabilities, and incentives to support performance, are easily recognizable. Yet they are easier to describe than to actually implement or replicate.

A cross-cutting conclusion of this book is that decision makers need better approaches on how they can make more informed decisions based on knowledge gained from implementation experience and research evidence. One way to view the challenge of using knowledge to influence decisions on implementation is as a process of institutional development and learning.

Notes

1. The term "decision maker" in most contexts in this book refers to the overlapping categories of policy makers, health professionals, planners, and funding and implementing agencies (often international).

2. The Disease Control Priorities Project 2 analyzes cost-effective interventions for 170 conditions (Jamison et al. 2006).

3. These include the Child Survival Series (2003); Neonatal Survival Series (2005); Maternal Series (2006); Reproductive Health Series (2006); and Undernutrition Series (2008). The first four of these series identify over 190 single interventions to implement (Kerber et al. 2007).

4. By unscientific but conventional practice, the level of statistical significance for concluding that there is a difference between groups, when in truth there is none, is often set at a probability of 5 percent (this is also called the type I or alpha error). The related probability of concluding that there is no difference when in truth there is a difference (also called type II or beta error) is often set at 20 percent. Whether decision makers and scientists believe that these levels of error are acceptable for a given question is a matter of widely differing opinion.

References

Bennett, A. 1995. *A Working Life: Child Labour through the Nineteenth Century.* (2nd ed.) Launceston: Waterfront Publications.

Bloom, G., C. Champion, H. Lucas, D.H. Peters, and H. Standing. 2008. *Making Health Markets Work For the Poor*. Institute for Development Studies and Future Health Systems Consortium. September.

Deaton, A. 2005. "Some Remarks on Randomization, Econometrics and Data." In *Evaluating Development Effectiveness*, ed. G.K. Pitman, O. Feinstein et al. New Brunswick, NJ: Transaction Publishers.

Eldridge, S., D. Ashby, C. Bennett, M. Wakelin, and G. Feder. 2008. "Internal and External Validity of Cluster Randomised Trials: Systematic Review of Recent Trials." *British Medical Journal* 336(7649): 876–80.

GAVI Alliance. 2007. *Revised Guidelines for GAVI Alliance Health System Strengthening (HSS) Applications*. Geneva: GAVI Alliance Secretariat.

Grahame-Smith, D. 1995. "Evidence-based Medicine: Socratic Dissent." *British Medical Journal* 310: 1126–1127.

Green, L.W., and R.E. Glasgow. 2006. "Evaluating the Relevance, Generalization, and Applicability of Research: Issues in External Validation and Translation Methodology." *Evaluation & The Health Professions* 29(1): 126–153.

Grimshaw, J.M., R.E. Thomas, G. MacLennan, C. Fraser, C. Ramsay, L. Vale et al. 2004. "Effectiveness and Efficiency of Guideline Dissemination and Implementation Strategies." *Health Technology Assessment* 8(6).

Habicht, J.P., C.G. Victora, and J.P. Vaughan. 1999. "Evaluation Designs for Adequacy, Plausibility, and Probability of Public Health Programme Performance and Impact." *International Journal of Epidemiology* 28: 10–18.

Heckman, J., and J. Smith. 1995. "Assessing the Case for Social Experiments." *The Journal of Economic Perspectives* 9: 85–110.

Jamison, D.T., J.G. Breman, A.R. Measham, G. Alleyne, M. Claeson, D.B. Evans, P. Jha, A. Mills, and P. Musgrove, eds. 2006. *Disease Control Priorities in Developing Countries*. (2nd ed.) Washington, DC: World Bank.

Janovsky, K., and D.H. Peters. 2006. *Improving Health Services and Strengthening Health Systems: Adopting and Implementing Innovative Strategies—An Exploratory Review in Twelve Countries*. WHO Making Health Systems Work, Working Paper No. 5, Geneva: World Health Organization.

Jha, P., A. Mills, K. Hanson, L. Kumaranayake, L. Conteh, C. Kurowski, S.N. Nguyen, V.O. Cruz, K. Ranson, L.M.E. Vaz, S. Yu, O. Morton, and J.D. Sachs. 2002. "Improving the Health of the Global Poor." *Science* 295(5562): 2036–2039.

Johns, B., and T.T. Torres. 2005. "Costs of Scaling Up Health Interventions: A Systematic Review." *Health Policy and Planning* 20(1): 1–13.

Kerber K., J. de Graft-Johnson, Z. Bhutta, P. Okong, A. Starrs, and J. Lawn. 2007. "Continuum of Care for Maternal, Newborn, and Child Health: From Slogan to Service Delivery." *Lancet* 370(9595): 1358–1369.

Ovretveit, J. 2003. *What is the Best Strategy for Improving Quality and Safety of Hospitals: A Review and Synthesis of the Evidence.* Copenhagen: WHO Regional Office for Europe.

Roberts, M.J., W. Hsiao, P. Berman, and M.R. Reich. 2008. *Getting Reform Right: A Guide to Improving Performance and Equity.* New York: Oxford University Press.

Ross-Degnan, D., R. Laing, B. Santoso, D. Ofori-Adjei, C. Lamoureux, and H. Hogerzeil. 1997. "Improving Pharmaceutical Use in Primary Care in Developing Counties: A Critical Review of Experience and Lack of Experience." Presented at the International Conference on Improving Use of Medicines, Chiang Mai, Thailand. April.

Smith, C. S., Pell, J. P. 2003. "Parachute use to prevent death and major trauma related to gravitational challenge: systematic review of randomised controlled trials". *British Medical Journal* 327: 1459–1461.

Smith, G.D., S. Ebrahim, and S. Frankel. 2001. "How Policy Informs the Evidence: 'Evidence-based' Thinking Can Lead to Debased Policy Making." *British Medical Journal* 322: 184–185.

Tan-Torres, T., M. Aikins, R. Black, L. Wolfson, R. Hutubessy, and D.B. Evans. 2005. "Achieving the Millennium Development Goals for Health: Cost Effectiveness Analysis of Strategies for Child Health in Developing Countries." *British Medical Journal* 331: 1177.

Victora, C.G., K. Hansen, J. Bryce, and J.P. Vaughan. 2004a. "Achieving Universal Coverage with Health Interventions." *Lancet* 364: 1541–48.

Victora, C.G., J.P. Habicht, and J. Bryce. 2004b. "Evidence-based Public Health: Moving Beyond Randomized Trials." *American Journal of Public Health* 94(3): 400–5.

Underhill, K., D. Operario, and P. Montgomery. 2007. "Systematic Review of Abstinence-Plus HIV Prevention Programs in High Income Countries." *PLoS Medicine* 4(9): 1471–1485.

World Bank. 1993. *World Development Report 1993: Investing in Health.* New York: Oxford University Press.

———. 2007. "Healthy Development: The World Bank Strategy for Health, Nutrition, and Population Results." Washington, DC.

World Health Organization (WHO). 2004. *The World Health Report 2004.* Geneva.

———. 2007. *Everybody's Business: Strengthening Health Systems to Improve Health Outcomes—WHO's Framework for Action.* Geneva.

CHAPTER 1

Review of Strategies to Strengthen Health Services

John Ovretveit, Banafsheh Siadat, David H. Peters, Anil Thota, and Sameh El-Saharty

Summary

Objective: To evaluate the published literature on strategies to strengthen the delivery of health services in LMICs.

Methods: A modified systematic review was made of electronic databases on publication, literature reviews, and bibliographies by type of strategy, implementation characteristics, validity of findings, and strength of evidence.

Key messages:
- The evidence base is weak for claiming success of any particular health services strengthening strategy across LMICs.
- How a strategy is implemented is as important as the type of strategy implemented.
- Strategies that are more effective in strengthening service delivery for the poor involve planning for benefits to reach the poor, ensuring regular measurement of impact on the poor, and providing oversight to ensure that the poor benefit.

(continued)

- Stakeholder involvement and consultation are necessary for effective implementation.
- Successful implementation is linked to interventions to identify and minimize constraints.
- There was no evidence that certain strategies are less dependent on the local environment and work in more countries than other strategies.
- Mobilization of adequate resources is linked to successful strategy implementation.
- The initial and continuous adaptation of the strategy to the local context is associated with more complete strategy implementation, and that adaptation is easier in small-scale interventions.
- Multiple strategies are more effective than single strategies, but risk of failure is greater.
- Moderate evidence suggests that strategies to strengthen disease-specific programs that are effective in one area can be successfully scaled up nationally.
- The evidence is inconclusive as to whether disease-specific programs are an effective way to strengthen health services.

Reasons for Conducting the Review

Action to strengthen health services is essential if people in LMICs are to have their basic health needs met. Since such strengthening is an increasing priority for countries and international agencies, it is important to ensure that new health care resources for these purposes are used effectively. This chapter summarizes some of the research into effective interventions and strategies for implementation, which is often either largely unknown to or unused by decision makers.

Objectives of the Review

This review of research concentrated on studies and reports describing the implementation of interventions that were designed to strengthen health services in LMICs. The specific objectives were to:

- Identify various strategies used to improve health services in low-income countries

- Determine the factors that helped and hindered implementation of the strategies reviewed
- Provide guidance to decision makers in designing and implementing strategies to deliver health services responsively and cost-effectively.

Methods Used

The review was based on methods described in more detail in the WHO Health Evidence Network reviews for policy makers (Ovretveit 2003a, b). It involved a systematic search of electronic databases, related literature reviews, and bibliographies of the literature (annex 1.1), using key terms (annex 1.2). Studies were selected for review according to their scope (for example, relevance in dealing with health system and health services strengthening interventions), as well as the quality of evidence provided. The review yielded 150 studies (annex 1.3) based on their inclusion of at least one of 15 approaches to strengthening health services, and use of research designs that focused on outcomes attributable to the strategy under investigation (categories D1 to D3 in table 4 in the *Overview*). The study designs were randomized controlled trials (RCTs), nonrandomized controlled trials (NRCTs), and time-series and uncontrolled before-after trials (BATs). They were classified by scale of implementation, type of health service provided, strategies employed, outcome measures, and implementation employed.

Studies were then summarized according to the following criteria: type of intervention and implementation strategy to improve or strengthen health services; macro and health systems environment; impact on health services resulting from the strategy in question; implementation process; validity of findings; and quality of data reported. A successful strengthening strategy was defined as one that was implemented and that improved the quantity or quality of health services. The strength of the evidence for each strategy investigated was then rated according to the study design (table 4 in the *Overview*) and categorized according to the strength of the evidence (table 5 in the *Overview*).

Main Findings

The review found three overlapping groups of research that characterize the majority of the evidence, including studies of:

- disease-specific strengthening strategies;

- scale-up programs (often disease-specific), which take an intervention from one area and attempt to reproduce it elsewhere or introduce it nationally;
- health service improvement reforms (for example, primary care), often involving various interventions.

The most common example of a primary health strengthening strategy (table 1.1) used in each category of study design was training of health workers, which was seen in 39.6 percent of the studies overall. Examples of this included training traditional birth attendants, community health workers, and often pharmacy staff to improve their dispensing practices. Educating individuals and households on healthy behavior was also commonly used (13.0 percent). Social marketing was used in about the same proportion as education (13.5 percent of all strategies), especially strategies that dealt with making the use of contraceptives more attractive.

An attempt was also made to note the scale at which the various interventions were carried out (table 1.2). It is clear that the majority of strategies are carried out on a relatively small scale, with the majority occurring at the level of one district or below. This limits the ability to use this literature to comment on strategies implemented on a large scale.

In examining results across different types of studies, the following summarizes key findings and factors to consider in selecting and implementing these different types of strategies.

Multiple strategies are more effective than single strategies, but risk of failure is greater. This work found that, with a reasonable degree of certainty for selected small-scale interventions, multiple-component strategies are slightly more effective than single-component strategies. Notably, multiple-action strategies, where components reinforce one another, were found to have a more significant, long-term effect than single-action strategies alone; however, the risks of failed intervention for multiple-action strategies are far greater. In sum, multiple-action strategies should only be used if the design and coordination can be done well. Such coordination involves dealing with difficulties in obtaining consensus and support, ensuring greater management capacity and oversight, the phasing in of individual components to make sure that existing resources and capacity are not overburdened, and ensuring that individual components do not undermine other components of the overall strategy.

Some of the single strategies that were found to be effective included the removal of financial barriers to access care, increases in the number of health workers, changes in physician behavior, and changes to drug procurement

Table 1.1 Primary Health Strengthening Strategy by Study Design

	Type of study design			
Primary strategy	Randomized controlled trials, % (n=33)	Nonrandomized controlled trials, % (n=52)	Uncontrolled before-after trials, % (n=65)	Total, % (N=150)
Training of health workers, managers, and auxiliary and support staff	38.7	50.8	32.5	39.6
Educating/training in healthy behavior, self-care, and appropriate health-seeking behavior	33.3	5.7	8.7	13.0
Pharmaceuticals—Logistics systems design and operations	11.2	5.7	3.7	5.8
Regulation	5.6	0.0	2.4	2.3
Social marketing	2.8	15	17.4	13.5
Contracting	2.8	1.9	3.7	3.0
Organization of community forums	2.8	0.0	0.0	0.6
Quality improvement programs	2.8	0.0	0.0	0.6
User vouchers	0.0	1.9	5.0	3.0
Franchising	0.0	7.6	0.0	2.4
Decentralization	0.0	3.8	0.0	1.2
Service agreement with nongovernmental organizations/providers	0.0	5.7	2.5	3.0
Raising revenues from developmental assistance	0.0	1.9	0.0	0.6

(continued)

Table 1.1 Primary Health Strengthening Strategy by Study Design (Continued)

Primary strategy	Type of study design			
	Randomized controlled trials, % (n=33)	Nonrandomized controlled trials, % (n=52)	Uncontrolled before-after trials, % (n=65)	Total, % (N=150)
Information on standards of care	0.0	0.0	6.3	3.0
Informing providers and communities about community perceptions	0.0	0.0	2.5	1.2
Disclosure of performance of service providers to the public	0.0	0.0	2.5	1.2
Collaborations between providers and with communities	0.0	0.0	2.5	1.2
Human resource performance management	0.0	0.0	2.5	1.2
Provider payment systems	0.0	0.0	1.3	0.6
Subsidies for service provision	0.0	0.0	1.3	0.6
Disease surveillance	0.0	0.0	1.3	0.6
Public-private partnerships	0.0	0.0	1.3	0.6
Provider-based accreditation	0.0	0.0	1.3	0.6
Vertically integrating services	0.0	0.0	0.6	0.6

Source: Authors.
Note: Some studies involved more than one primary strategy.

Table 1.2   Scale of Implementation

Scale of implementation: Where intervention carried out	Randomized controlled trials, % (n=33)	Nonrandomized controlled (n=52)	Uncontrolled before-after trials, % (n=65)	Total (N=150)
In one district/administrative division or less	69.7	55.8	38.5	51.3
In two or more districts or administrative divisions	12.1	30.8	43.1	32
In one province or state	9.1	3.9	6.2	6.1
In two or more provinces	3.0	7.7	4.6	5.3
Nationwide	6.1	1.8	7.6	5.3

Source: Authors.

systems. There was moderate evidence that some of the aforementioned strategies can be effective in a number of settings. However, the overall evidence is not strong and, possibly because of the multiple interventions within each of these strategies, some were found to be more successful than others. With regard to health professionals, strategies to increase the number of health workers, including the use of paid or unpaid community health workers, had positive results, particularly for the poor. Over the short term and within a number of settings, this work found moderate evidence that strategies involving strengthening accountability and linking financing to performance measures and accountability (for example, through contracting) were effective. As regards the payment of incentives to health workers to increase the quantity and quality of services, the review found moderate evidence of strategies of this type to be successful.

The evidence was inconclusive as to whether disease-specific programs are an effective way to strengthen health services. However, there was also only weak evidence that such programs divert resources from other programs and distort overall health services away from local needs. This begs the question: do these programs significantly strengthen health systems beyond their specific area of interest? Again, there is weak, inconclusive evidence on this issue. Furthermore, the effectiveness of the strategy depends on how the strategy is implemented. As an example, careful implementation of certain types of HIV/AIDS programs can also strengthen other services, but here, too, the research is limited and cannot be generalized.

Strategies to strengthen disease-specific programs that are effective in one area can be successfully scaled up nationally. There is some moderate evidence that actions to strengthen disease-specific programs can be successfully scaled up. In fact, more studies have been found on successful scale-up programs than those shown to be unsuccessful. However, this may be due to publication bias toward the reporting of successful scaled-up interventions. This work also found that "success" depends on how the implementation itself was carried out, certain enabling factors in the environment, and the type of disease-specific programs: complex, multiple-component programs appear to be less successful when scaled up, but this may be due to limited capacity to ensure continual coordination.

For the poor, the implementation process is as important as the type of strategy implemented. Overall evidence exists to support the notion that, of all the fully implemented strategies, some are more effective in strengthening service delivery for the poor. What appear to be important are interventions that focus on addressing the needs of the poor, that ensure regular measurement of impact on the poor, and that provide oversight to ensure that the poor benefit. Failed strategies have lacked supportive implementation conditions or been poorly managed, though the 150 studies reviewed were likely to have significant amounts of resources to ensure full implementation. Notably, in those few studies with many positive outcomes, an assessment of both needs and constraints was conducted and, subsequently, plans to minimize constraints were found in 66 percent of the randomized interventions; however, many interventions that did not use this approach also had positive outcomes. Notably, however, the available research often did not describe to what extent these plans to minimize constraints were implemented, preventing a more thorough conclusion.

The initial and continuous adaptation of the strategy to the local context is associated with more complete strategy implementation; and adaptation is easier in small-scale interventions. In Ghana, for example, a scaled-up child and maternal health services strengthening pilot used an approach adapted for the national context using peer demonstration, diffusion, and teamwork. Adapting strategies to local conditions in this way proved to be more important in the multicultural context of Ghana, particularly when compared to Bangladesh, which is more homogeneous (Phillips et al. 2006).

Various approaches are used to adapt an intervention. One common approach involves a pilot, feedback, further modification of the intervention, followed by regional or national dissemination. An approach that involves more phases may be even more effective: if time and resources allow, the initial pilot may be followed by additional pilots at the same time within different contexts within a country, allowing for more detailed guidance for decision makers. There is evidence that implementation effectiveness is increased by providing continuous feedback to the strategy team and leaders about needs, constraints, implementation progress, and impact.

Stakeholder involvement and consultation are necessary for effective implementation. Consultation and consensus building require the participation of multiple stakeholders (including local communities), which in turn, require education about the strengthening intervention itself if they are to contribute effectively. This helps shape priorities, guide the strengthening approach, and create local ownership. It also shows that each level of the health system and local government needs to play its part in strengthening health care services. To do so, the review suggests that each health system level will need to be developed through adequate training of personnel, who are then held accountable for their role.

There was no evidence that certain strategies are less dependent on the local environment and work in more countries than other strategies. However, it was found that successful implementation was linked to undertaking interventions to identify and minimize the constraints. The review found studies of successful implementation where efforts to identify and minimize constraints were undertaken. In appraising the available research, this review found that if decision makers took action to ensure that as many enabling conditions as possible were met, this would increase the likelihood of implementation of the strategy. However, it would also be necessary for decision makers to use local research to investigate and address other specific factors that may prevent or hinder implementation of the strategy locally, and encourage those that facilitate it.

The mobilization of adequate resources is linked to the successful implementation of the strategy. The research reviewed shows that the availability of resources (for example, human and financial resources, and leadership) profoundly influences all strengthening strategies. Therefore, decision makers would benefit in drawing lessons on strengthening strategies from situations that share similar resource characteristics. Accordingly, they should not implement a strategy if they are uncertain that the "right" resources are available. Overall, this work found that strategies to maintain or increase the number of health workers are likely to strengthen health services delivery in low-income countries. However, additional management skills for implementing the strengthening changes are also needed. For most strategies, managers at all levels need to be developed and given time to plan and implement strengthening interventions (rather than solely manage routine operations), with some managers dedicated full time to implementing the relevant intervention. Aspects of leadership associated with successful strengthening include a clearly communicated mandate from top management that gives authority, resources, and accountability to leaders and teams throughout the organization, as well as respected "change champions" and implementation teams.

An attempt was also made to associate different approaches to strategy implementation directly with the level of success of implementation. In more than half the studies (57.3 percent), the outcomes measured were all positive, while 27.3 percent of interventions had outcomes that were mostly positive. Hence approximately 85 percent of the studies analyzed had a majority of positive outcomes. Table 1.3 shows the distribution of the proportion of positive outcomes by study design. Nearly all studies (96 percent) had at least one positive outcome. However, the role of publication bias—where studies with negative findings are less likely to be submitted or published (Olson et al. 2002; Stern and Simes 1997)—should be considered.

Cross-tabulations of the key approaches to implementing strengthening strategies were used to identify whether some approaches were more likely to be associated with a majority of positive outcomes, compared to a majority of negative outcomes (table 1.4).

For studies with strong designs (RCTs), there was no implementation approach that had a statistically significant difference (at the level of $p<0.05$) in the chance of attaining mostly positive outcomes, though "flexibility and modification through stakeholder feedback" ($p=0.11$) and the development of "constraints reduction plans" ($p=0.12$) approached this level. The case with D2 studies (NRCTs) was similar, though "ensuring resource availability" was close ($p=0.08$). When

Table 1.3   Direction of Outcomes from Reviewed Literature

Proportion of positive outcomes	Randomized controlled trials, % (n=33)	Nonrandomized controlled trials, % (n=52)	Uncontrolled before-after trials, % (n=65)	Total, % (N=150)
All outcomes positive	75.8	48.1	55.4	57.3
Majority (but not all) outcomes positive	12.1	30.8	32.3	27.3
Majority outcomes negative	9.1	17.3	7.7	11.4
No outcomes positive	3	3.8	4.6	4

Source: Authors.

Table 1.4 Aspects of Health Strategy Implementation and Their Association with Positive Outcomes

	Randomized controlled trials (D1 studies) (n=33)		Nonrandomized controlled trials (D2 studies) (n=52)		Uncontrolled before-after trials (D3 studies) (n=65)		All studies (N=150)	
	Odds ratio	P value	Odds ratio	P value	Odds ratio	P value	Odds ratio	P value
Assessment of needs and constraints	..		..		..		2.8	0.4
Constraints reduction plans	6.7	0.1	1.4	0.7	7.3	0.06	2.7	0.03
Development of leaders	1.1	1.0	0.8	0.7	..		1.4	0.8
Development of a management structure	..		0.8	0.7	..		1.7	0.3
Broad-based support of various stakeholders	..		1.9	0.7	5.5	0.1	3.9	0.03
Consultation and engagement of powerful interest groups	2.8	0.6	1.7	0.5	..		3.8	0.009
Representation from powerful interest groups	2.4	0.6	1.4	0.7	..		3	0.03
Coordination and community organization	..		1.5	0.7	..		4.6	0.01
Flexibility and modification through stakeholder feedback	..		1.4	0.7	5.1	0.1	3.4	0.03

(continued)

Table 1.4   Aspects of Health Strategy Implementation and Their Association with Positive Outcomes (Continued)

	Randomized controlled trials (D1 studies) (n=33)		Nonrandomized controlled trials (D2 studies) (n=52)		Uncontrolled before-after trials (D3 studies) (n=65)		All studies (N=150)	
	Odds ratio	P value	Odds ratio	P value	Odds ratio	P value	Odds ratio	P value
Local adaptation of the intervention	9.3	0.2	..		16.5	0.01	4.3	0.05
Addresses institutional and policy constraints	1.1	1.0	0.5	0.3	..		1.0	1.0
Ensures sufficient resources	2.9	0.4	4.1	0.8	18	0.003	6.8	0.0006
Reduces corruption	..		..		..		..	
Coordination of multiple-action strategies at different levels	0.9	1	1.2	0.7	5.5	0.1	1.4	0.4
Financial incentives for individuals or teams based on monitored outputs	0.5	0.5	2.6	0.3	2.3	0.7	1.7	0.4

Source: Authors.

Note: .. means indeterminate odds ratio (zero cases in one); p values determined by Fisher's exact test.

uncontrolled studies were considered, six implementation approaches had p values ≤0.05 to demonstrate a statistically significant difference in the chance of attaining mostly positive outcomes. When all studies were combined, eight implementation approaches had statistically significant p values, including:

- flexibility and modification through stakeholder feedback (p=0.03)
- constraints reduction plans (p=0.03)
- local adaptation (p=0.05)
- broad-based support of stakeholders (p=0.03)
- coordination and community organization (p=0.01)
- ensuring resource availability (p=0.0006)
- consultation at various stages (p=0.009)
- representation from various groups (p=0.03).

Main Limitations

This review found significant limitations to the research in this field. In summary, it found that there is little research giving enough information needed by decision makers about the results, implementation actions, and factors that helped or hindered implementation of a health services strengthening intervention in a developing country. Many studies do not give sufficient detail of the strategies or interventions pursued or whether they were fully implemented. In addition, different strategies are often given the same label. Strategies often involve multiple components that are not specified, nor studied in a way that would indicate which component is essential, or where there are synergies between components.

Few studies examine factors beyond the health system or the intervention itself that may influence the results being examined. A further limitation is the degree to which the studies' results can be attributed to the strengthening actions. Few studies use designs that could increase certainty of attribution of short- or long-term results to the strategy, such as time-series comparisons or assessments by a cross-section of informed observers. More and better research and evaluation of health services strategies in developing countries are greatly needed. Significant learning could also be gained from the rich but unsystemized experience of those overseeing or managing programs, some of which is documented in evaluation reports, case studies, lessons learned, best practices, and pooled expert opinions.

Table 1.5 Summary of Recommendations Based on Review

Theme	Recommendation	Implications (and level of research support)
Assessment and planning		
Use of research evidence	Use available research capacity and evidence to conduct a thorough assessment of needs and constraints, etc.	Strengthening programs that use the available research capacity and evidence to address health system needs, constraints, and results can better guide planning and implementation, and allow for adaptation to local conditions (S3).
Constraints reduction plan	Apply existing research frameworks to assess and address constraints. Identify health system challenges and develop a specific plan to minimize constraints.	The evidence is moderate that the assessment of constraints, and the development of a plan to address constraints, were factors in the successful implementation of some specific strengthening interventions (S2).
Contracting out specific services	Switch to outside providers for certain noncore services.	This measure can work in different circumstances, but evidence about effects is conflicting (S3).
Drug logistics	Finance, develop, and implement a strategy to ensure that health facilities have a continuous supply of essential drugs and provide training in drug prescribing.	There is conflicting evidence of success in implementing drug supply improvements and sustainable funding (S3). Implementation is very dependent on the situation and may have negative results if personnel cannot prescribe essential drugs properly.
Leadership support and management structure		
Leadership support	Develop competent and committed leaders to implement a strategy through leadership training and careful selection.	There is moderate evidence that strengthening strategies often fail due to leadership without skills (S2). However, there is weak evidence that effective leadership development is necessary for implementing strengthening strategies (S4). The "right" leadership includes a clearly communicated mandate from top management that gives authority, resources, and accountability to leaders and teams throughout the organization, as well as respected "change champions" and implementation teams (S4).
Management structure	Develop management structure to implement the strategy while providing routine services.	Moderate evidence exists that strengthening strategies are less successful when implemented under a management structure with weak delegation authorities and accountability (S2).

Stakeholder involvement and consultation

Broad-based consultation	Develop broad-based support of multiple stakeholders. Consult and involve interest groups at all stages.	Limited evidence is seen that implementation of interventions will be more effective with broad-based consensus-building and consultation of key actors (S3). Limited evidence exists that some strategies have failed, in part, due to consultations organized in order to gain support and input regarding the details of the implementation process (S3).
Representation	Develop and use representation from powerful groups who will support or oppose implementation.	There is limited evidence that most strategies are difficult to implement due to "organizational inertia." Moderate evidence that some strategies are blocked or accelerated by powerful interest groups (S3).
Coordination and community organization	Create and use formal networks and community groups to help design, conduct, and monitor the implementation process.	Limited evidence exists that coordination with community groups and other agencies is effective in designing, implementing, and sustaining interventions (S3).
Flexibility and modification	Obtain continuous feedback and input from all stakeholder levels.	Continuous review and modification of the strategy are necessary (through local pilots, for example), particularly when the strategy is adapted to the local context (S4).
Local adaptation	Adapt the intervention to the local context, drawing on the analysis of constraints, as well as previous research and experts in the field.	There is moderate evidence that most interventions require local adaptation. Leaders will need detailed advice/consultations from local experts to formulate the implementation process (S3).
Policy and institutional constraints	Identify and address current and impending policy and institutional constraints.	Implementers should be mindful of evolving policy and institutional constraints, which can be more serious than resource constraints (S5).
Resource availability		
Financial resources	Ensure sufficient financial and human resources are available and can be made available to continuously support the implementation process.	Limited evidence exists that the financial and human resources required are often underestimated, in part because the implementation process becomes longer than anticipated (S3).

(continued)

Table 1.5 Summary of Recommendations Based on Review *(Continued)*

Theme	Recommendation	Implications (and level of research support)
	Increase finance to ministry of health if the public health system has been historically underfunded and there is reason to believe that financial resources will be effectively spent on health care.	Limited evidence is seen that countries with good governance have been able to effectively spend on health reforms or specific programs (S3). There is evidence that increasing financial resources can be an effective means to create the conditions for other successful interventions (for example, infrastructure improvements, leadership and management support).
	Create financial incentives for health workers to conduct specific tasks that are immediately required and for which there will be minor negative effects resulting from workers' time being allocated from other activities.	The evidence is moderate that financial incentives can increase the task performance of health workers and organizations (S2), but potential negative side effects can occur if the strategy is not designed or implemented well.
Human resources	Consider salary increases, particularly in situations with low employee morale or low compensation.	The evidence is limited (S3), but there is a strong rationale in many LMIC situations.
	Increase workforce in total and possibly specific cadres (for example, midwives, doctors).	The evidence is limited (S3), but there is a strong rationale in many LMIC situations.
Governance structure	Reduce the opportunities for corruption in transferring resources.	Studies show limited evidence that corruption above a certain level reduces resources and increases the time needed for health services strengthening (S3). There is evidence that implementers will need to understand how the governance structure affects both the type of strengthening strategies most likely to be effective, and the implementation process. Decision makers can learn most from other settings that share similar governance characteristics (S5).
	Understand fully the governance structure's impact on strengthening strategies. Learn from other settings with similar characteristics.	
Coordination of multiple-action strategies	Use actions of different types and levels if the management capacity and health systems can continuously coordinate them.	There is some evidence that multiple actions at various levels can be more effective than single actions, but only if carefully planned and coordinated throughout the implementation process. There is some evidence that more complex strategies cannot be adequately managed by some LICs (S3).

Source: Authors.

Note: The level of research support is based on the criteria in table 5 in the *Overview*: S1 = strong; S2 = moderate; S3 = limited; S4 = evidence of implementation only; S5 = descriptive studies only.

Implications for Decision Makers

The review found a weak evidence base for claiming success of any particular health services strengthening strategy in one LMIC. There is even less evidence to expect the same results in another country, and most evidence points to the need to adapt any strategy to the local context. Although this provides considerable room for additional research, the focus of this review is on the implications for decision making.

The research gives a basis for preliminary suggestions on how decision makers can try to strengthen health services. Table 1.5 presents recommendations, based on the review, that are intended to guide decision makers in designing and implementing strategies to strengthen health services delivery.

References

Chen, L., T. Evans, S. Anand, et al. 2004. "Human Resources for Health: Overcoming the Crisis." *Lancet* 364: 184–90.

Olson, C.M., D. Rennie, D. Cook, et al. 2002. "Publication Bias in Editorial Decision Making." *Journal of the American Medical Association* 287: 2825–8.

Ovretveit, J. 2003a. *What is the Best Strategy for Improving Quality and Safety of Hospitals: A Review and Synthesis of the Evidence.* Copenhagen: WHO Regional Office for Europe.

———. 2003b. "Grading Evidence for Decision-makers: Issues and Methods in Assessing the Scientific Quality of Research and Summarizing Strength of Evidence for Public Health Research Reviews." Discussion document for WHO Health Evidence Network, Copenhagen, available from Karolinska Institutet, Medical Management Centre, Stockholm.

Phillips, J.F., T.C. Jones, F.K. Nyonator, and S.R. Ravikumar. 2006. "Evidence-based Scaling-up of Health and Family Service Innovations in Bangladesh and Ghana." In *Scaling-up Health Service Delivery: From Pilot Innovations to Policies and Programmes*, ed. R. Simmons, P. Fajans, and L. Ghiron. Geneva: World Health Organization.

Stern, J.M., and R.J. Simes. 1997. "Publication Bias: Evidence of Delayed Publication in a Cohort Study of Clinical Research Projects." *British Medical Journal* 315: 640–5.

Travis, P., S. Bennett, A. Haines, T. Pang, Z. Bhutta, A.A. Hyder, N.R. Pielemeier, A. Mills, and T. Evans. 2004. "Overcoming Health-systems Constraints to Achieve the Millennium Development Goals." *Lancet* 364 (9437): 900–906.

Annex 1.1 Electronic Databases Searched

- PubMed (http://www.ncbi.nlm.nih.gov/entrez/query.fcgi)
- CINAHL (http://www.cinahl.com/)
- Eldis/HRC Health Systems Resource Guide (Open access at: http://www.eldis.org/healthsystems/)
- Cochrane Library (http://www.cochrane.org/index0.htm)
- Campbell Collaboration (http://www.campbellcollaboration.org/Fralibrary.html)
- European Observatory for Health Systems and Health Policy (http://www.euro.who.int/observatory)
- Best Evidence (ACP Journal Club) (http://www.acponline.org/catalog/journals/acpjc.htm)
- York Database of Abstracts of Reviews of Effects (DARE) (http://www.york.ac.uk/inst/crd/darehp.htm)
- Web of Science (http://sub3.isiknowledge.com/error/Error?Domain= isiknowledge.com&Params=DestApp%3DWOS%26Func%3DFrame &Error=IPError&Src=IP&PathInfo=%2F&RouterURL=http%3A%2F %2Fisiknowledge.com&IP=69.251.2.250)
- Management Sciences for Health "The managers resource" (http://erc.msh.org/)

Annex 1.2 Key Search Terms

The health services strengthening review included an in-depth search of the following terms: "health services" OR "delivery of health care" OR one or more of the following search terms and country codes.

Other Key Search Terms

quality improvement; quality management systems; total quality management; continuous quality improvement; quality assurance, health care; quality of health care; quality collaborative; quality indicator comparisons; benchmarking; balanced scorecard; re-engineering; quality strategy; patient safety; patient risk management

community based services; community driven services; community mobilization; community empowerment; coalitions; community based organizations; local nongovernmental organizations; consumer groups; consumer advocacy; consumer courts; consumer protection; conditional cash transfers; demand side financing; demand creation; vouchers; co-payment; co-production; peer support; community scorecards contracting; regulation; accreditation; licensing; compact; service agreements; public-private partnership; stewardship; oversight; certificate of need

Countries

afghanistan OR bangladesh OR benin OR bhutan OR burkina faso OR burundi OR cambodia OR cameroon OR central african republic OR chad OR comoros OR congo OR the democratic republic of congo OR cote d'ivoire OR eritrea OR ethiopia OR the gambia OR ghana OR guinea OR guinea-bissau OR haiti OR india OR kenya OR democratic republic of korea OR kyrgyzstan republic OR lao pdr OR lesotho OR liberia OR madagascar OR malawi OR mali OR mauritania OR moldova OR mongolia OR mozambique OR myanmar OR nepal OR nicaragua OR niger OR nigeria OR north korea OR pakistan OR papua new guinea OR rwanda OR sao tome and principe OR senegal OR sierra leone OR solomon islands OR somalia OR sudan OR tajikistan OR tanzania OR timor leste OR togo OR uganda OR uzbekistan OR vietnam OR yemen OR republic of yemen OR zaire OR zambia OR zimbabwe OR albania OR algeria OR angola OR armenia OR azerbaijan OR belarus OR bolivia OR bosnia and herzegovina OR brazil OR bulgaria OR cape verde OR china OR colombia OR cuba OR djibouti OR dominican republic OR ecuador OR egypt OR arab republic of egypt OR el salvador OR fiji OR georgia OR guatemala OR guyana OR honduras OR indonesia OR iran OR islamic republic of iran OR iraq OR jamaica OR jordan OR kazakhstan OR kiribati OR macedonia OR fyr of macedonia OR former yugoslav republic of macedonia OR maldives OR marshall islands OR micronesia OR federated states of micronesia OR morocco OR namibia OR paraguay OR peru OR philippines OR romania OR samoa OR serbia and montenegro OR sri lanka OR suriname OR swaziland OR syrian arab republic OR syria OR thailand OR tonga OR tunisia OR turkmenistan OR ukraine OR vanuatu OR west bank and gaza OR american samoa OR antigua and barbuda OR argentina OR barbados OR belize OR botswana OR chile OR costa rica OR croatia OR czech republic OR dominica OR equatorial guinea OR estonia OR gabon OR grenada OR hungary OR latvia OR lebanon OR libya OR lithuania OR malaysia OR mauritius OR mayotte OR mexico OR northern mariana islands OR oman OR palau OR panama OR poland OR russian federation OR seychelles OR slovak republic OR south africa OR st. kitts and nevis OR st. lucia OR st. vincent and the grenadines OR trinidad and tobago OR turkey OR uruguay OR venezuela OR bolivariana republic of venezuela

OR developing countries OR less developed countries OR third-world countries OR under-developed countries OR poor countries OR less developed countries OR under developed countries OR less developed nations OR third world nations OR under developed nations OR developing nations OR poor nations OR poor economies OR third world economies OR developing economies OR under developed economies OR less developed economies OR burma OR czechoslovakia OR democratic republic of congo OR french guiana OR east timor OR laos OR north korea OR ivory coast OR republic of georgia OR republic of yemen OR republic of zaire OR slovakia OR soviet union OR surinam OR ussr OR west samoa OR yugoslavia OR zaire OR asia OR west indies OR polynesia OR micronesia OR middle east OR africa OR latin america OR central america OR south america OR caribbean OR west indies region OR hispanico OR southeast asia OR sub-saharan africa OR eastern europe OR the Balkans

Annex 1.3 Studies Reviewed

Abdulla, S., J.A. Schellenberg, R. Nathan, et al. 2001. "Impact on Malaria Morbidity of a Programme Supplying Insecticide Treated Nets in Children Aged under Two Years in Tanzania: Community Cross-sectional Study." *British Medical Journal* 322: 270–3.

Adu-Sarkodie, Y., M.J. Steiner, J. Attafuah, and K. Tweedy. 2000. "Syndromic Management of Urethral Discharge in Ghanaian Pharmacies." *Sexually Transmitted Infections* 76(6): 439–442.

Agha, S., A.M. Karim, A. Balal, and S. Sossler. 2003. "A Quasi-experimental Study to Assess the Performance of a Reproductive Health Franchise in Nepal." Commercial Market Strategies, Washington, DC.

Agha, S. 2002. "A Quasi-experimental Study to Assess the Impact of Four Adolescent Sexual Health Interventions in Sub-Saharan Africa." *International Family Planning Perspectives* 28(2): 67–118.

Agha, S., A. Karlyn, and D. Meekers. 2001. "The Promotion of Condom Use in Non-regular Sexual Partnerships in Urban Mozambique." *Health Policy and Planning* 16: 144–51.

Akpala, C.O. 1994. "An Evaluation of the Knowledge and Practices of Trained Traditional Birth Attendants in Bodinga, Sokota State, Nigeria." *Journal of Tropical Medicine and Hygiene* 97: 46–50.

Alford. S., N. Cheetham, and D. Hauser. 2005. "Science and Success in Developing Countries: Holistic Programs that Work to Prevent Teen Pregnancy, HIV and Sexually Transmitted Infections." Advocates For Youth, Washington, DC.

Alisjahbana, A., C. Williams, R. Dharmayanti, D. Hermawan, B.E. Kwast, and M. Koblinsky. 1995. "An Integrated Village Maternity Service to Improve Referral Patterns in a Rural Area in West-Java." *International Journal of Gynecology & Obstetrics* 48(suppl. 1): S83–S94.

Angeles-Agdeppa, I., L. S. Paulino, A. C. Ramos, U. M. Etorma, T. Cavalli-Sforza, and S. Milani. 2005. "Government-industry Partnership in Weekly Iron-Folic Acid Supplementation for Women of Reproductive Age in the Philippines: Impact on Iron Status." *Nutrition Reviews* 2: 116–125.

Angunawela, I.I., V.K. Diwan, and G. Tomson. 1991. "Experimental Evaluation of the Effects of Drug Information on Antibiotic Prescribing: A Study in Outpatient Care in an Area of Sri Lanka." *International Journal of Epidemiology* 20: 558–64.

El Arifeen, S., L.S. Blum, D.M.E. Hoque, E.K. Chowdhury, R. Khan, R.E. Black, et al. 2004. "Integrated Management of Childhood Illness (IMCI) in Bangladesh: Early Findings from a Cluster-randomised Study." *Lancet* 364(9445): 1595–1602.

Araujo, G., L. Araujo, B. Janowitz, S. Wallace, and M. Potts. 1983. "Improving obstetric care in northeast Brazil." *PAHO Bulletin* 17: 233–242.

Bailey, P.E, J.A. Szaszdi, and L. Glover. 2002. "Obstetric Complications: Does Training Traditional Birth Attendants Make a Difference?" *Revista panamericana de salud pública (Pan American Journal of Public Health)* 11: 15–23.

Bang, A.T., R.A. Bang, S.B. Baitule, M.H. Reddy, and M.D. Deshmukh. 1999. "Effect of Home-based Neonatal Care and Management of Sepsis on Neonatal Mortality: Field Trial in Rural India." *Lancet* 354(9194): 1955–61.

Bashir, A. 1991. "Maternal Mortality in Pakistan. A Success Story of the Faisalabad District." *IPPF Medical Bulletin* 25: 1–3.

Begum, J.A, I.A. Kabir, and A.Y. Mollah. 1990. "The Impact of Training Traditional Birth Attendants in Improving MCH Care in Rural Bangladesh." *Asia-Pacific Journal of Public Health* 4: 142–4.

Berggren, G.G, W. Berggren, A. Verly, et al. 1983. "Traditional Midwives, Tetanus Immunization, and Infant Mortality in Rural Haiti." *Tropical Doctor* 13: 79–87.

Berman, P., and L. Rose. 1996. "The Role of Private Providers in Maternal and Child Health and Family Planning Services in Developing Countries." *Health Policy and Planning* 11(2): 142–155.

Bexell, A., E. Lwando, B. von Hofsten, S. Tembo, B. Eriksson, and V. K. Diwan. 1996. "Improving Drug Use Through Continuing Education: A Randomized Controlled Trial in Zambia." *Journal of Clinical Epidemiology* 49(3): 355–357.

Bhandari, N., R. Bahl, S. Mazumdar, J. Martines, R. E. Black, and M. K. Bhan. 2003. "Effect of Community-based Promotion of Exclusive Breastfeeding on

Diarrheal Illness and Growth: A Cluster Randomized Controlled Trial." *Lancet* 361(9367): 1418–1423.

Bhutta, Z.A., I. Gupta, H. de'Silva, D. Manandhar, S. Awasthi, S.M.M. Hossain, et al. 2004. "Maternal and Child Health: Is South Asia Ready for Change?" *British Medical Journal* 328(7443): 816–819.

Black, R. E., S. S. Morris, and J. Bryce. 2003. "Where and Why are 10 million Children Dying Every Year?" *Lancet* 361(9376): 2226–2234.

Brieger, W., L. Salako, R. Umeh, P. Agomo, B. Afolabi, and A. Adeneye. "Promoting Pre-packaged Drugs for Prompt and Appropriate Treatment of Febrile Illnesses in Rural Nigerian Communities." *International Quarterly of Community Health Education* 2002–2003, 21(1): 19–40.

Briggs, C.J., and P. Garner. "Strategies for Integrating Primary Health Services in Middle- and Low-income Countries at the Point of Delivery." *Cochrane Database of Systematic Reviews* 2006, Issue 2. Art. No.: CD003318. DOI: 10.1002/14651858.CD003318.pub2.

Burkhalter, B.R. 1998. "Employer-based Maternal and Child Health Model in Malawi." In *Community-based Approaches to Child Health: BASICS Experience to Date*, ed. M. Rasmuson, N. Bashir, and N. Keith. Arlington, VA: Basic Support for Institutionalizing Child Survival Project (BASICS).

Chakraborty, S., S.A. D'Souza, and R.S. Northrup. 2000. "Improving Private Practitioner Care of Sick Children: Testing New Approaches in Rural Bihar." *Health Policy and Planning* 15: 400–407.

Chalker, J., S. Ratanawijitrasin, N.T.K. Chuc, M. Petzold, and G. Tomson. 2005. "Effectiveness of a Multi-component Intervention on Dispensing Practices at Private Pharmacies in Vietnam and Thailand: A Randomized Controlled Trial." *Social Science & Medicine* 60(1): 131–141.

Chipfakacha, V. 1993. "Prevention of Sexually Transmitted Disease: The Shurugwi Sex-workers Project." *South African Medical Journal* 83: 40–1.

China Tuberculosis Control Collaboration. 1996. "Results of Directly Observed Short-course Chemotherapy in 112842 Chinese patients with smear-positive tuberculosis." *Lancet* 347: 358–362.

Chongsuvivatwong, V., L. Mo-Suwan, K. Tayakkanonta, K. Vitsupakorn, and R. McNeil. 1996. "Impacts of Training of Village Health Volunteers in Reduction of Morbidity from Acute Respiratory Infections in Southern Thailand." *The Southeast Asian Journal of Tropical Medicine and Public Health* 27(2): 333–338.

Chowdhury, A.M.R., S. Chowdhury, N. Islam, A. Islam, and J.P. Vaughan. 1997. "Control of Tuberculosis by Community Health Workers in Bangladesh." *Lancet* 350, 169–172.

Chowdhury, A.M.R., A. Alam, S.A. Chowdhury, and J. Ahmed. 1992. "Tuberculosis Control in Bangladesh." *Lancet* 339, 1181–1182.

Chowdhury, A.M.R., F. Karin, S.K. Sarkar, et al. 1997. "The Status of ORT in Bangladesh: How Widely is it Used?" *Health Policy and Planning* 12: 58–66.

Chukudebelu, W., A. Ikeme, J. Okaro et al. 1997. "Involving the Private Sector in Improving Obstetric Care: Anambra State, Nigeria. The Enugu PMM Team." *International Journal of Gynaecology and Obstetrics* 59: S107–12.

Commission on Macroeconomics and Health. 2002. "Improving Health Outcomes of the Poor." Working Group Report, World Health Organization, Geneva.

Crabbe, F., J. P. Tchupo, T. Manchester, et al. 1998. "Prepackaged Therapy for Urethritis: The "MSTOP" Experience in Cameroon." *Sexually Transmitted Infections* 74: 249–52.

Curtale, F., B. Siwakoti, C. Lagrosa, M. LaRaja, and R. Guerra. 1995/4. "Improving Skills and Utilization of Community Health Volunteers in Nepal." *Social Science & Medicine* 40(8): 1117–1125.

Daga, S.R., A.S. Daga, R.V. Dighole, R.P. Patil, and H.L. Dhinde. 1992. "Rural Neonatal Care: Dahanu Experience." Indian Pediatrics 29: 189–93.

Daga, A.S., S.R. Daga, R.V. Dighole, R.P. Patil, and M.R. Patil. 1997. "Evaluation of Training Programme for Traditional Birth Attendants in Newborn Care." *Indian Pediatrics* 34: 1021–4.

Dange Chettri G., K. Kafle, S. Karkee, V. Rajubhandari, and B. Humagain. 2004. "Effect of regulatory intervention on drug availability in Nepal." *Proceedings of International Conferences on Improving Use of Medicines (ICIUM)*. March 30–April 2, Chiang Mai, Thailand.

Dehne, K., J. Wacker, and J. Cowley. 1995. "Training Birth Attendants in the Sahel." *World Health Forum* 16: 415–9.

Delacollete, C., P. van der Stuyft, and K. Molima. 1996. "Using Community Health Workers for Malaria Control: Experience from Zaire." *Bulletin of the World Health Organization* 74 (4): 423–430.

Denis, M. B. 1998. "Improving Compliance with Quinine + Tetracycline for Treatment of Malaria: Evaluation of Health Education Interventions in Cambodian Villages." *Bulletin of the World Health Organization*, 79(suppl. 1): 43–49.

Eichler, R., P. Auxila, and J. Pollock. 2001a. "Output-based Health Care: Public Policy for the Private Sector." The World Bank Group Private Sector and Infrastructure Network. World Bank, Washington, DC.

Eichler, R., P. Auxila, and J. Pollock. 2001b. "Performance-based Payment to Improve the Impact of Health Services: Evidence from Haiti." *The World Bank Institute Online Journal*. Washington, DC: Flagship Program on Health Sector Reform and Sustainable Financing, World Bank Institute.

Egger, M., J. Pauw, A. Lopatatzidis, D. Medrano, F. Paccaud, and G.D. Smith. 2000. "Promotion of Condom Use in a High-risk Setting in Nicaragua: A Randomized Controlled Trial." *Lancet* 355(9221): 2101–2105.

Eloundou-Enyegue, P., D. Meekers, A. Calves. 1998. *From Awareness to Adoption: The Effect of AIDS Education and Condom Social Marketing on Condom Use in Tanzania (1993–1996)*. Washington, DC: Population Services International.

Fauveau, V., K. Stewart, S.A. Khan, and J. Chakraborty. 1991. "Effect on Mortality of Community-based Maternity-care Programme in Rural Bangladesh." *Lancet* 338(8776): 1183–1186.

Ford, K., D.N. Wirawan, P. Fajans, et al. 1996. "Behavioral Interventions for Reduction of Sexually Transmitted Disease/HIV Transmission among Female Commercial Sex Workers and Clients in Bali, Indonesia." *AIDS* 10: 213–22.

Fraser-Hurt, N., and E. Lyimo. 1998. "Insecticide-treated Nets and Treatment Service: A Trial Using Public and Private Sector Channels in Rural United Republic of Tanzania." *Bulletin of the World Health Organization* 76: 607–15.

Fullerton, J., A. Fort, and K. Johal. 2003. "A Case/comparison Study in the Eastern Region of Ghana on the Effects of Incorporating Selected Reproductive Health Services on Family Planning Services." *Midwifery* 19(1): 17–26.

Garcia, P.J., E. Gotuzzo, J.P. Hughes, and K.K. Holmes. 1998. "Syndromic Management of STDs in Pharmacies: Evaluation and Randomized Intervention Trial." *Sexually Transmitted Infections* 74 (supp. 1): S153–S158.

Gloyd, S., F. Floriano, M. Seunda, M.A. Chadreque, J.M. Nyangezi, and A. Platas. 2001. "Impact of Traditional Birth Attendant Training in Mozambique: A Controlled Study." *Journal of Midwifery & Women's Health* 46(4): 210–216.

Goel, P., J. Makhulo, and G. Mwangi. 1994. "Working with Pharmacists in Kenya." *Dialogue on Diarrhoea* (55).

Grabowsky, M., N. Farrell, W. Hawley, J. Chimumbwa, S. Hoyer, A. Wolkon, and J. Selanikio. 2005. "Integrating Insecticide-treated Bednets into a Measles Vaccination Campaign Achieves High, Rapid and Equitable Coverage with Direct and Voucher-based Methods." *Tropical Medicine & International Health* 10(11): 1151–1160.

Green, M., I.F. Hoffman, A. Brathwaite et al. 1998. "Improving Sexually Transmitted Disease Management in the Private Sector: The Jamaica Experience." *AIDS* 12: S67–72.

Greenwood, A., A. Bradely, P. Bypass et al. 1990. "Evaluation of a Primary Health Care Programme in The Gambia. I. The Impact of Trained Traditional Birth Attendants on the Outcome of Pregnancy." *Journal of Tropical Medicine and Hygiene* 93: 87–97.

Greer, G., A. Akinpelumi, L. Madueke, B. Plowman, B. Fapohunda, Y. Tawfik, R. Holmes, J. Owor, U. Gilpin, C. Clarence, et al. 2004. "Improving Management of Childhood Malaria in Nigeria and Uganda by Improving Practices of Patent Medicine Vendors." Arlington: BASICS II and USAID.

Grosskurth, H., J. Todd, E. Mwijarubi, P. Mayaud, A. Nicoll, G. ka-Gina, et al. 1995/8/26. "Impact of Improved Treatment of Sexually Transmitted Diseases on HIV Infection in Rural Tanzania: Randomized Controlled Trial." *Lancet* 346(8974): 530–536.

Guyatt, G.H, D.L. Sackett, J.C. Sinclair, R. Hayward, D.J. Cook, and R.J. Cook. 1995. "Users' Guides to the Medical Literature. IX. A Method for Grading Health Care Recommendations. Evidence-based Medicine Working Group." *Journal of the American Medical Association* 274(22): 1800–1804.

Hadiyono, J.E.P., S. Suryawati, S.S. Danu, Sunartono, and B. Santoso. 1996. "Interactional Group Discussion: Results of a Controlled Trial Using a Behavioral Intervention to Reduce the Use of Injections in Public Health Facilities." *Social Science & Medicine* 42(8): 1177–1183.

Haider, R., A. Ashworth, I. Kabir, and S.R. Huttly. 2000. "Effect of Community-based Peer Counselors on Exclusive Breastfeeding Practices in Dhaka, Bangladesh: A Randomized Controlled Trial." *Lancet* 356(9242): 1643–1647.

Haines, A., S. Kuruvilla, and M. Borchert. 2004. "Bridging the Implementation Gap between Knowledge and Action for Health." *Bulletin of the World Health Organization* 82(10): 724–31.

Hanson, K., K. Ranson, V. Oliveira-Cruz, and A. Mills. 2003. "Expanding Access to Priority Health Interventions: A Framework for Understanding the Constraints to Scaling-up." *Journal of International Development* 15(1): 1–14.

Helitzer-Allen, D.L., D.A. McFarland, J.J. Wirima, and A.P. Macheso. 1993. "Malaria Chemoprophylaxis Compliance in Pregnant Women: A Cost-effectiveness Analysis of Alternative Interventions." *Social Science & Medicine* 36: 403–407.

Helitzer-Allen, D.L., A. Macheso, J. Wirima, and C. Kendall. 1994. "Testing Strategies to Increase Use of Chloroquine Chemoprophylaxis during Pregnancy in Malawi." *Acta Tropica* 58: 255–266.

Hill, J.P. 1992. "A Simple Scheme to Improve Compliance in Patients Taking Tuberculosis Medication." *Tropical Doctor* 22: 161–163.

Homedes, N., and A. Ugalde. 2001. "Improving the Use of Pharmaceuticals through Patient and Community Level Interventions." *Social Science & Medicine* 52(1): 99–134.

Huntington, D., and A. Aplogan. 1994. "The Integration of Family Planning and Childhood Immunization Services in Togo." *Studies in Family Planning* 25(3): 176–183.

Ibrahim, S.A., M.I. Omer, I.K. Amin, A.G. Babiker, and H. Rushwan. 1992. "The Role of the Village Midwife in Detection of High Risk Pregnancies and Newborns." *International Journal of Gynecology and Obstetrics*, 39, 117–122.

Islam, M. A., S. Wakai, et al. 2002. "Cost-effectiveness of Community Health Workers in Tuberculosis Control in Bangladesh." *Bulletin of the World Health Organization* 80(6): 445–50.

Jacobs, B., F.S. Kambugu, J.A. Whitworth, et al. 2003. "Social Marketing of Pre-packaged Treatment for Men with Urethral Discharge (Clear Seven) in Uganda." *International Journal of STD and AIDS* 14: 216–21.

Janowitz, B., M. Suazo, D.B. Fried, J.H. Bratt, and P.E. Bailey. 1992. "Impact of Social Marketing on Contraceptive Prevalence and Cost in Honduras." *Studies in Family Planning* 23: 110–7.

Johns, B., T.T. Torres, and on behalf of WHO-CHOICE. 2005. "Costs of Scaling Up Health Interventions: A Systematic Review." *Health Policy and Planning* 20(1): 1–13.

Kambo, I.P., R.N. Gupta, A.S. Kundu, B.S. Dhillon, H.M. Saxena, and B.N. Saxena. 1994. "Use of Traditional Medical Practitioners to Deliver Family Planning Services in Uttar Pradesh." *Studies in Family Planning* 25(1): 32–40.

Kaona, F. A., and M. Tuba. 2003. "Improving Ability to Identify Malaria and Correctly Use Chloroquine in Children at Household Level in Nakonde District, Northern Province of Zambia." *Malaria Journal* 2(1): 43.

Karim, R., S. A. Lamstein, M. Akhtaruzzaman, KM. Rahman, and N. Alam. 2003. "The Bangladesh Integrated Nutrition Project Community-based Nutrition Component Endline Evaluation." Institute of Nutrition and Food Sciences, University of Dhaka, Bangladesh and International Food and Nutrition Center, Tufts University.

Kaufman, J., Jing F. 2002. "Privatisation of Health Services and the Reproductive Health of Rural Chinese Women." *Reproductive Health Matters* 10: 108–16.

Kenya, P.R., S. Gatiti, L. N. Muthami, R. Agwanda, H. A. Mwenesi, M. N. Katsivo, et al. 1990. "Oral Rehydration Therapy and Social Marketing in Rural Kenya." *Social Science & Medicine* 31(9): 979–987.

Kidane, G., and R. H Morrow. 2000. "Teaching Mothers to Provide Home Treatment of Malaria in Tigray, Ethiopia: A Randomized Trial." *Lancet* 356(9229): 550–555.

Ladipo, O.A., R. McNamara, G.E. Delano, E. Weiss, and E.O. Otolorin. 1990. "Family Planning in Traditional Markets in Nigeria." *Studies in Family Planning* 21: 311–21.

Lavadenz, F., N. Schwab, and H. Straatman. 2001. "Redes publicas, descentralizadas y comunitarias de salud en Bolivia." *Revista panamericana de salud pública (Pan American Journal of Public Health)* 9: 182–89.

Lehmann, U., I. Friedman, and D. Sanders. 2004. "Review of the Utilization and Effectiveness of Community-based Health Workers in Africa." JLI Working Paper 4–1, Joint Learning Initiative on Human Resources for Health and Development.

Lewin, S. A., J. Dick, P. Pond, M. Zwarenstein, G. Aja, B. van Wyk, X. Bosch-Capblanch, and M. Patrick. 2005. "Lay Health Workers in Primary and

Community Health Care." *The Cochrane Database of Systematic Reviews* 1(2): Art No: CD004015. DOI: 10.1002/14651858. CD004015.

Loevinsohn, B., and A. Harding. 2005. "Buying results? Contracting for Health Service Delivery in Developing Countries." *Lancet* 366(9486): 676–681.

Luby, S., N. Zaidi, S. Rehman, and R. Northrup. 2002. "Improving Private Practitioner Sick-child Case Management in Two Urban Communities in Pakistan." *Tropical Medicine & International Health* 7: 210–19.

Mahmud, H., A. Ullah Khan, and S. Ahmed. 2002. "Mid-term Health Facility Survey—Urban Primary Health Care Project." Dhaka: Mitra and Associates.

Manandhar, D. S., D. Osrin, B. P. Shrestha, N. Mesko, J. Morrison, K. M. Tumbahangphe, et al. 2004. "Effect of a Participatory Intervention with Women's Groups on Birth Outcomes in Nepal: Cluster-randomised Controlled Trial." *Lancet* 364(9438): 970–979.

Mantra, I. B., and J. Davies. 1989. "In Rural Indonesia Social Marketing of Oral Rehydration Salts: The Mothers' Perspective." *Hygie* 8(4): 26–31.

Marek, T., I. Diallo, B. Ndiaye, and J. Rakotosalama. "Successful Contracting of Prevention Services: Fighting Malnutrition in Senegal and Madagascar." *Health Policy and Planning* 1999; 14: 382–89.

Marsh, V. M., W. M. Mutemi, A. Willetts, K. Bayah, S. Were, A. Ross, and K. Marsh. 2004. "Improving Malaria Home Treatment by Training Drug Retailers in Rural Kenya." *Tropical Medicine & International Health* 9(4): 451–460.

Mathur, N. B., A. K. Gargye, and V. J. Rajput. 1983. "Knowledge, Attitude and Practice of Perinatal Care Amongst Traditional Birth Attendants (DAIS) Trained vs. Untrained." *Indian Pediatrics* 20: 837–42.

Mayhew, S., Nzambi, K., Pepin, J., and Adjei, S. 2001. "Pharmacists' Role in Managing Sexually Transmitted Infections: Policy Issues and Options for Ghana." *Health Policy and Planning* 16(2): 152–160.

McGinn, T., H. Aboagye-Owusu, R. Dugan, M. Nudanu, and D. Lauro. 1990. "Private Midwives: A New Approach to Family Planning Service Delivery in Ghana." *Midwifery* 6: 117–24.

McPake, B., and A. Mills. 2000. "What Can We Learn from International Comparisons of Health Systems and Health System Reform?" *Bulletin of the World Health Organization* 78(6): 811–20.

Meek, S., J. Hill, and J. Webster. 2001. *The Evidence Base for Interventions to Reduce Malaria Mortality in Low and Middle-Income Countries.* Commission on Macroeconomics and Health Working Paper Series, Paper No. WG5: 6.

Meekers, D. 2001. "The Role of Social Marketing in Sexually Transmitted Diseases/HIV Protection in 4600 Sexual Contacts in Urban Zimbabwe." *AIDS* 15: 285–7.

Meekers, D., S. Agha, and M. Klein. 2005. "The Impact on Condom Use of the '100% Jeune' Social Marketing Program in Cameroon." *Journal of Adolescent Health* 36(6): 530.

Meuwissen, L. E., A. C. Gorter, and A. J. A. Knottnerus. 2006. "Impact of Accessible Sexual and Reproductive Health Care on Poor and Underserved Adolescents in Managua, Nicaragua: A Quasi-experimental Intervention Study." *Journal of Adolescent Health* 38(1): 56.e1–56.e9.

Miles, S. H., and R. B. Maat. 1984. "A Successful Supervised Outpatient Short-course Tuberculosis Treatment Program in an Open Refugee Camp on the Thai-Cambodian Border." *American Review of Respiratory Diseases*, 130, 827–830.

Miller, L., F. Jami-Imam, M. Timouri, and J. Wijnker. 1995. "Trained Traditional Birth Attendants as Educators of Refugee Mothers." *World Health Forum* 16: 151–6.

Mills, A., R. F. Brugha, K. Hanson, and B. McPake. 2002. "What Can be Done about the Private Health Sector in Low-income Countries?" *Bulletin of the World Health Organization* 80(4): 325–330.

Mtango, F. D. E., and D. Neuvians. 1986. "Acute Respiratory Infections in Children under Five Years: Control Project in Bagamoyo district, Tanzania." *Transactions of the Royal Society of Tropical Medicine and Hygiene* 80(6): 851–858.

Müller, O., K. Cham, S. Jaffar, and B. Greenwood. 1997. "The Gambian National Impregnated Bednet Programme: Evaluation of the 1994 Cost Recovery Trial." *Social Science & Medicine* 44(12): 1903–1909.

Murthy, K.J.R., T.R. Frieden, A. Yazdani, and P. Hreshikesh. 2001. "Public-private Partnership in Tuberculosis Control: Experience in Hyderabad, India." *The International Journal of Tuberculosis and Lung Disease*; 5: 354–59.

Mushi, A.K., J.R. Schellenberg, H. Mponda, and C. Lengeler. 2003. "Targeted Subsidy for Malaria Control with Treated Nets Using a Discount Voucher System in Tanzania." *Health Policy and Planning*, 18(2): 163–171.

Muturi, J. 2005. "Lessons Learnt in Training Retail Sellers on Correct Use of OTC Anti-malaria Drugs in Kenya." In *Interventions to Improve the Role of Medicine Sellers in Malaria Case Management for Children in Africa*, ed. W.R. Brieger, A. Unwin, M. Green, and S. Meek. Arlington: Malaria Consortium and BASICS.

Nathan, R., H. Masanja, H. Mshinda, J.A. Schellenberg, D. de Savigny, C. Lengeler, M. Tanner, and C.G. Victora. 2004. "Mosquito Nets and the Poor: Can Social Marketing Redress Inequities in Access?" *Tropical Medicine & International Health* 9(10): 1121–1126.

Neuman, A.K., D.D. Nicholas, M.B. Ammonoo-Acquah, M. Peasah, and D. L. Boyd. 1986. "Evaluation of a Programme to Train Traditional Birth Attendants in Ghana." In *The Potential of the Traditional Birth Attendant*, ed. A. Mangay-Maglacas and J. Simons, 51–60. Geneva: The World Health Organization.

Newman, C., M. Ambegaokar, M. Abbey, A. Muhawenimana, and P. Combary. 2001. "Evaluation of the GRMA/PRIME Self-directed Learning, Client Provider Interaction and Adolescent Reproductive Health Initiative." University of North Carolina at Chapel Hill, School of Medicine, Program for International Training in Health.

Nganda, B., J. Wang'ombe, K. Floyd, and J. Kangangi. 2003. "Cost and Cost-effectiveness of Increased Community and Primary Care Facility Involvement in Tuberculosis Care in Machakos District, Kenya." *The International Journal of Tuberculosis and Lung Disease* 7(9) suppl. 1: S14–20.

Nunn, P., A. Harries, P. Godfrey-Faussett, R. Gupta, D. Maher, and M. Raviglione. "The Research Agenda for Improving Health Policy, Systems Performance, and Service Delivery for Tuberculosis Control: A WHO Perspective." *Bulletin of the World Health Organization* 80(6): 471–476.

Nuwaha, F. 1999a. "High Compliance in an Ambulatory Tuberculosis Treatment Programme in a Rural Community of Uganda." *International Journal of Tuberculosis and Lung Disease*, 3, 79–81.

———. 1999b. "Control of Tuberculosis in Uganda: A Tale of Two Districts." *International Journal of Tuberculosis and Lung Disease*, 3, 224–230.

Nyamuryekung'e, K., U. Laukamm-Josten, B. Vuylsteke, C. Mbuya, C. Hamelmann, A. Outwater, et al. 1997. "STD Services for Women at Truck Stop in Tanzania: Evaluation of Acceptable Approaches." *East African Medical Journal* 74(6): 343–347.

O'Rourke, K. 1995. "The Effect of Hospital Staff Training on Management of Obstetrical Patients Referred by TBAs." *International Journal of Gynaecology and Obstetrics* 48: S95–102.

Ogedengbe, O.K., O.F. Giwa-Osagie, C.A. Usifoh, and O. Solanke. 1998. "The Impact of the Lagos Manual Vacuum Aspiration (MVA) Training Courses on Medical Education." *West African Journal of Medicine* 17: 210–2.

Ogunbanjo, B.O., M.C. Asuzu, E.E. Edet, and A.O. Osoba. 1986. "Reinforcement of Health Education and Counseling by Doctors in Treatment and Control of Sexually Transmitted Disease." *Genitourinary Medicine* 62, 53–55.

Okello, D, K. Floyd, F. Adatu, R. Odeke, and G. Gargioni. 2003. Cost and cost-effectiveness of community-based care for tuberculosis patients in rural Uganda. *The International Journal of Tuberculosis and Lung Disease* 7(9) suppl. 1: S72–9.

Okonofua, F.E., P. Coplan, S. Collins, F. Oronsaye, D. Ogunsakin, J.T. Ogonor, et al. 2003. "Impact of an Intervention to Improve Treatment-seeking Behavior and Prevent Sexually Transmitted Diseases among Nigerian Youths." *International Journal of Infectious Diseases* 7(1): 61–73.

Oliveira-Cruz, V., K. Hanson, and A. Mills. 2003. "Approaches to Overcoming Constraints to Effective Health Service Delivery: A Review of the Evidence." *Journal of International Development* 15(1): 41–65.

Olson, C.M., D. Rennie, D. Cook, et al. 2002. "Publication Bias in Editorial Decision Making." *Journal of the American Medical Association* 287: 2825–8.

Oshiname, F.O., and W.R. Brieger. 1992. "Primary Care Training for Patent Medicine Vendors in Rural Nigeria." *Social Science & Medicine* 35(12): 1477–1484.

Ovretveit, J., D. Peters, and B. Siadat. 2006. "Strengthening Health Services in Low Income Countries: Lessons from a Rapid Review of Research." Draft.

Palmer, L. 2003. *Private Sector Providers: Do they Behave the Way they Say they Do?* Bath: Futures Group.

Paramasivan, R., R.T. Parthasarathy, and S. Rajasekaran. 1993. "Short-course Chemotherapy: A Controlled Study of Indirect Defaulter Retrieval Method." *Indian Journal of Tuberculosis* 40, 185–190.

Patouillard, E., C. Goodman, C. Hanson, and A. Mills. 2007. "Can Working with the Private Sector Improve Utilization of Quality Health Services by the Poor? A systematic review of the literature." Draft.

Peters, D.H. 2005. "Health Services Delivery: Lessons from Low- and Middle-income Countries Concept Note." World Bank.

Peters, D.H., G.G. Mirchandani, and P.M. Hansen. 2004. "Strategies for Engaging the Private Sector in Sexual and Reproductive Health: How Effective are They?" *Health Policy and Planning* 19(suppl. 1): i5–21.

Podhipak, A., W. Varavithya, P. Punyaratabandhu, K. Vathanophas, and R. Sangchai. 1993. "Impact of an Educational Program on the Treatment Practices of Diarrheal Diseases among Pharmacists and Drugsellers." *The Southeast Asian Journal of Tropical Medicine and Public Health* 24(1): 32–39.

Preker, A.S., G. Carrin, D. Dror, M. Jakab, W. Hsiao, and D. Arhin-Tenkorang. 2002. "Effectiveness of Community Health Financing in Meeting the Cost of Illness." *Bulletin of the World Health Organization* 80(2): 143–50.

Qingjun, L., J. Duan, L. Tang, X. Zhang, J. Liang, A. Hay, S. Shires, and V. Navaratnam. 1998. "The Effect of Drug Packaging on Patients' Compliance with Treatment for Plasmodium Vivax Malaria in China." *Bulletin of the World Health Organization* 79(suppl. 1): 21–27.

Ramadas, K., R. Sankaranarayanan, B. J. Jacob, G. Thomas, T. Somanathan, C. Mahé, et al. 2003. "Interim Results from a Cluster Randomized Controlled Oral Cancer Screening Trial in Kerala, India." *Oral Oncology* 39(6): 580–588.

Ratanajamit, C., Chongsuvivatwong, V., and Geater, A. 2002. "A Randomized Controlled Educational Intervention on Emergency Contraception among Drugstore Personnel in Southern Thailand." *Journal of the American Medical Women's Association* 57(4): 196–199.

Ronsmans, C., A. Endang, S. Gunawan, A. Zazri, J. McDermott, M. Koblinsky, and T. Marshall. 2001. "Evaluation of a Comprehensive Home-based Midwifery

Programme in South Kalimantan, Indonesia." *Tropical Medicine & International Health*, 6, 799–810.

Ross-Degnan, D., S.B. Soumerai, P.K. Goel, J. Bates, J. Makhulo, N. Dondi, et al. 1996. "The Impact of Face-to-face Educational Outreach on Diarrhea Treatment in Pharmacies." *Health Policy and Planning* 11(3): 308–318.

Saade, C., M. Bateman, and D.B. Bendahmane. 2001. *The Story of a Successful Public-private Partnership in Central America: Handwashing for Diarrhoeal Disease Prevention*. Arlington, VA: Basic Support for Child Survival Project (BASICS II), the Environmental Health Project, UNICEF, USAID and World Bank.

Sandiford, P., A. Gorter, and M. Salvetto. 2002. "Vouchers for Health: Using Voucher Schemes for Output-based Aid." *Public Policy for the Private Sector*, an online journal of the World Bank.

Sanders, D., and A. Haines. 2006. "Implementation Research is Needed to Achieve International Health Goals." *PLoS Med* 3(6): e186.

Santoso, B. 1996. "Small Group Intervention vs. Formal Seminar for Improving Appropriate Drug Use." *Social Science & Medicine* 42(8): 1163–1168.

Schaider, J., S. Ngonyani, S. Tomlin, R. Rydman, and R. Roberts. 1999. "International Maternal Mortality Reduction: Outcome of Traditional Birth Attendant Education and Intervention in Angola." *Journal of Medical Systems* 23: 99–105.

Schellenberg, J.R.A., S. Abdulla, R. Nathan, O. Mukasa, T. J. Marchant, N. Kikumbih, et al. 2001. "Effect of Large-scale Social Marketing of Insecticide-treated Nets on Child Survival in Rural Tanzania." *Lancet* 357(9264): 1241–1247.

Schellenberg, J.R.A., T. Adam, H. Mshinda, H. Masanja, G. Kabadi, O. Mukasa, et al. "Effectiveness and Cost of Facility-based Integrated Management of Childhood Illness (IMCI) in Tanzania." *Lancet* 364(9445): 1583–1594.

Schellstede, W.P., and R.L. Ciszewski. 1984. "Social Marketing of Contraceptives in Bangladesh." *Studies in Family Planning* 15: 30–9.

Schwartz, J.B., and I. Bhushan. 2004. "Improving Immunization Equity through a Public-private Partnership in Cambodia." *Bulletin of the World Health Organization* 82: 661–667.

Sengupta, G., and P. Chatterjee. 1986. "Health Education for Tuberculosis Drug Defaulters." *Nursing Journal of India* 67: 91–93, 112.

Shrestha, A., T.T. Kane, and H. Hamal. 1990. "Contraceptive Social Marketing in Nepal: Consumer and Retailer Knowledge, Needs and Experience." *Journal of Biosocial Science* 22: 305–22.

Shwe, T., L. Myint, and A. Soe. 1998. "Influence of Blisterpackaging on the Efficacy of Artesunate+Mefloquine over Artesunate Alone in Community-based Treatment of Non-severe Falciparum Malaria in Myanmar." *Bulletin of the World Health Organization* 79(suppl. 1): 35–41.

Sigonda-Ndomondo, M., O. Kowero, E. Alphonce, R. Mbwasi, R. Shirima, C. Frankiewicz, M. Taylor, N. Heltzer, and M. Clark. 2003. "Accredited Drug Dispensing Outlets: A Novel Public-Private Partnership." *Proceedings of the Conference on Strategies for Enhancing Access to Medicines (SEAM)*. December. Dar es Salaam: Management Sciences for Health.

Smith, J.B., N.A. Coleman, J.A. Fortney, J.D. Johnson, D.W. Blumhagen, and T.W. Grey. 2000. "The Impact of Traditional Birth Attendant Training on Delivery Complications in Ghana." *Health Policy and Planning* 15(3): 326–331.

Somse, P., M.K. Chapko, J.B. Wata, et al. 1998." Evaluation of an AIDS Training Program for Traditional Healers in the Central African Republic." *AIDS Education and Prevention* 10: 558–64.

Stanton, B. F., L. Xiaoming, J. Kahihuata, A. M. Fitzgerald, S. Neumbo, G. Kanduuomber, et al. 1998. "Increased Protected Sex and Abstinence among Namibian Youth Following a HIV Risk-reduction Intervention: A Randomized Longitudinal Study." *AIDS* 12(18): 2473–2480.

Stenson, B., L. Syhakhang, C.S. Lundborg, B. Eriksson, and G. Tomson. 2001. "Private Pharmacy Practice and Regulation: A randomized Trial in Lao P.D.R." *International Journal of Technology Assessment* 17: 579–589.

Stephenson, R., A.O. Tsui, S. Sulzbach, P. Bardsley, G. Bekele, T. Giday, R. Ahmed, G. Gopalkrishnan, and B. Feyesitan. 2004. "Franchising Reproductive Health Services." *Health Services Research* 39: 2053–2080.

Stern, J.M., and R.J. Simes. 1997. "Publication Bias: Evidence of Delayed Publication in a Cohort Study of Clinical Research Projects." *British Medical Journal* 315: 640–5.

Stoeckel, J., A.A. Fisher, M. Viravaidya, and R.N. Pattalung. 1986. "Maintaining Family Planning Acceptance Levels through Development Incentives in Northeastern Thailand." *Studies in FamilyPlanning* 17: 36–43.

Swaminathan, M., A. Naidu, and T.A. Krishan. 1986. "An Evaluation of *Dai* Training in Andhra Pradesh." In *The Potential of the Traditional Birth Attendant*, ed. A. Mangay-Maglacas and J. Simons, 22–34. Geneva: World Health Organization.

Tawfik, Y., J. Nsungwa-Sabitii, G. Greer, J. Owor, R. Kesande, and S. Prysor-Jones. 2006. "Negotiating Improved Case Management of Childhood Illness with Formal and Informal Private Practitioners in Uganda." *Tropical Medicine & International Health* 11: 967–973.

Tavrow, P, J. Shabahang, and S. Makama. 2003."Vendor-to-vendor Education to Improve Malaria Treatment by Private Drug Outlets in Bungoma District, Kenya." *Malaria Journal* 2: 10.

Touchette, P., E. Douglass, J. Graeff, I. Monoang, M. Mathe, and L.W. Duke. 1994. "An Analysis of Home-based Oral Rehydration Therapy in the Kingdom of Lesotho." *Social Science & Medicine* 39: 425–432.

Tuladhar, S.M., S. Mills, S. Acharya, et al. 1998. "The Role of Pharmacists in HIV/STD Prevention: Evaluation of An STD Syndromic Management Intervention in Nepal." *AIDS* 12: S81–7.

Tumwikirize, W.A., P.J. Ekwaru, K. Mohammed, J.W. Ogwal-Okeng, and O. Aupont. 2004. "Impact of a Face-to-face Educational Intervention on Improving the Management of Acute Respiratory Infections in Private Pharmacies and Drug Shops in Uganda." *East African Medical Journal* (suppl.): 25–32.

Vernon, R., G. Ojeda, and M.C. Townsend. 1988. "Contraceptive Social Marketing and Community-based Distribution Systems in Colombia." *Studies in Family Planning* 19: 354–60.

Victora, C.G., J. Habicht, and J. Bryce. 2004. "Evidence-based Public Health: Moving Beyond Randomized Trials." *American Journal of Public Health* 94: 400–405.

Walker, D., H. Muyinda, S. Foster, J. Kengeya-Kayondo, and J. Whitworth. 2001. "The Quality of Care by Private Practitioners for Sexually Transmitted Diseases in Uganda." *Health Policy and Planning* 16(1): 35–40.

Waters, H., L. Hatt, and D. Peters. 2003. "Working with the Private Sector for Child Health." *Health Policy and Planning* 18(2): 127–137.

Wawer, M.J., N.K. Sewankambo, D. Serwadda, T.C. Quinn, L.A. Paxton, N. Kiwanuka, et al. 1999. "Control of Sexually Transmitted Diseases for AIDS Prevention in Uganda: A Randomised Community Trial." *Lancet* 353(9152): 525–535.

Westphal, M.F., J.A. Taddei, S.I. Venancio, and M.C. Bogus. 1995. "Breast-feeding Training for Health Professionals and Resultant Institutional Changes." *Bulletin of the World Health Organization* 73(4): 461–468.

Williams, B., and F. Yumkella. 1986. "An Evaluation of the Training of Traditional Birth Attendants in Sierra Leone and their Performance after Training." *WHO Offset Publication* 95: 35–50.

Williamson, N.E, J.P. Parado, and E.G. Maturan. 1983. "Providing Maternal and Child Health-family Planning Services to a Large Rural Population: Results of the Bohol Project, Philippines." *American Journal of Public Health* 73: 62–71.

World Health Organization. 2003. "The Multi-country Evaluation of IMCI Effectiveness, Cost and Impact." MCE Progress Report, May 2002–April 2003. Department of Child and Adolescent Health and Development, Geneva.

Xiong, W., M.R. Philips, H. Xiong, W. Ruiwen, D. Quinquing, J. Kleinman, and A. Kleinman. 1994. "Family-based Intervention for Schizophrenic Patients in China: A Randomized Controlled Trial. *British Journal of Psychiatry* 65: 239–247.

Zhang, L.-X., G.-Q. Kan, and C. Liu. 1989. "A Model of Fully Supervised Chemotherapy for Pulmonary Tuberculosis in the Tuberculosis Programme in a Rural Area in China." *Bulletin of the International Union Against Tuberculosis and Lung Disease* 64: 20–21.

Zhang, L.-X., and G.-Q. Kan. 1992. "Tuberculosis Control Programme in Beijing." *Tubercle and Lung Disease* 73: 162–166.

Zhang, M., W. Mingtad, L. Jianjun, and M.R. Phillips. 1994. "Randomised-controlled Trial of Family Interventions for 78 First-episode Male Schizophrenic Patients: An 18-month study in Suzhou, Jiangsu." *British Journal of Psychiatry* 165(suppl. 24): 96–10.

CHAPTER 2

Review of Strategies to Strengthen the Performance of Health Organizations

Anbrasi Edward, David H. Peters, Amy Daniels, Yong Rang, and Toru Matsubayashi

Summary

Objective: To develop and analyze a database of studies that define strategies to improve health organization performance and to identify strategies with demonstrated effectiveness in improving organizational outcome measures, both clinical and managerial.

Methods: A systematic review was conducted of published literature from electronic databases addressing the performance of health organizations in LMICs. Studies were classified according to strength and quality of study design, and outcomes summarized. Median effect sizes were calculated from RCTs and NRCTs.

Key messages:

- The strategies for improving the performance of health organizations, including human resource strategies, are not likely reproducible in detail across countries.

(continued)

- Many methods seem to improve overall organizational performance—there are no blueprints.
- Strategies involving organizational change had widely variable results.
- Provider-based performance improvement strategies seemed to hold the most promise, with a large effect size.
- The types of strategies were usually not the same, even when carrying similar labels.
- Although conclusions are plausible, it is unrealistic to claim probabilistic statements about the magnitude of change attributable to particular strategies.
- It was impossible to tell which approaches are more successful or sustainable, given the small number of studies involved, and the fact that few organizational changes were really comparable to each other.

Reasons for Conducting the Review

In the quest to improve the health of populations, organizations that provide health services play a critical role. The way in which health services are organized and delivered determines the overall performance of the health system and impacts the health of the population (Berwick 2004). Despite enormous investments in the health sector by national governments and funding agencies, the returns have not been satisfactory in achieving the targets for the MDGs. Although there has been considerable debate about the obstacles to be overcome in order to improve the performance of health systems (Travis et al. 2004), relatively little is known about the strategies that health services organizations can, in fact, take to overcome them.

Many different types of organizations deliver health services in LMICs. These include ministries of health, not-for-profit nongovernmental organizations (NGOs), and private for-profit organizations. They may also have a wide-ranging scope of services and scale of operations, ranging from a single clinic providing a limited set of health services, to networks of providers of different levels of services, to entire countries. A plethora of published and gray literature covers the multiple small-scale and fragmented initiatives that, addressing specific deficiencies, have been implemented by health services organizations. Many of these initiatives involved a specific disease-control program or a particular department of a health facility or health ministry. However, there has not been a systematic synthesis of the empirical evidence on which approaches are effective in improving overall performance of a health organization in LMICs. Most disease-control projects or programs examine a limited range of results related to their specific interests, and do not look at how their activities may contribute to success or failure of other programs or parts of the organization.

Although there are many examples of successes of short-term measures from categorical programs, such as those related to disease-control programs, systemwide deficiencies impede the overall performance of ministries of health and other organizations, and therefore have less impact on other health conditions or on broader measures of organizational performance related to efficiency or equity. The international community is increasingly concerned about how categorical programs can affect other parts of a health system (McKinsey & Company 2005; Stillman and Bennett 2005); alternative approaches concerned with improving the overall performance of health organizations are not well known. Many assessments of organizations focus on a narrow range of clinical results or on a set of managerial processes. If health organizations are to provide a platform for implementing better targeted priority health programs, more needs to be known about how they can improve their overall ability to deliver services and improve health outcomes. A more balanced assessment of health services organizations is required, one that can more broadly represent their performance.

Myriad factors are known to affect the ways in which organizations provide care in accordance with clinical standards. These result in deficiencies in diagnosis, treatment, counseling, and recording of clinical results. Efforts have been made to improve clinical outcomes and performance using many innovative strategies, and benchmarking successes from the industrial economies. However, it is not clear which of these strategies, if any, can be reproduced across different types of health organizations in LMICs.

Other system constraints involve the inputs into organizations, including human and financial resources, or the lack of infrastructure that exacerbate the ability of health organizations to provide care. Some of the major determinants of the performance of any organization are its management and organizational structures. Major efforts have been undertaken to establish a conceptual framework of health systems performance assessment and to foster further development of tools to measure the components (Murray et al. 2003). Decision makers in LMICs require appropriate decision-making tools to determine the appropriate, cost-effective choices.

The World Health Organization (WHO) has paid some attention to the question of making health systems work (WHO 2005). It highlights various concerns common to central decision makers, including insufficient managerial expertise and the lack of information on how health systems could perform better. It recommends multiple strategies for systems strengthening.

However, systematic evidence about which approaches will work better is still needed, so that government and health organization decision makers can make appropriate choices.

Objectives of the Review

The purpose of this review is to assess the global evidence from published literature on strategies intended to improve the delivery of health services and related aspects of performance of organizations from the public health sector, NGOs, and other private sector health organizations in LMICs. The specific objectives are to

- develop and analyze a database of studies that define strategies to improve the performance of health organizations, defined by a balance of both clinical and managerial outcomes; and
- identify strategies that have demonstrated effectiveness in improving organizational outcome measures, both clinical and managerial.

Methods Used

The review method described by Grimshaw et al. (2004) was adapted and modified for performing the systematic review, as briefly described in the *Overview* (in the section, *Systematic review methods*). In this review, the first stage of review of articles on performance of health organizations involved an analysis of the frameworks used to assess organizational performance in order to identify how determinants and outcomes of health organizations would be systematically reviewed (annex 2.1), which were compared by an external panel of experts and incorporated in the study protocol (see annex 2.2 for key terms searched). A simple conceptual framework was then devised for measuring organizational performance in

LMICs for this analysis (figure 2.1). Studies that examined strategies to address organizational performance were included. Outcome measures were categorized into clinical and managerial measures, and studies that reported on both were included (listed in annex 2.3).

The following major criteria were applied to determine if a study was to be included in the review:

- The study described strategies at a national, state, or local level, but not strategies pursued only at an individual health facility.
- It described measurable indicators of performance of the organization that represents the entire organization, or at least two or more different departments, services, or programs of the organization.
- The study described measurable performance (of the health organization) that addresses at least three dimensions of performance: two or more clinical and one or more managerial. The indicators (or composite indicator) would be included in the outcome domains described in table 2.1.
- RCTs, NRCTs, uncontrolled BATs, time-series studies, case-control trials, or cross-sectional studies comparing two or more groups based

Figure 2.1   Conceptual Framework for Health Organization Performance Review

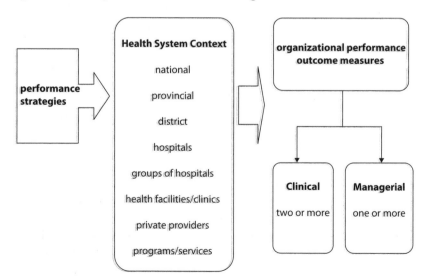

Source: Authors.

Table 2.1   Classification of Clinical and Managerial Outcomes

Clinical outcome	Managerial outcome
1. Composite population health measures (disability-adjusted life years, quality-adjusted life years)	1. Health care coverage, utilization, accessibility
2. Mortality, case fatality	2. Financial performance (funding, cost-effectiveness, subsidies, return on assets)
3. Morbidity, health status, cure rate	3. Patient and client perspective (adherence, satisfaction, perceived service quality, behavior)
4. Disease incidence and/or prevalence	
5. Complications (nosocomial infection, postsurgical wound infection)	4. Staff or internal perspectives (staff turnover, provider satisfaction, provider knowledge, human resource issues)
6. Technical efficiency of care (accuracy of screening, diagnosis, treatment, counseling, compliance/adherence to clinical or evidence-based standards, safety, rate of medication error, postsurgical wound infection)	5. Managerial efficiency (production efficiency, efficiency gains, reduced wastage, allocative efficiency, accessibility, coverage, overcrowding, physician/ nonphysician ratios, providers per 1,000 population, admissions, cross-sectoral indicators, stockouts)
7. Other (percentage of bacterial resistance)	6. Other (equity, market share, mission, strategy)

Source: Authors.

on outcome measures were included for review. A study that provided only cross-sectional or descriptive data with no comparison groups was excluded from the review. Hence a study that was cross-sectional with no measure of performance outcome prior to the intervention or no comparison group was also excluded.

• Since the review focused on strategies that improved organizational performance, a study that only reported impact on a specific disease or service department and did not include the entire organization or other service department was excluded.

The search strategy resulted in 127,438 citations to be screened for possible relevance. The resulting 10,891 titles and abstracts were then reviewed independently by two trained reviewers to assess whether they met the inclusion criteria, resulting in 1,493 possible papers for full text review, of which 1,224 papers could be located. Of the total number of papers reviewed, only 94 met the inclusion criteria for detailed abstraction and analysis, but since some of them reported findings in several countries, the total number of studies included was 98. As described in the *Overview*, studies were classified according to the strength of the study design, the quality of the study, and the outcomes that were found. For making consistent comparisons about outcomes across studies, a median effect size was calculated from the RCTs and NRCTs, which is consistent with making inferences about the probability and plausibility of findings (also discussed in the *Overview*).

Main Findings

The most obvious finding is that among the vast amount of health literature, remarkably little research measures multiple dimensions of performance of health organizations in LMICs. The final database of studies covered a wide range of strategies, and included 11 RCTs, 20 NRCTs, 27 uncontrolled BATs, 24 case-control studies, and 5 time-series studies.

A wide variety of organizational strategies were used to try to improve performance, as shown in table 2.2. Human resource strategies were the most common, followed by management of inputs. Studies assessing public oversight strategies were least likely to be assessed. Although strategies to reorganize public providers are very commonly pursued, the fact that only 14 of the studies evaluated them suggests that they are not frequently exposed to rigorous evaluation.

Strategies were also delivered in multiple combinations. Fifty-six percent of all the studies reported using multiple strategies during the study period, with up to eight specific strategies recorded in some studies. Each study essentially demonstrated, individually, that it used a set of strategies that is a different trial and that is not replicated elsewhere, while together the set of studies demonstrated many different ways to improve performance of organizations in different contexts. None of the strategies for improving the performance of health organizations was reproduced across studies in a way allowing for combining results at a detailed level. More important, the strategies are likely not reproducible. Unlike a simple intervention (such as a pill in medicine or a single intervention in public health), the types of strategies that are used to improve multiple dimensions of performance of an organization (as defined in a minimal way in the review) are not the same, as they evolve differently and are implemented differently, even when they have similar labels. About half the studies (47 percent) were designed to specifically overcome constraints identified by their organization.

Nearly all the published papers reported positive findings for the priority outcomes. Even among those studies with stronger designs (RCTs,

Table 2.2   Number of Studies Employing Specific Strategies to Improve Performance (All Studies)

Organizational strategy	Frequency	% of studies
Public oversight strategies		
Contracting out	3	2
Enforcement approaches	3	2
Accreditation	3	2
Accountability	1	1
Provider strategies: Human resources		
Training of health provider (in-service and on the job)	51	52
Peer learning	4	3
Team building and peer support	2	1
Career or personal development	1	1
Provider strategies: Performance improvement or input management		
Guidelines, standards	16	10
Supervision	10	7
Medical audit	1	1
Provision of additional financial resources	1	1
Financial management	4	3
Pharmaceutical management	3	2
Total quality management	2	1
Critical pathway/clinical pathway	2	1
Monitoring health status/health information	2	1
Quality assurance	1	1
Continuous quality improvement	1	1
Quality design	1	1
Facility management systems	1	1
Job aids/reminders/decision support	1	1
Provider strategies: Public provider reorganization		
Decentralization	8	5
Integration of service delivery	4	3
Vertical program introduction	1	1
Redesign/Re-engineering	1	1
Household and community empowerment		
Community education	9	6
Community capacity for care	6	3
Community driven services	4	3
Community mobilization/empowerment	4	3
Client provider interaction	1	1
Health education of patients	1	1
Community based health info system	1	1

Source: Authors.
Note: Studies may employ more than one type of specific strategy.

NRCTs, and BATs), 93 percent had positive outcomes. Given that many studies employed multiple strategies and examined multiple outcomes, these findings are remarkable. This high rate of positive results raises suspicions of publication bias (Dickersin 1990; Ioannidis 2005; Rosenthal 1979; Sackett 1979; Scargle 2000), and limits our ability to even crudely test if some broad strategic areas are more successful than others.

An analysis of studies of the strongest study designs (RCTs and NRCTs) showed a wide range of effect sizes, most of which were positive, though only small numbers of studies were available to compare each type of strategy (table 2.3). As a group, provider-based performance improvement strategies seemed to hold the most promise with a large effect size (which was statistically significant at $p<0.05$). This group of strategies included efforts to improve supervision and introduce guidelines for health care providers. In-service training also looked promising, particularly among the RCTs. Finding that training can be successful is not particularly surprising in the context of efforts to improve the performance of health organizations. Of course, the content, quality, duration, and modality of training are likely to be very different across settings, and would not be expected to have simply reproducible effects.

It is also useful to know how strategies to change health organizations are directed. Are they driven from top leadership in the organization, or do they involve bottom-up processes from managers and staff in the organization? Do they represent radical changes from the way the organization has functioned in the past, or are they introduced incrementally? Where information was available, the majority of health organizations and strategies were identified as donor driven or top-down, and seldom engaged the managers of the health systems or front-line providers (table 2.4). None of the studies described the changes as originating from either clients or from front-line workers. Most of the studies involved an incremental rather than radical change to the organization. Unfortunately, it is not possible to tell which approaches are more successful or sustainable, given the small number of studies involved, and the fact that few organizational changes are really comparable to each other.

Main Limitations

Systematic reviews have several inherent limitations and weaknesses, and therefore the findings have to be interpreted with caution when one generalizes the effectiveness of the strategies employed. As a body of research, the quality of papers examined was not very strong, as the

Table 2.3 Median Effect Sizes for Strategies Used to Improve Organizational Performance

Detailed strategy	(n)	Randomized controlled trials		Nonrandomized controlled trials		Total	
		Median effect size (%)	P value	Median effect size (%)	P value	Median effect size (%)	P value
Public oversight strategies	4	-14		-0.5		-14.5	
Contracting out	1			-0.5		-0.5	
Enforcement approaches	3	-14				-14	
Provider strategy: Human resources	25	42.6	0.22	-0.24	0.70	42.36	0.74
Training of health provider (in-service and on the job)	23	88.59	0.004	-0.238	0.70	88.35	0.43
Peer learning	2	-46				-46	
Provider strategy: Performance improvement or input management	11	63.3		12.92	0.55	76.22	0.02
Guidelines, standards	4	41.8		0.625		42.43	
Supervision	5	21.5		2.32		23.82	0.28
Financial management	2			9.97		9.97	
Provider strategy: Public provider reorganization	5			-4.5		-4.5	
Decentralization	3			-4.48		-4.48	
Redesign/re-engineering	2			-0.023		-0.023	
Household and community empowerment	7	0.20		-3.87	0.39	-3.67	1.00
Community education	1	0.202				0.202	
Community capacity for care	6			-3.87	0.39	-3.87	0.28

Source: Authors.

Note: P values were determined from a nonparametric test (Mann-Whitney) because of highly skewed data, comparing use of strategy to nonuse of strategy when there were more than five studies with a strategy. More than one strategy could be employed per study.

Table 2.4   Approach to Organizational Change (RCTs and NRCTs Only)

Approach used	(n)	Total Median effect size (%)	P value
Top-down origin	25	2.50	.5
Bottom-up origin	2	0.93	.9
Not described	4	−1.06	.6
Incremental change in implementation	20	3.00	.4
Radical change in implementation	6	1.84	.6
Not described	5	−2.10	.1

Source: Authors.
Note: P values were determined from a nonparametric test (Mann-Whitney) because of highly skewed data; this test compared use of an approach to its nonuse.

Table 2.5   Quality of Studies Reviewed (All Studies)

Quality of study design factor	%
Controlled for confounding factors	24
Reported characteristics of control and treatment groups	29
Characteristics of control and treatment groups similar	23
Blinded assessment of outcome	4
Completeness of dataset	27
Concealment of allocation	2
Follow-up of patients	3
Follow-up of health organization	23
Intervention independent of other changes	1
Intervention unlikely to affect data collection	24
Outcomes at baseline: no difference between the groups	
Baseline values reported	6
Qualitative description reported indicating no differences	4
Statistical tests reported indicating no differences	5
Protection against contamination	11
Reliable outcome measure	51
Described limitations to generalizability	27
Analysis appropriate for sampling method	35
Cost data reported	27

Source: Authors.

majority of papers failed to describe the factors needed to assess the quality of their data (table 2.5). Even among those with stronger designs, such as the RCTs and NRCTs, most failed to describe the details of the study's design and of the strategies' implementation. Although the conclusions are still plausible in that the strategies employed led to positive results, it is unrealistic to claim probabilistic statements about the magnitude of change that can be attributed to particular strategies.

Nearly all the studies reported positive outcomes (97 percent), even if the median effect size of the primary outcomes was not positive. The suspicion of publication bias is not new, and it is important to recognize that its effects tend to be more important when there are few studies that have been conducted in the field, and where each study analyzes different interventions or outcomes (Dickersin 1990; Ioannidis 2005; Rosenthal 1979; Sackett 1979; Scargle 2000).

There are also many studies on health services in LMICs that were not included in this review. Many of the studies that were removed in the screening process involved popular programs and health services that did not look across other health services or aspects of organizational performance. Categorical programs with extensive donor funding, such as HIV/AIDS, family planning, tuberculosis (TB), and child and reproductive health, have a considerable literature, but in most cases the research focuses on the disease aspects of the program rather than the organizations that deliver care.

The published studies are likely to have support from donor agencies and academic institutions, and documents on organizational interventions in LMICs are unlikely to be available to the public, as these are government documents and seldom posted for public consumption. Most reports on performance of health systems and organizations are likely to be available at the country level or from the multinational agencies supporting these efforts. Although attempts were made to contact several of these, the response rate was unsatisfactory and therefore the gray literature, which might have provided useful insights into the effectiveness and utility of the performance strategies, was excluded from this review.

Misclassification of strategies is a concern in this type of review. The review team made efforts to standardize the commonly used strategies and terms through the use of a glossary, training of reviewers, and independent analysis of studies followed by comparison and discussion with the team leader and advisory committee. Even during the data abstraction phase there was considerable ambiguity between authors' perceptions or specific organizational norms and universally accepted definitions. Even with these cross-checks, it was apparent that most strategies and their outcomes are unique to the type of health service organization and context in which they occur. Inferences must be drawn cautiously before they are generalized.

In addition to these inherent methodological limitations, Smith (1993) cautions on the interpretations of performance as they may be based on management incentives. He also addresses the issues of "tunnel vision" where organizations tend to focus on certain clinical areas to the detriment of others, of pursuit of narrow objectives within a single organizational unit, of myopia or a focus on short-term issues with no consideration of long-term sustainability, and of misinterpretation of data due to errors in reporting.

Implications for Decision Makers

This review suggests that there are no blueprints for improving the performance of health organizations in LMICs. Although there are not nearly as many studies examining how to improve overall organizational performance as there are studies on specific health interventions or outcomes, the studies reviewed here suggest there are many ways to improve overall organizational performance. There do not seem to be specific strategies or program variables that lead to success. The public sector, NGOs, the private sector, and partnerships have all been seen to make improvements, and each strategy seems particular to the context in which it has been implemented. Both targeted and broad-based approaches work, along with single components and multiple strategies. Strategies relying on government oversight, strengthening human resources, strengthening management systems, public sector reorganization, community empowerment, and financing systems have all been shown to work.

Strategies involving organizational change have widely variable results. As seen in the literature, organizations tend to take on significant institutional change for one of four reasons: the organization is experiencing serious performance problems, new programs and/or product lines are developed, there is a change in leadership, or there are changes in the environment that directly influence internal policies (Leatt et al. 1997).

Whereas it was difficult to assess these factors in the research, they clearly have implications for the possibilities of success. An organizational change strategy is unlikely to be reproducible in much detail across countries, and its implementation would also be highly dependent on the leadership, organizational culture, and level of trust within the organization. Recognizing this factor suggests that leaders of change should think carefully about their own context, and be careful to monitor what happens within their organizations and their environment as change occurs. In this respect, the types of models listed in annex 2.1 may be helpful for organization managers to think about where to intervene and to monitor effects, both within their organization and among key stakeholders and markets.

In recent years, there has been more emphasis on promoting and monitoring change across the health sector, which usually involves several types of health services organizations. In particular, sectorwide approaches (SWAps) have been organized to introduce change with a national scope (Cassels 1997; HLSP Institute 2005). Similar to the strategies reviewed here, the types of organizational changes promoted through SWAps are highly specific to the country context. Whereas most SWAps involve routine review (usually annual) of sector progress, it is not clear that these approaches have been consistently used to promote change across the sector. Other innovative approaches for monitoring strategies in the sector have involved the adaptation of the balanced scorecard, which has been effectively used to identify and solve a range of organizational and service delivery problems at national and provincial levels for several years in Afghanistan (Peters et al. 2007; Hansen et al. 2008; see also chapter 9).

These studies represent only a small fraction of the number of times these organizational improvement strategies have actually been used in health organizations in LMICs. One important implication is that most organizational reform efforts are not being well evaluated and reported. If policy makers and managers are to learn from the past and current efforts, more consistent and better quality evaluation will be needed. What these studies have in common is the measurement of successful results. Although it is not clear that the lack of negative findings is due to publication bias against those studies that do not find improvement, it also appears that the measurement of outcomes is itself a critical part of success.

References

Arah, O.A., G.P. Westert, J. Hurst, and N.S. Klazinga. 2006. "A Conceptual Framework for the OECD Health Care Quality Indicators Project." *International Journal for Quality in Health Care* 18(suppl. 1): 5–13.

Berwick, D.M. 2004. "Lessons from Developing Nations on Improving Health Care." *British Medical Journal* 328(7448): 1124–1129.

Cassels, A. 1997. "A Guide to Sector Wide Approaches to Health Development: Concepts, Issues, and Working Arrangements." World Health Organization, Geneva. http://libdoc.who.int/hq/1997/WHO_ARA_97.12.pdf.

Dickersin, K. 1990. "The Existence of Publication Bias and Risk Factors for Its Occurrence." *JAMA* 263 (10): 1385–1359.

Donabedian, A. 1998. "The Quality of Care: How Can It Be Assessed?" *JAMA.* 260: 1743–1748.

Ferlie, E.B, and S.M. Shortell. 2001. "Improving the Quality of Health Care in the United Kingdom and the United States: A Framework for Change." *The Milbank Quarterly* 79(2): 281–315.

Goldstein, S.M., and S.B. Schweikhart. 2005. "Empirical Support for the Baldridge Award Framework in U.S. Hospitals." *Health Care Management Review* 27 (1): 36–42.

Grimshaw, J.M, R.E. Thomas, G. MacLennan, C. Fraser, C.R. Ramsay, L. Vale, et al. 2004. "Effectiveness and Efficiency of Guideline Dissemination and Implementation Strategies." *Health Technology Assessment* (Winchester, England) 8(6):iii-iv, 1–72.

Handler, A., M. Issel, and B. Turnock. 2001. "A Conceptual Framework to Measure Performance of the Public Health System." *American Journal of Public Health* 91(8): 1235–1239.

Hansen, P.M., D.H., Peters, H. Niayesh, L.P. Singh, V. Dwivedi, and G. Burnham. 2008. "Measuring and Managing Progress in the Establishment of Basic Health Services: The Afghanistan Health Sector Balanced Scorecard." *International Journal of Health Planning and Management* 23: DOI: 10.1002/hpm.931.

HLSP Institute. 2005. "Sector Wide Approaches: A Resource Document for UNFPA Staff." HLSP Institute, London. http://www.unfpa.org/upload/lib_pub_file/626_filename_swap-unfpa-resource-2005%20.pdf.

Ioannidis, J.P.A. 2005. "Why Most Published Research Findings Are False." *PLoS Med* 2(8): e124 doi: 10.1371/journal.pmed.0020124.

Kaplan, R.S, and D.S. Norton. *The Balanced Scorecard.* 1996. Boston: Harvard Business School Press.

Leatt, P., G.R. Baker, P.K. Halverson, and C. Aird. 1997. "Downsizing, Reengineering, and Restructuring: Long-term Implications for Healthcare Organizations." *Frontiers of Health Services Management* 13(4): 3–37.

Lusthaus, C., M.H. Adrien, G. Anderson et al. 2002. *Organizational Assessment. A Framework for Improving Performance.* Washington, DC and Ottawa, Ontario: Inter-American Development Bank and International Development Research Centre.

Maxwell, R.J. 1984. "Perspectives in NHS Management." *British Medical Journal* 288: 1470–1472.

McKinsey & Company. 2005 *Global Health Partnerships: Assessing Country Consequences.* http://www.hlfhealthmdgs.org/Documents/GatesGHPNov2005.pdf

Murray, C.J.L., and D.B. Evans, eds. 2003. *Health Systems Performance Assessment. Debates, Methods and Empiricism.* Geneva: World Health Organization.

Ovretveit, J. 2006. *Strengthening Health Services in Low Income Countries. Implementation and Results.* World Bank Draft Document, Stockholm: Karolinska Institute MMC.

Peters, D.H., A.A. Noor, L.P. Singh, F.K. Kakar, P.M. Hansen, and G. Burnham. 2007. "A Balanced Scorecard for Health Services in Afghanistan." *Bulletin of the World Health Organization* 85: 146–151.

Rosenthal, R. 1979. "The File Drawer Problem and Tolerance for Null Results." *Psychological Bulletin* 86 (3): 638–641.

Sackett, D. L. 1979. "Bias in Analytic Research." *Journal of Chronic Diseases* 32: 1–2.

Scargle, J. D. 2000. Publication Bias: The "File-Drawer Problem' in Scientific Inference." *Journal of Scientific Exploration* 14 (2): 94–106.

Smith, P. 1993. "Outcome-related Performance Indicators and Organizational Control in the Public Sector." *British Journal of Management* 4 (3): 135–151.

Stillman, K., and S. Bennett. 2005. "System-wide Effects of the Global Fund: Interim Findings from Three Country Studies." The Partners for Health Reform*plus* Project, Abt Associates Inc., Bethesda, Maryland.

Travis, P., S. Bennett, A. Haines, T. Pang, Z. Bhutta, A. Hyder, N. Pielemeier, A. Mills, and T. Evans. 2004. "Overcoming Health-systems Constraints to Achieve the Millennium Development Goals." *Lancet* (364): 900–06.

Vallejo, P., R.M. Saura, R. Sunol, V. Kazandjian, V. Urena, and J. Mauri. 2006. "A Proposed Adaptation of the EFQM Fundamental Concepts of Excellence to Health Care Based on the PATH framework." *International Journal for Quality in Health Care* 18(5): 327–35.

Veillard, J., F. Champagne, N. Klazinga, V. Kazandjian, O.A. Arah, and A.L. Guisset. 2005. "A performance assessment framework for hospitals: the WHO regional office for Europe PATH project." *International Journal for Quality in Health Care* 17(6): 487–96.

World Health Organization (WHO). 2003. *Measuring Hospital Performance to Improve the Quality of Care in Europe: A Need for Clarifying the Concepts and Defining the Main Dimensions.* Copenhagen: WHO Regional office for Europe.

———. 2005. "Making Health Systems Work." Working Papers 1–3. Geneva.

Annex 2.1 Outcome Measures of Selected Health Organization Performance Models

Model	Performance outcome measures
Baldridge Framework (Goldstein and Schweikhart 2005)	Health care and services delivery; patient and customer focus; financial and market results; human resources; organizational effectiveness; leadership; and social response
Balanced Score Card (Kaplan and Norton 1996)	Customers, and financial and business processes; and learning and growth

(continued)

Model	Performance outcome measures
Donabedian (1998)	Structure, process, and outcome in clinical care; financial, and human resources management; and effectiveness, productivity, and efficiency
European Foundation for Quality Management (WHO 2003)	People satisfaction; customer satisfaction; impact on society; business results
Adapted EFQM based on PATH (Vallejo et al. 2006)	Customer focus; safety; leadership and constancy of purpose; clinical effectiveness; responsive governance; staff; results orientation; and partnership development
IDB and IDRC Institutional and Organizational Assessment (Lusthaus et al. 2002)	Effectiveness in fulfillment of mission (achievements, organizational productivity, clients served, quality of services, and service performance); efficiency in fulfilling mission (rates, costs/services, turnover, absenteeism, outputs, administrative efficiency); relevance (adaptation to mission, meeting stakeholder needs, adaptation to environment); financial viability (diversification of funding sources, profitability over time [for-profit] and surplus over time [non-profit])
Maxwell Expanded (Maxwell 1984)	Effectiveness; efficiency; equity; equality; appropriateness; acceptability; accessibility; responsiveness; economy; choice; and ethical considerations
UK Performance Assessment Frame work (Ferlie and Shortell 2001)	Effective delivery of appropriate health care; efficiency; patient and carer experience; health outcome; fair access to services; and health improvement
WHO Health System Performance (Murray and Evans 2005)	Overall health; distribution of health; overall level of responsiveness (how it meets clients expectations, interpersonal relationships, waiting times); distribution of responsiveness; and financial contribution
WHO Euro Hospital Performance (Veillard et al. 2005)	Clinical effectiveness (re-admission rate, mortality, complication rate, appropriateness, length of stay disease specific, quality improvement, evidence-based processes); safety (hospital-acquired infections, falls, bed sores); patient centeredness (waiting time, equity of access, patient rights, patient perception); production efficiency (disease-specific length of stay); staff orientation (turnover rate, absentee rate); and responsive governance
Handler et al. (2001)	Efficiency; effectiveness; and equity
OECD Health Care Quality Indicators Project (Arah et al. 2006)	Organizational motivation (history, mission, culture, incentives/rewards); environment (administrative, political, social/cultural, economic, stakeholder); organizational capacity (strategy, leadership, structure, human resources, financial management, infrastructure, program management, process management. interorganizational linkages); and organizational performance (effectiveness, efficiency, relevance, and economic and financial viability)

Source: Complied by authors.

Annex 2.2 Key Search Terms

The following delineates the key search terms used for the performance review:

Type of Health Organization or Health Provider

ambulatory care OR CBO OR "community based" OR organization OR "community health practitioners" OR "community health services" OR "community health" OR "volunteers" OR "community health workers" OR "community-based organization" OR "district health system" OR "district hospital" OR "doctors" OR "faith-based organization" OR FBO OR "health care organization" OR "health center" OR "health facility" OR "health personnel" OR "health posts" OR "health service organization" OR "health systems" OR "health workers" OR hospital OR "managed care" OR "medical students" OR "midwives" OR "ministry of health" OR "ministry of public health" OR NGO OR "nongovernmental organization" OR "nurse midwives" OR "nurse practitioners" OR paramedical OR "pharmaceutical services" OR pharmacy OR physicians OR "primary health care" OR "primary health centre" OR "private voluntary organizations" OR providers OR "provincial health system" OR PVO OR "registered nurses" OR "traditional birth attendants" OR "traditional health workers" OR "trained birth attendants"

Strategies or interventions. accountability OR accreditation OR "action learning" OR "adherence" OR "alternative health delivery" OR Audit OR authorization OR "automatic stop order" OR autonomization OR "balanced scorecard" OR "banning drug" OR "banning formulation" OR benchmarking OR branding" OR "branding private" OR providers OR "capital finance" OR capitation OR "capitation fee" OR "career development" OR "career experience" OR "career management" OR "case management map" OR "certificate of need" OR "client provider interaction" OR "client satisfaction" OR "clinical decision support system" OR "clinical guidelines" OR "clinical pathways" OR "clinical peer review" OR "clinical practice" OR coalitions OR collaboratives OR "commercial health insurance" OR communication OR "community capacity for care" OR "community driven services" OR "community education" OR "community empowerment" OR "community engagement" OR "community financing" OR "community governance" OR "community improvement" OR "community information" OR "community input" OR "community insurance" OR "community management" OR "community mobilization" OR "community partnership" OR "community scorecards" OR "community-based health insurance" OR "community-based services" OR compact OR competence OR compliance OR "computer based training" OR "computerized medical records" OR "computerized standardized medical records" OR "conditional cash transfers" OR "consultation fee" OR "consumer advocacy" OR "consumer courts" OR "consumer groups" OR "consumer management" OR "consumer protection" OR "consumer ratings" OR "contacting-out services" OR "continuing education" OR "continuous quality improvement" OR contracting OR "contracting with incentives" OR "contracting-in services" OR "contracting-out services" OR "control of corruption" OR cooperation OR co-payment OR COPE OR co-production OR "cost benefit" OR coverage OR "critical pathway" OR "cross functional teams" OR "culture" OR "customer strategies" OR decentralization OR "decision rights" OR deconcentration OR delegation OR "delegation of authority" OR "demand creation" OR "demand side financing" OR DHMT OR "disability benefits" OR dissemination OR "district health management teams" OR "district management teams" OR "drug therapeutic committee" OR "drug utilization evaluation" OR "drug utilization review" OR DTPS OR education OR "employee benefit management" OR "employee recognition program" OR "employee relations" OR "employee relationship management" OR "employer-based health insurance" OR "employment benefits" OR "enforcement approaches" OR "enterprise-based health insurance" OR "essential drug" OR "estate management" OR "ethical considerations" OR "evidence based guidelines" OR "evidence based practice" OR "external environment" OR "external financial management" OR "external management" OR "facilities maintenance" OR "facilities management systems" OR "facilities rebuild" OR "facilities repair" OR "facility structural factor" OR "fair access" OR fairness OR "federal grant" OR "fee exemptions" OR "fee for service" OR "fee increases" OR "fee per drug item" OR "fee reduction" OR "financial discipline" OR "financial incentives" OR "financial management" OR financing OR franchising OR "full time work" OR "functional teams" OR "funding mechanism" OR "generic substitution" OR "global health initiatives" OR governance OR "government effectiveness" OR "government financing" OR guidelines OR "health care costs" OR "health education" OR "health information systems" OR "health insurance" OR "health professional education" OR "health service performance reporting" OR "health systems research" OR holidays OR "hours of work" OR "human adaptability" OR "human performance improvement" OR "human resource" OR "in service training" OR "incentive payment" OR incentives

OR "information access" OR "institutional capacity" OR institutionalization OR "insurance premiums" OR "integration of service delivery" OR "integration of services" OR "interdisciplinary care" OR "internal financial management" OR "internal management" OR "inventory management" OR "job aids" OR "Just in time training" OR "Justice" OR "kit systems" OR "lead teams" OR leadership OR "lean sigma" OR "legal status" OR licensing OR "local grant" OR "macroenvironment strategies" OR "maintenance systems" OR "management information systems" OR "management infrastructure" OR "managerial decision rights" OR manpower OR "market environment" OR "market exposure" OR marketing OR "maternity benefits" OR "maternity leave" OR "medical audit OR "medical education" OR "medical equipment" OR "inventory management" OR "medical equipment systems" OR "medical savings account" OR "medical technology assessment systems" OR mentoring OR "mentoring program" OR "mid level cadres" OR "minimum wage" OR "mobilizing private funds" OR "monitoring health status" OR motivation OR "night work" OR "nursing education" OR "occupational safety management" OR "on the job training" OR organization OR "organizational climate" OR "out of pocket payment" OR oversight OR "overtime work" OR ownership OR "paramedical education" OR "part time work" OR "partnership defined quality" OR "patient bill of rights" OR "patient involvement" OR "patient provider interaction" OR "patient provider relationship" OR "patient risk management" OR "patient safety" OR "patient satisfaction" OR "pay for performance" OR "payment mechanism" OR "PDCA cycle" OR "peer learning" OR "peer review" OR "peer support" OR "people management" OR "performance based pay" OR "performance collaborative" OR "performance improvement" OR "performance incentive" OR "performance measurement" OR "performance monitoring" OR "performance-based pay" OR "personal development" OR "personal health savings" OR "personnel development" OR "pharmaceutical management" OR "pharmacology education" OR "physician education" OR "physician/non-physician ratios" OR "PI teams" OR "policy and strategy resources" OR "policy resources" OR "political stability" OR "pooling revenue" OR "positive deviance" OR "preadmission criteria" OR "pre-packaging" OR prepayment OR "pre-service training" OR "preventive health care" OR "printed management information register" OR "printed management information system" OR "prior authorization" OR "private financing" OR "private health insurance" OR "problem solving" OR "process improvement" OR productivity OR promotion OR "provider patient interaction" OR "provision of facility" OR "provision of medical equipment" OR "public financing" OR "public goods" OR "public private partnership" OR qualification OR "quality assessment" OR "quality assurance" OR "quality award" OR "quality circles" OR "quality collaboratives" OR "quality design OR quality improvement OR quality indicator OR quality management systems OR quality of health care" OR "quality prize" OR "quality strategy" OR "quality system" OR "randomized trials" OR "rationing decisions" OR redesign OR "redress mechanisms" OR reengineering OR "reform design" OR register OR registration OR regulation OR "regulatory approaches" OR "regulatory quality" OR "regulatory strategies" OR reminders OR reorganization OR report cards OR "residual claimant status" OR "responsive governance" OR "retirement benefits" OR "revolving drug fund" OR "risk management" OR "risk pooling" OR "sanctions based on provider qualifications" OR "sanctions based on services" OR sanitation OR "scaling up" OR "sector wide approach" OR "service agreement" OR "service delivery" OR "shift work" OR "sick leave" OR "six sigma" OR "skill mix" OR "social function" OR "social health insurance" OR "social insurance" OR "social marketing" OR "social responsibility" OR "span of control" OR specialists OR "staff management" OR "staff orientation" OR "staff training" OR staffing OR "standard treatment guidelines" OR "standardized medical technology lists" OR "standardized procurement systems" OR standards OR "state funded health care system" OR "state grant" OR stewardship OR "strategic planning" OR "structure redesign" OR "structured prescribing" OR "structured stock ordering" OR subsidies OR supervision OR "supervision with feedback" OR "supply chain management" OR "support supervision" OR SWAP OR "system redesign" OR "tax-based health insurance" OR taxes OR "team based problem solving" OR "team building" OR teams OR "technology assessment" OR "total quality management" OR training OR "training personnel" OR "treatment quality" OR "unconditional cash transfer" OR upgrade OR "user fees" OR vaccination OR "vertical programs" OR "vocational guidance" OR "vocational training" OR "voluntary health insurance" OR vouchers OR "wage scales" OR wages OR "work hour management" OR "work load" OR "work load management" OR "working condition improvement" OR "working conditions"

Organizational outcomes. Absenteeism OR Acceptability OR accessibility OR accountability OR "accountability of managers" OR "accountability of staff" OR adherence OR "adverse event" OR "allocative efficiency" OR appropriateness OR "bond rating" OR "client satisfaction" OR "clinical effectiveness" OR communication OR "community empowerment" OR "community engagement" OR "community improvement" OR "community mobilization" OR co-morbidity OR competence OR compliance OR connectedness OR "constancy of purpose" OR "consumer protection" OR "consumer ratings" OR "continuity of care" OR "continuous quality improvement" OR "control of corruption" OR "coordination of care" OR "cost effectiveness" OR "cost of recruiting" OR cost-benefit OR cost-effective OR culture OR "customer focus" OR "debt/equity ratio" OR decentralization OR "decision rights" OR deconcentration OR "demand creation" OR "diagnostic accuracy" OR "diagnostic quality" OR "drug interaction" OR economic OR "economic viability" OR economy OR effectiveness OR efficiency OR "employee relations" OR equality OR equity OR "fair access" OR fairness OR "federal grant" OR "fee increases" OR "fee reduction" OR "financial contribution" OR "financial discipline" OR "governance effectiveness" OR "government effectiveness" OR "health care costs" OR "health care coverage" OR "health expenditure" OR "health insurance" OR "health knowledge" OR attitudes OR practice OR "hours of work" OR "iatrogenic injury" OR impact OR incentives OR "information access" OR "information mastery" OR "institutional capacity" OR integration OR "integration of services" OR justice OR leadership OR "length of stay" OR "local grant" OR "management information systems" OR "managerial efficiency" OR "market share" OR "maternity benefits" OR" medication error" OR "occupational safety" OR "operating margins" OR "organizational climate" OR "organizational effectiveness" OR "organizational efficiency" OR overcrowding OR oversight OR "partnership development" OR "patient bill of rights" OR "patient centeredness" OR "patient experience" OR "patient safety" OR "patient satisfaction" OR "peer support" OR "performance improvement" OR "personal development" OR "personnel development" OR "process improvement" OR "production efficiency" OR "productive efficiency" OR productivity OR "provider satisfaction" OR "provision of facility" OR "provision of medical equipment" OR "public goods" OR "public private partnership" OR quality OR "quality assurance" OR "quality collaboratives" OR "quality design" OR "quality "improvement" OR "quality indicator" OR "quality management systems" OR "quality of health care" OR "rationing decisions" OR readmission OR reengineering OR regulation OR "regulatory quality" OR relevance OR reorganization OR "responsive governance" OR responsiveness OR "retirement benefits" OR "return on assets" OR "revolving drug fund" OR "risk pooling" OR safety OR sanitation OR "scaling up" OR "service agreements" OR "service delivery" OR "sick leave" OR "skill mix" OR "social functions" OR "span of control" OR "staff satisfaction"

OR "standard treatment guidelines" OR "state grant" OR stewardship OR "structured prescribing" OR "structured stock ordering" OR subsidies OR "supervision with feedback" OR "technical efficiency" OR timeliness OR "total quality management" OR "treatment quality" OR turnover OR "turnover rate" OR utilization OR voice OR wages OR "work load" OR "working condition improvement" OR "working conditions"

Countries. afghanistan OR bangladesh OR benin OR bhutan OR burkina faso OR burundi OR cambodia OR cameroon OR central african republic OR chad OR comoros OR congo OR the democratic republic of congo OR cote d'ivoire OR eritrea OR ethiopia OR the gambia OR ghana OR guinea OR guinea-bissau OR haiti OR india OR kenya OR democratic republic of korea OR kyrgyzstan republic OR lao pdr OR lesotho OR liberia OR madagascar OR malawi OR mali OR mauritania OR moldova OR mongolia OR mozambique OR myanmar OR nepal OR nicaragua OR niger OR nigeria OR north korea OR pakistan OR papua new guinea OR rwanda OR sao tome and principe OR senegal OR sierra leone OR solomon islands OR somalia OR sudan OR tajikistan OR tanzania OR timor lester OR togo OR uganda OR uzbekistan OR vietnam OR yemen OR republic of yemen OR zaire OR zambia OR zimbabwe OR albania OR algeria OR angola OR armenia OR azerbaijan OR belarus OR bolivia OR bosnia and herzegovina OR brazil OR bulgaria OR cape verde OR china OR colombia OR cuba OR djibouti OR dominican republic OR ecuador OR egypt OR arab republic of egypt OR el salvador OR fiji OR georgia OR guatemala OR guyana OR honduras OR indonesia OR iran OR islamic republic of iran OR iraq OR jamaica OR jordan OR kazakhstan OR kiribati OR macedonia OR fyr of macedonia OR former yugoslav republic of macedonia OR maldives OR marshall islands OR micronesia OR federated states of micronesia OR morocco OR namibia OR paraguay OR peru OR philippines OR romania OR samoa OR serbia and montenegro OR sri lanka OR suriname OR swaziland OR syrian arab republic OR syria OR thailand OR tonga OR tunisia OR turkmenistan OR ukraine OR vanuatu OR west bank and gaza OR american samoa OR antigua and barbuda OR argentina OR barbados OR belize OR botswana OR chile OR costa rica OR croatia OR czech republic OR dominica OR equatorial guinea OR estonia OR gabon OR grenada OR hungary OR latvia OR lebanon OR libya OR lithuania OR malaysia OR mauritius OR mayotte OR mexico OR northern mariana islands OR oman OR palau OR panama OR poland OR russian federation OR seychelles OR slovak republic OR south africa

OR st. kitts and nevis OR st. lucia OR st. vincent and the grenadines OR trinidad and tobago OR turkey OR uruguay OR venezuela OR bolivariana republic of venezuela OR developing countries OR less developed countries OR third-world countries OR under-developed countries OR poor countries OR less developed countries OR under developed countries OR less developed nations OR third world nations OR under developed nations OR developing nations OR poor nations OR poor economies OR third world economies OR developing economies OR under developed economies OR less developed economies OR burma OR czechoslovakia OR democratic republic of congo OR french guiana OR east timor OR laos OR north korea OR ivory coast OR republic of georgia OR republic of yemen OR republic of zaire OR slovakia OR soviet union OR surinam OR ussr OR west samoa OR yugoslavia OR zaire OR asia OR west indies OR polynesia OR micronesia OR middle east OR africa OR latin america OR central america OR south america OR caribbean OR west indies region OR hispanico OR southeast asia OR sub-saharan africa OR eastern europe OR the Balkans

Annex 2.3 Studies Reviewed

Abel, R. 1992. "RUHSA—A Model Primary Health Care Programme." *Journal of Tropical Pediatrics* 38(5): 270–272.

Aleman, J., I. Brannstrom, J. Liljestrand, R. Pena, L.A. Persson, and J. Steidinger. 1998. "Saving More Neonates in Hospital: An Intervention towards a Sustainable Reduction in Neonatal Mortality in a Nicaraguan Hospital." *Tropical Doctor* 28(2): 88–92.

Amaral, J., E. Gouws, J. Bryce, A.J. Leite, A.L. Cunha, and C.G. Victora. 2004. "Effect of Integrated Management of Childhood Illness (IMCI) on Health Worker Performance in Northeast-Brazil." *Cadernos de saude publica* 20(suppl. 2): S209–219.

Anand, K., B.K. Patro, E. Paul, and S.K. Kapoor. 2004. "Management of Sick Children by Health Workers in Ballabgarh: Lessons for Implementation of IMCI in India." *Journal of Tropical Pediatrics* 50(1): 41–47.

Anokbonggo, W.W., J.W. Ogwal-Okeng, C. Obua, O. Aupont, and D. Ross-Degnan. 2004. "Impact of Decentralization on Health Services in Uganda: A Look at Facility Utilization, Prescribing and Availability of Essential Drugs." *East African Medical Journal* (suppl.): S2–7.

Anh, N.N., and T.T. Tram. 1995. "Integration of Primary Health Care Concepts in a Children's Hospital with Limited Resources." *Lancet* 346(8972): 421–424.

El Arifeen, S., L.S. Blum, D.M.E. Hoque, E.K. Chowdhury, R. Khan, P.R.E. Black, et al. 2004. "Integrated Management of Childhood Illness (IMCI) in

Bangladesh: Early Findings from a Cluster-randomised Study." *Lancet* 364(9445): 1595–1602.

Armstrong Schellenberg, J., J. Bryce, D. de Savigny, T. Lambrechts, C. Mbuya, L. Mgalula, et al. 2004. "The Effect of Integrated Management of Childhood Illness on Observed Quality of Care of Under-fives in Rural Tanzania." *Health Policy and Planning* 19(1): 1–10.

Armstrong Schellenberg, J., T. Adam, H. Mshinda, H. Masanja, G. Kabadi, O. Mukasa, et al. 2004. "Effectiveness and Cost of Facility-based Integrated Management of Childhood Illness (IMCI) in Tanzania." *Lancet* 364(9445): 1583–1594.

Arole, R. 2001. "Community-based Health and Development: The Jamkhed Experience." *Health Promotion Journal of Australia* 11(1): 5–9.

Atkinson, S., L. Fernandes, A. Caprara, and, J. Gideon. 2005. "Prevention and Promotion in Decentralized Rural Health Systems: A Comparative Study from Northeast Brazil." *Health Policy and Planning* 20(2): 69–79.

Bang, A., R. Bang, S. Baitule, M. Reddy, M. Deshmukh. 1999. "Effect of Home-based Neonatal Care and Management of Sepsis on Neonatal Mortality Field Trial in Rural India." *Lancet* 334: 1955–61.

Bang, A.T., R.A. Bang, H.M. Reddy, M.D. Deshmukh, and S.B. Baitule. 2005. "Reduced Incidence of Neonatal Morbidities: Effect of Home-based Neonatal Care in Rural Gadchiroli, India." *Journal of Perinatology* 25: S51–61.

Bantar, C., B. Sartori, E. Vesco, C. Heft, M. Saul, F. Salamone, et al. 2003. "A Hospitalwide Intervention Program to Optimize the Quality of Antibiotic Use: Impact on Prescribing Practice, Antibiotic Consumption, Cost Savings, and Bacterial Resistance." *Clinical Infectious Diseases* 37(2): 180–186.

Bexell, A., E. Lwando, B. Von Hofsten, S. Tembo, B. Eriksson, and V.K. Diwan. 1996. "Improving Drug Use through Continuing Education: A Randomized Controlled Trial in Zambia." Journal of Clinical Epidemiology 49(3):355–357.

Bhatia, K., and Cleland, C. 2005. "Health Care of Female Outpatients in South-central India: Comparing Public and Private Sector Provision." *Health Policy and Planning* 19(6): 402–409.

Bhutta, Z. A., I. Khan, S. Salat, F. Raza, and H. Ara. 2004. "Reducing Length of Stay in Hospital for Very Low Birthweight Infants by Involving Mothers in a Stepdown Unit: An Experience from Karachi (Pakistan)." *British Medical Journal* 329(7475): 1151–1155.

Birrell, G., and K.G. Birrell. 2000. "Assessment of a 1-year Teaching Programme in Zanzibar, Tanzania." *Lancet* 356(9235): 1084.

Bitran, R. 1995. "Efficiency and Quality in the Public and Private Sectors in Senegal." *Health Policy and Planning* 10(3): 271–283.

Bitran, R., S. Brewster, and B. Ba. 1994. "Costs, Financing, and Efficiency of Health Providers in Senegal. A Comparative Analysis of Public and Private Providers.

Phase 2 and 3: Field Work, Research Results, and Policy Recommendations." USAID, Health Financing and Sustainability Project.

Boller, C., K. Wyss, D. Mtasiwa, and M. Tanner. 2003. Quality and Comparison of Antenatal Care in Public and Private Providers in the United Republic of Tanzania." *Bulletin of the World Health Organization* 81(2): 116–122.

Bradley, J., and, S. Igras. 2005. "Improving the Quality of Child Health Services: Participatory Action by Providers." *International Journal for Quality in Health Care* 17(5): 391–399.

Bryce, J., E. Gouws, T. Adam, R.E. Black, J.A. Schellenberg, F. Manzi, et al. 2005. "Improving Quality and Efficiency of Facility-based Child Health Care through Integrated Management of Childhood Illness in Tanzania." *Health Policy and Planning* 20(suppl. 1): i69–i76.

Bukonda, N., P. Tavrow, H. Abdallah, K. Hoffner, and J. Tembo. 2002. "Implementing a National Hospital Accreditation Program: The Zambian Experience." *International Journal of Quality in Health Care* 14(suppl. 1): 7–16.

Catacutan, A.R. 2006. "The Health Service Coverage of Quality-certified Primary Health Care Units in Metro-Manila, The Philippines." *Health Policy and Planning* 21(1): 65–74.

Cavalcante, M.D.A., O.B. Braga, C.H. Teofilo, E. N. Oliveira, and A. Alves. 1991. "Cost Improvements through the Establishment of Prudent Infection Control Practices in a Brazilian General Hospital, 1986–1989." *Infection Control & Hospital Epidemiology* 12(11): 649–653.

Chalker, J. 1995. "Effect of a Drug Supply and Cost Sharing System on Prescribing and Utilization: A Controlled Trial from Nepal." *Health Policy and Planning* 10(4): 423–430.

———. 1998. "Improving Quality of Care in Hai Phong Province." *Essential Drugs Monitor* (25–26), 15–17.

Chalker, J., S. Ratanawijitrasin, N.T.K. Chuc, M. Petzold, and, G. Tomson. 2005. "Effectiveness of a Multi-Component Intervention on Dispensing Practices at Private Pharmacies in Vietnam and Thailand: A Randomized Controlled Trial." *Social Science and Medicine* 60(1): 131–141.

Chaudhary, N., P.N. Mohanty, and, M. Sharma. 2005. "Integrated Management of Childhood Illness (IMCI) Follow-up of Basic Health Workers." *Indian Journal of Pediatrics* 72(9): 735–739.

Chopra, M., S. Patel, K. Cloete, D. Sanders, and S. Peterson. 2005. "Effect of an IMCI intervention on Quality of Care across Four Districts in Cape Town, South Africa." *Archives of disease in childhood* 90(4): 397–401.

Chuc, N.T., M. Larsson, N.T. Do, V.K. Diwan, G.B. Tomson, and T. Falkenberg. 2002. "Improving Private Pharmacy Practice: A Multi-intervention Experiment in Hanoi, Vietnam." *The Journal of Clinical Epidemiology* 55(11): 1148–1155.

Cufino Svitone, E., R. Garfield, M. Ines Vasconcelos, and V. Araujo Craveiro. 2000. "Primary Health Care Lessons from the Northeast of Brazil: The Agentes de Saude Program." *Pan American Journal of Public Health* 7(5): 293–302.

de Noronha, J.C., and T.R.D. Pereira. 1998. "Health Care Reform and Quality Initiatives in Brazil." *Joint Commission Journal on Quality Improvement* 24(5): 251–263.

de Oliveira, T.C., and M.L.M. Branchini. 1999. "Infection Control in a Brazilian Regional Multihospital System." *American Journal of Infection Control* 27(3): 262–269.

Emond, A., J. Pollock, N. da Costa, T. Maranhão, and A. Macedo. 2002. "The Effectiveness of Community-based Interventions to Improve Maternal and Infant Health in the Northeast of Brazil." *Pan American Journal of Public Health* 12(2): 101–110.

Farid-ul-Hasnain, S., S.M. Israr, and S. Jessani. 2005. "Assessing the Effects of Training on Knowledge and Skills of Health Personnel: A Case Study from the Family Health Project in Sindh, Pakistan." *Journal of Ayub Medical College Abbottabad* 17(4): 26–30.

Foord, F. 1995. "Gambia: Evaluation of the Mobile Health Care Service in West Kiang District." *World Health Statistics Quarterly* 48(1): 18–22.

Foreit, K.G., D. Haustein, M. Winterhalter, and E. La Mata. 1991. "Costs and Benefits of Implementing Child Survival Services at a Private Mining Company in Peru." *American Journal of Public Health* 81(8): 1055–1057.

Fort, A. L., and L. Voltero. 2004. "Factors Affecting the Performance of Maternal Health Care Providers in Armenia." *Human Resources for Health* 2(1): 8.

Fu, D., H. Fu, P. McGowan, Y.E. Shen, L. Zhu, H. Yang, et al. 2003. "Implementation and Quantitative Evaluation of Chronic Disease Self-management Programme in Shanghai, China: Randomized Controlled Trial." *Bulletin of the World Health Organization* 81(3): 174–182.

Gouws, E., J. Bryce, J. Habicht, J. Amaral, G. Pariyo, J. A. Schellenberg, et al. 2004. "Improving Antimicrobial Use among Health Workers in First-level Facilities: Results from the Multi-Country Evaluation of the Integrated Management of Childhood Illness Strategy." *Bulletin of the World Health Organization* 82(7): 509–515.

Greenwood, A.M., A.K. Bradley, P. Byass, B.M. Greenwood, R.W. Snow, S. Bennett, et al. 1990. "Evaluation of a Primary Health Care Programme in The Gambia. I. The Impact of Trained Traditional Birth Attendants on the Outcome of Pregnancy." *Journal of Tropical Medicine and Hygiene* 93(1):58–66.

Greenwood, B.M., A.K. Bradley, P. Byass, A.M. Greenwood, A. Menon, R.W. Snow, et al. 1990. "Evaluation of a Primary Health Care Programme in The Gambia. II. Its Impact on Mortality and Morbidity in Young Children." *Journal of Tropical Medicine and Hygiene* 93(2):87–97.

Guiscafre, H., H. Martinez, M. Palafox, S. Villa, P. Espinosa, R. Bojalil, et al. 2001. "The Impact of a Clinical Training Unit on Integrated Child Health Care in Mexico." *Bulletin of the World Health Organization* 79(5): 434–441.

Hermida, J., and, M.E. Robalino. 2002. "Increasing Compliance with Maternal and Child Care Quality Standards in Ecuador." *International Journal for Quality in Health Care* 14(suppl. 1): 25–34.

Holloway, K.A., B.R. Gautam, and, B.C. Reeves. 2001. "The Effects of Different Kinds of User Fees on Prescribing Quality in Rural Nepal." *Journal of Clinical Epidemiology* 54(10): 1065–1071.

Huang, J., D. Jiang, X. Wang, Y. Liu, K. Fennie, J. Burgess, et al. 2002. "Changing Knowledge, Behavior, and Practice Related to Universal Precautions among Hospital Nurses in China." *Journal of Continuing Education in Nursing* 33(5): 217–224.

Huicho, L., M. Davila, F. Gonzales, C. Drasbek, J. Bryce, and C.G. Victora. 2005. "Implementation of the Integrated Management of Childhood Illness Strategy in Peru and its Association with Health Indicators: An Ecological Analysis." *Health Policy and Planning* 20(suppl. 1): i32-i42.

Jeffery, H.E., M. Kocova, F. Tozija, D. Gjorgiev, M. Pop-Lazarova, K. Foster, et al. 2004. "The Impact of Evidence-based Education on a Perinatal Capacity-building Initiative in Macedonia." *Medical Education* 38(4): 435–447.

Jitapunkul, S., C. Nuchprayoon, S. Aksaranugraha, D. Chaiwanichsiri, B. Leenawat, W. Kotepong, et al. 1995. "A Controlled Clinical Trial of Multidisciplinary Team Approach in the General Medical Wards of Chulalongkorn Hospital." *Journal of the Medical Association of Thailand* 78(11): 618–623.

Kanji, N., P. Kilima, N. Lorenz, and P. Garner. 1995. "Quality of Primary Outpatient Services in Dar-es-Salaam: A Comparison of Government and Voluntary Providers." *Health Policy and Planning* 10: 186–190.

Kelley, E., C. Geslin, S. Djibrina, and M. Boucar. 2001. "Improving Performance with Clinical Standards: The Impact of Feedback on Compliance with the Integrated Management Of Childhood Illness Algorithm in Niger, West Africa." *International Journal of Health Planning and Management* 16(3): 195–205.

Kilic, Y.A., F.A. Agalar, M. Kunt, and M. Cakmakci. 1998. "Prospective, Double-blind, Comparative Fast-tracking Trial in an Academic Emergency Department during a Period of Limited Resources." *European Journal of Emergency Medicine* 5(4): 403–406.

Luby, S., N. Zaidi, S. Rehman, and R. Northrup. 2002. "Improving Private Practitioner Sick-child Case Management in two Urban Communities in Pakistan." *Tropical Medicine & International Health* 7(3): 210–219.

Magnani, R.J., J.C. Rice, N.B. Mock, A.A. Abdoh, D.R. Mercer, and K. Tankari. 1996. "The Impact of Primary Health Care Services on Under-five

Mortality in Rural Niger." *International Journal of Epidemiology* 25(3): 568–577.

Mahe, A., O. Faye, H.T. N'Diaye, H.D. Konare, I. Coulibaly, S. Keita, et al. 2005. "Integration of Basic Dermatological Care into Primary Health Care Services in Mali." *Bulletin of the World Health Organization* 83(12): 935–941.

Manandhar, D.S., D. Osrin, B.P. Shrestha, et al. 2004. "Effect of a Participatory Intervention with Women's Groups on Birth Outcomes in Nepal: Cluster-randomised Controlled trial." *Lancet* 364: 970–979.

Mercer, A., M.H. Khan, M. Daulatuzzaman, and, J. Reid. 2004. "Effectiveness of an NGO Primary Health Care Programme in Rural Bangladesh: Evidence from the Management Information System." *Health Policy and Planning* 19(4): 187–198.

Meyer, J.C., R.S. Summers, and H. Möller. 2001. "Randomized, Controlled Trial of Prescribing Training in a South African Province." *Medical Education* 35(9): 833–840.

Mills, A., N. Palmer, L. Gilson, D. McIntyre, H. Schneider, E. Sinanovic, et al. 2004. "The Performance of Different Models of Primary Care Provision in Southern Africa." *Social Science and Medicine* 59(5): 931–943.

Mukhopadhyay, S.P., A.K. Halder, and, K.K. Das. 1990. "Dr. P. C. Sen Memorial Oration: A Study of Utilisation of Family Planning Services through MCH Package Care in Rural Areas of West Bengal." *Indian Journal of Public Health* 34(3): 147–151.

Mukti, A.G., C. Treloar, Suprawimbarti, A.H. Asdie, K. D'Este, N. Higginbotham, et al. 2000. "A Universal Precautions Education Intervention for Health Workers in Sardjito and PKU Hospital Indonesia." *The Southeast Asian Journal of Tropical Medicine and Public Health* 31(2): 405–411.

Muller, M. 2000. "The Quality of Nursing Service Management in South African Hospitals." *Curationis* 23(2): 63–69.

Needleman, J., and M. Chawla. 1996. "Hospital Autonomy in Zimbabwe." Harvard University. Draft.

Obua, C., J.W. Ogwal-Okeng, P. Waako, O. Aupont, and D. Ross-Degnan. 2004. "Impact of an Educational Intervention to Improve Prescribing by Private Physicians in Uganda." *East African Medical Journal* (suppl.): S17–24.

Odusanya, O.O., and M.A. Oyediran. 2004. "The Effect of an Educational Intervention on Improving Rational Drug Use." *The Nigerian Postgraduate Medical Journal* 11(2): 126–131.

Omaswa, F., G. Burnham, G. Baingana, H. Mwebesa, and R. Morrow. 1997. "Introducing Quality Management into Primary Health Care Services in Uganda." *Bulletin of the World Health Organization* 75(2): 155–161.

Ozkurt, Z., S. Erol, A. Kadanali, M. Ertek, K. Ozden, and M.A. Tasyaran. 2005. "Changes in Antibiotic Use, Cost and Consumption after an Antibiotic

Restriction Policy Applied by Infectious Disease Specialists" *Japanese Journal of Infectious Diseases* 58: 338–343.

Pagaiya, N., and P. Garner. 2005. "Primary Care Nurses Using Guidelines in Thailand: A Randomized Controlled Trial." *Tropical Medicine & International Health* 10(5): 471–477.

Pariyo, G.W., E. Gouws, J. Bryce, and, G. Burnham. 2005. "Improving Facility-based Care for Sick Children in Uganda: Training is Not Enough." *Health Policy and Planning* 20(suppl. 1): i58-i68.

Peck, R., D.W., Fitzgerald, B. Liautaud, M.M. Deschamps, R.I. Verdier, M.E. Beaulieu, et al. 2003. "The Feasibility, Demand, and Effect of Integrating Primary Care Services with HIV Voluntary Counseling and Testing: Evaluation of a 15-year Experience in Haiti, 1985–2000." *Journal of Acquired Immune Deficiency Syndromes* 33(4): 470–475.

Perks, C., M.J. Toole, and, K. Phouthonsy. 2006. "District Health Programmes and Health-sector Reform: Case Study in the Lao People's Democratic Republic." *Bulletin of the World Health Organization*, 84(2): 132–138.

Perry, H., N. Robison, D. Chavez, O. Taja, C. Hilari, D. Shanklin, et al. 1998. "The Census-based, Impact-oriented Approach: Its Effectiveness in Promoting Child Health in Bolivia." *Health Policy and Planning* 13(2): 140–151.

Peters, D. H., and S. Becker. 1991. "Quality of Care Assessment of Public and Private Outpatient Clinics in Metro Cebu, The Philippines." *International Journal of Health Planning and Management* 6(4): 273–286.

Salinas, A. M., I. Coria, H. Reyes, and M. Zambrana. 1997. "Effect of Quality of Care on Preventable Perinatal Mortality." *International Journal of Quality in Health Care* 9(2): 93–99.

Sasichay-Akkadechanunt, T., C.C. Scalzi, and A.F. Jawad. 2003. "The Relationship between Nurse Staffing and Patient Outcomes." *Journal of Nursing Administration* 33(9): 478–485.

Simoes, E.A.F., T. Desta, T. Tessema, T. Gerbresellassie, M. Dagnew, and S. Gove. 1998. "Performance of Health Workers after Training in Integrated Management of Childhood Illness in Gondar, Ethiopia." *Bulletin of the World Health Organization* 75(suppl. 1): 43–53.

Singhal, N., D.D. McMillan, F.L. Cristobal, R.S. Arciaga, W. Hocson, J. Franco, et al. 2001. "Problem-based Teaching of Birth Attendants in the Philippines." *Health Care for Women International* 22(6): 569–583.

Solomon, N.M. 2005. "Health Information Generation and Utilization for Informed Decision-making in Equitable Health Service Management: The Case of Kenya Partnership for Health Program." *SOURCE International Journal for Equity in Health* 4: 24 Jun.

Sriratanaban, J., and Wanavanichkul, Y. 2004. "Hospitalwide Quality Improvement in Thailand." *Joint Commission Journal on Quality & Safety* 30(5): 246–256.

Starling, C.E.F., B.R.G.M. Couto, and S.M.C. Pinheiro. 1997. "Applying the Centers for Disease Control and Prevention and National Nosocomial Surveillance System Methods in Brazilian Hospitals." *American Journal of Infection Control* 25(4): 303–311.

Suwangool, P., P. Moola-Or, A. Waiwatana, C. Sitthi-Amorn, S. Israsena, and M. Hanvanich. 1991. "Effect of a Selective Restriction Policy on Antibiotic Expenditure and Use: An Institutional Model." *Journal of The Medical Association of Thailand* 74(7): 272–275.

Thamlikitkul, V., S. Danchaivijitr, S. Kongpattanakul, and S. Ckokloikaew. 1998. "Impact of an Educational Program on Antibiotic Use in a Tertiary Care Hospital in a Developing Country." *Journal of Clinical Epidemiology* 51(9): 773–778.

Trap, B., C.H. Todd, H. Moore, and R. Laing. 2001. "The Impact of Supervision on Stock Management and Adherence to Treatment Guidelines: A Randomized Controlled Trial." *Health Policy and Planning* 16(3): 273–280.

Tuan, T., V.T.M. Dung, I. Neu, and M.J. Dibley. 2005. "Comparative Quality of Private and Public Health Services in Rural Vietnam." *Health Policy and Planning* 20(5): 319–327.

Uys, L.R., A. Minnaar, B. Simpson, and S. Reid. 2005. "The Effect of Two Models of Supervision on Selected Outcomes." *Journal of Nursing Scholarship* 37(3): 282–288.

Vang, C., G. Tomson, S. Kounnavong, T. Southammavong, A. Phanyanouvong, R. Johansson, et al. 2006. "Improving the Performance of Drug and Therapeutics Committees in Hospitals—A Quasi-experimental Study in Laos." *European Journal of Clinical Pharmacology* 62(1): 57–63.

Velema, J.P., S.M. Alihonou, T. Gandaho, and F.H. Hounye. 1991. "Childhood Mortality among Users and Non-users of Primary Health Care in a Rural West African Community." *International Journal of Epidemiology* 20(2): 474–479.

Wilkinson, D. 1997. "Reducing Perinatal Mortality in Developing Countries." *Health Policy and Planning* 12(2): 161–165.

Wouters, A. 1995. "Improving Quality through Cost Recovery in Niger." *Health Policy and Planning* 10(3): 257–270.

Xi, B., and A. Lu. 1999. "A Job Description-based Health Worker Training Model for Rural China." *Education for Health* 12(2): 149–158.

Xu, Z. 1995. "China: Lowering Maternal Mortality in Miyun County, Beijing." *World Health Statistics Quarterly* 48(1): 11–14.

CHAPTER 3

Review of Strategies to Improve Health Care Provider Performance

Alexander K. Rowe, Samantha Y. Rowe, Marko Vujicic, Dennis Ross-Degnan, John Chalker, Kathleen A. Holloway, and David H. Peters

Summary

Objective: To develop a database of studies on improving health care provider (HCP) performance in LMICs; to identify recommendations and guidance on ways to improve HCP performance on the basis of the strength of research evidence from LMICs; and to identify a research agenda to fill critical knowledge gaps on how to improve the performance of HCPs in LMICS.

Methods: A systematic literature search was conducted of electronic databases, document inventories, and Web sites of organizations involved in HCP performance. Data were independently abstracted. Effect sizes were assessed for each primary outcome for each study or, in studies with more than one primary outcome, median effect sizes were calculated as a summary measure of the study.

(continued)

Key messages (based on preliminary results):

- Diverse strategies have been implemented across LMICs to improve HCP performance.
- Most strategies, including the common ones such as training only, had small effect sizes (improvements of less than 10 percentage points).
- Most strategies had multiple components, but there was no clear relationship between the number of components in a strategy and the strategy's effect size.
- Strategies with the same label often had heterogeneous effects.
- Effect size seemed to vary by scale of implementation, with strategies implemented at state, province, or national level generally more successful than those carried out at the district level or lower.
- Methodological differences (for example, different study settings, outcomes, and strategies) complicated comparisons across studies.

Reasons for Conducting the Review[1]

Each year in LMICs, millions of children and adults die prematurely despite interventions such as drugs, vaccines, and other technologies (insecticide-treated nets, for example) that can prevent such deaths. Low coverage by these interventions is a critical public health problem and a major obstacle to achieving the Millennium Development Goals. Health care providers (HCPs)—doctors, nurses, community health workers, and others who deliver health services—are a key part of almost any strategy for increasing coverage of health interventions (WHO 2006). However, performance is often inadequate, as documented in studies from LMICs concerning child health (Bryce et al. 2003; Naimoli 2001; Peters and Becker 1991; Rowe et al. 2001), sexually transmitted diseases (Bitera et al. 2002), family planning and obstetrics (Goldman and Glei 2003), mental disorders (Abas et al. 2003; Prince et al. 2007; WHO 2007), injuries (Bickler and Rode 2002), diabetes (Whiting et al. 2003), malaria (Ofori-Adjei and Arhinful 1996; Rowe et al. 2000; Rowe et al. 2003; Zurovac et al. 2004), illnesses managed by private sector health workers (Brugha and Zwi 1998; Mills et al. 2002), and medicine use (Hogerzeil et al. 1993; Ross-Degnan et al. 1997; WHO 2001). Not only can improving HCP performance directly save lives of patients seen by HCPs, but some studies suggest that improving performance might increase use of health services (Arifeen et al. 2004). Many strategies have been used to improve HCP performance, and a systematic review of the evidence on the effectiveness and costs of these strategies is valuable for guiding policy. Whereas past reviews have been useful, they have important shortcomings, largely because they did not include LMICs, or only examined a few specific interventions. Thus, an updated and more comprehensive review is needed that includes new research.

Objectives of the Review

The objectives of this review are to:

- develop a database of studies on improving HCP performance in LMICs for use by decision makers, managers, and researchers;
- identify recommendations and guidance on ways to improve HCP performance on the basis of the strength of research evidence from LMICs (that is, guidance on how to implement clinical guidelines in LMICs);
- identify a research agenda to fill critical knowledge gaps on how to improve the performance of HCPs in LMICs.

Methods Used

The review searched 15 electronic databases, document inventories and Web sites of 18 organizations involved in HCP performance, and other sources to identify published and unpublished studies that tested strategies to improve HCP performance in LMICs. The databases used are noted in annex 3.1, the key search terms are provided in annex 3.2, and the studies reviewed are listed in annex 3.3.

The definition of HCPs for this review includes the following: facility- or community-based health workers, pharmacists, shopkeepers who sell medicines, and private sector health workers with some medical training, but it excludes household providers (for example, the patient's family). Studies could be of HCP practices (such as diagnosis or treatment) or patient outcomes (mortality, for example) related to any health condition.

The term "strategy" describes all the interventions for improving HCP performance in a given study group, and "component" describes individual interventions included in the strategy. For example, the strategy "training only" has one component, and "training plus supervision" has two components.

Study designs were classified as "adequate" (type D1 and D2 studies or time-series studies shown in the *Overview*, table 4) or "inadequate" (type D3 and D4 study designs that are not time-series studies in that table). The primary analysis was restricted to studies with adequate designs. As with the other systematic reviews, data were independently abstracted by two researchers into a database and reconciled. Effect sizes were also assessed for each primary outcome for each study, which equaled the percentage point change in a performance indicator of an intervention group minus the change in the comparison group. When a study had more than one primary outcome, we calculated a median effect size as a summary measure of the study (see the *Overview* for a further description of methods).

Main Findings

The review has not yet been completed. As of February 2008, about 40,000 citations had been screened, nearly 800 reports identified for abstraction, and abstraction and data entry completed for 160 reports. Notably, beginning in August 2007, data abstraction was prioritized such that reports of studies with adequate designs were abstracted first. The 160 reports for which data abstraction was completed were for 127 distinct studies (some studies had results in more than one report) that tested 167 strategies.[2] The studies were from over 40 countries and examined HCP practices for more than 15 health conditions (including antenatal care, diarrhea, and malaria). The geographic focus of HCP research has been in Africa and Southeast Asia (50 percent of all studies were in those regions). Europe (2 percent) and the Americas (16 percent) made up only a small portion. Strategies for improving HCP performance typically had multiple components, and the most commonly studied components were training, supervision, printed materials for HCPs, community activities, team problem solving, provision of commodities, and job aids (table 3.1). By far the most common component that has been evaluated in the scientific literature is training, which is included in over 80 percent of all HCP strategies.

Of the 127 studies abstracted, 75 had an adequate design (D1, D2, or D3 time-series-type study), although this frequency was influenced by the decision to focus on studies with adequate designs. Fifty-six of these 75 studies compared an intervention group to a nonintervention group.

Table 3.1   Types of Strategy Components Used to Improve Health Care Provider Performance (Preliminary Results)

Strategy component	% of 127 studies in which the component was evaluated
Training	82
Supervision/feedback	48
Printed materials for HCPs	33
Community activities (such as home visits)	30
Group process/team problem solving	27
Provision of commodities	25
Job aids	23
Printed materials for patients	17
Incentives/budget support	12
Contracting	3
Marketing of health services	2
Other	38

Source: Authors.

As some studies tested more than one strategy, the 56 studies evaluated a total of 74 strategies. Preliminary analyses of these 56 studies revealed that most strategies had small median effect sizes (<10 percentage points), although some had large effects (>25 percentage points) (figure 3.1).

Most studies tested strategies with multiple components; however, there was no clear relationship between the number of components in a strategy and the strategy's effect size (figure 3.2). This finding echoes results of a review of studies from primarily high-income countries (Grimshaw et al. 2004).

Are there any clear winners in terms of which strategies work better to improve HCP performance? Figure 3.3 shows the median effects according to the type of strategy used. First, it was found that very diverse strategies had been implemented across countries to improve HCP performance. This is consistent with other findings in this book (chapters 1, 3, and 8) and results from other reviews (Grimshaw et al. 2004; Ross-Degnan et al. 1997). Second, the largest effects were seen with community activities (also noted by Ross-Degnan et al. 1997), in combination with other strategy components. However, this result is somewhat difficult to interpret because "community activities" are partly defined by the setting in which interventions are implemented rather than only the strategy itself. Additionally, these studies often reported the impact on mortality; and while such outcomes are clearly important

Figure 3.1   Distribution of 74 Median Effect Sizes (1 per Strategy Tested) from 56 Studies of Adequate Design (Preliminary Results)

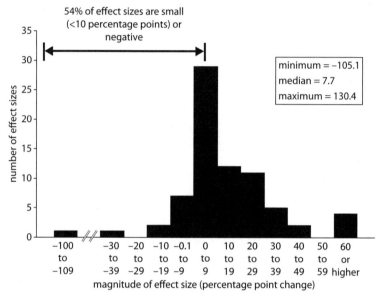

Source: Authors.

Figure 3.2   Distribution of 74 Median Effect Sizes from 56 Studies of Adequate Design Stratified by Number of Components in the Strategy (Preliminary Results)

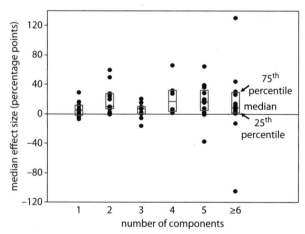

Source: Authors.

Figure 3.3   Summary of Distribution of Median Effect Size for Selected Strategies from 56 Studies of Adequate Design Testing Strategies Alone or in Combination with Other Strategies (Preliminary Results)

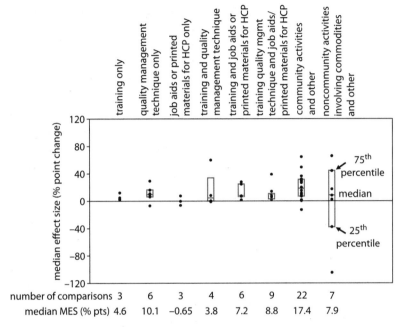

| number of comparisons | 3 | 6 | 3 | 4 | 6 | 9 | 22 | 7 |
| median MES (% pts) | 4.6 | 10.1 | −0.65 | 3.8 | 7.2 | 8.8 | 17.4 | 7.9 |

Source: Authors.

from a public health perspective, they do not show how well HCPs actually adhered to guidelines.

A third finding was that strategies that involved training alone or job aids or printed materials alone, which are commonly used in LMICs, had small effects. Fourth, we found that three strategies—training only, training plus job aids or printed materials, and training plus job aids or printed materials plus quality management techniques—resulted in only positive effects, with a fairly wide variation. Indeed, in most cases, strategies with the same label had quite heterogeneous effects. Fifth, when specific types of components are combined, there was much more potential for a larger positive effect size. This finding suggests that the types of components combined, rather than simply the number of components, is related to effect size. For example, combining printed materials for HCPs or job aids with training, or printed materials for HCPs or jobs aids with training and quality management techniques, results in a larger median effect compared to training alone or printed materials for HCPs or job aids alone. Lastly, there were some differences in effect according to the scale of implementation. Strategies implemented at a state, province, or national level had universally positive median effects (from 3 percent to 130 percent), whereas those implemented at a district or lower level had much greater variation (from −105 percent to 66 percent).

Main Limitations

First, methodological differences (for example, different study settings, outcomes, and strategies) complicated comparisons across studies. Thus, a true meta-analysis of studies was not possible, and it is difficult to know to what degree study results can be generalized to real-world settings on a larger scale. Second, few studies reported costs or cost-effectiveness. Third, the database has some missing details, as reports often lacked key details and contacting authors has been difficult. Fourth, the median effect size is a crude summary measure that can mask larger variation in effects. Fifth, the statistical precision of the results is difficult to assess, as many studies did not use appropriate analyses and obtaining datasets for these studies was not feasible. Sixth, comparisons between strategy types should be interpreted with caution because of the small samples of effect sizes within most of the types. Finally, these are preliminary results based on incomplete data, so clearly the investigators must complete the review. In addition to completing the database, other analytical approaches will be used (for example, stratifying by a variety of potential predictors of effect size, assessing the incremental effect of adding one strategy component onto another, and investigating studies with particularly large effect sizes).

Implications for Decision Makers

One important implication is that there is not a simple solution to improving the performance of HCPs in LMICs. It also seems that similar strategies can have very different results, implying that care is needed in monitoring the effects of any strategy to improve HCP performance. Stand-alone simple strategies, such as a training course or providing job aids alone, seem to have the smallest effects on performance, and may be least worthwhile to pursue. Taking on more complex strategies seems to produce more diverse responses, both positive and negative. This suggests that it will be important for each country or health organization to try to match the complexity or number of strategies with its capabilities.

This review also shows that the research base is biased toward training interventions. There is a clear need to build up the evidence base for less traditional human resource reforms such as changing the incentive mechanisms for health workers, or changing accountability systems.

For decision makers and consumers of information, these preliminary results suggest that strategies often adopted to improve health worker performance (for example, training alone) might be relatively ineffective. Whatever strategy is pursued, program managers should monitor performance over time to assess how well they are working (and if not, why not). This evidence suggests that managers need to be flexible, so that if one strategy is not working, another one can be tried.

For researchers, these preliminary results suggest that more coordinated work on identifying affordable and effective strategies is needed, with greater attention paid to building on existing studies and to conducting research that can be more easily generalized to large-scale real-world settings. Additionally, standardization of outcomes and methods for estimating effect sizes, precision, and cost-effectiveness (as well as standardization of reporting results) would improve future attempts to synthesize the evidence base.

Notes

1. This chapter is a preliminary analysis of an ongoing work that is planned to be completed by late 2009.
2. Not all 167 strategies were different (for example, three studies evaluated the effect of training only).

References

Abas, M., F. Baingana, J. Broadhead, E. Iacoponi, and J. Vanderpyl. 2003. "Common Mental Disorders and Primary Health Care: Current Practice in Low-income Countries." *Harvard Review of Psychiatry* 11: 166–73.

El Arifeen, S., L.S. Blum, D.M.E. Hoque, E.K. Chowdury, R. Khan, R.E. Black, et al. 2004. "Integrated Management of Childhood Illness (IMCI) in Bangladesh: Early Findings from a Cluster-randomised Study." *Lancet* 364: 1595–1602.

Bickler, S.W, and H. Rode. 2002. "Surgical Services for Children in Developing Countries." *Bulletin of the World Health Organization* 80: 829–835.

Bitera, R, M. Alary, B. Masse, et al. 2002. ["Quality of disease management of sexually transmitted diseases: investigation of care in six countries in West Africa"]. *Santé* 12: 233–9.

Brugha, R., and A. Zwi. 1998. "Improving the Quality of Private Sector Delivery of Public Health Services: Challenges and Strategies." *Health Policy and Planning* 13: 107–120.

Bryce, J., S. el Arifeen, G. Pariyo, C.F. Lanata, D. Gwatkin, J.P. Habicht, et al. 2003. "Reducing Child Mortality: Can Public Health Deliver? *Lancet* 362: 159–164.

Goldman, N., and D.A. Glei. 2003. "Evaluation of Midwifery Care: Results from a Survey in Rural Guatemala." *Social Science & Medicine* 56: 685–700.

Grimshaw, J.M., R.E. Thomas, G. MacLennan, et al. 2004. "Effectiveness and Efficiency of Guideline Dissemination and Implementation Strategies." *Health Technology Assessment* 8.

Hogerzeil, H. V., Bimo, D. Ross-Degnan, et al. 1993. "Field Tests for Rational Drug Use in Twelve Developing Countries." *Lancet* 342(8884): 1408–10.

Mills, A, R. Brugha, K. Hanson, and B. McPake. 2002. "What Can be Done about the Private Health Sector in Low-income Countries?" *Bulletin of the World Health Organization* 80: 325–30.

Naimoli, J. 2001. "Theoretical and Empirical Advances in Research on the Implementation of an Integrated Approach to Managing Childhood Illness in Outpatient Facilities in Developing Countries." Doctoral dissertation. Cambridge, MA: Harvard School of Public Health.

Ofori-Adjei, D., and D.K. Arhinful. 1996. "Effect of Training on the Clinical Management of Malaria by Medical Assistants in Ghana." *Social Science & Medicine* 42: 1169–76.

Peters, D. H., and S. Becker "Quality of Care Assessment of Public and Private Outpatient Clinics in Metro Cebu, The Philippines." *International Journal of Health Planning and Management* 1991, 6: 273–286.

Prince, M., V. Patel, S. Saxena, M. Maj, J. Maselko, M.R. Phillips, and A. Rahman. 2007. "No Health without Mental Health." *Lancet* 370: 859–77.

Ross-Degnan, D., R. Laing, B. Santoso, D. Ofori-Adjei, C. Lamoureux, and H. Hogerzeil. 1997. "Improving Pharmaceutical Use in Primary Care in Developing Counties: A Critical Review of Experience and Lack of Experience." Paper presented at the International Conference on Improving Use of Medicines, Chiang Mai, Thailand.

Rowe, A.K., M.J. Hamel, W.D. Flanders, R. Doutizanga, J. Ndoya, and M.S. Deming. 2000. "Predictors of Correct Treatment of Children with Fever seen at Outpatient Health Facilities in the Central African Republic." *American Journal of Epidemiology* 151(10): 1029–1035.

Rowe, A.K, F. Onikpo, M. Lama, F. Cokou, and M. S. Deming. 2001. "Management of Childhood Illness at Health Facilities in Benin: Problems and their Causes." *American Journal of Public Health* 91: 1625–1635.

Rowe, A.K., M. Lama, F. Onikpo, and M.S. Deming. 2003. "Risk and Protective Factors for Two Types of Error in the Treatment of Children with Fever at

Outpatient Health Facilities in Benin. *International Journal of Epidemiology* 32: 296–303.

Whiting, D.R., L. Hayes, and N.C. Unwin. 2003. "Diabetes in Africa. Challenges to Health Care for Diabetes in Africa." *Journal of Cardiovascular Risk* 10: 103–10.

World Health Organization (WHO). 2001. "Interventions and Strategies to Improve the Use of Antimicrobials in Developing Countries." Drug Management Program. Geveva. Document: WHO/CDS/CSR/DRS/2001.9.

———. 2006. "*The World Health Report 2006: Working Together for Health.* Geneva.

———. 2007. *Atlas: Nurses in Mental Health 2007.* Geneva.

Zurovac, D., A. K. Rowe, S. A. Ochola, et al. 2004. "Predictors of the Quality of Health Worker Treatment Practices for Uncomplicated Malaria at Government Health Facilities in Kenya." *International Journal of Epidemiology* 33: 1080–91.

Annex 3.1 Databases Searched

The following were searched: 15 electronic databases (for published studies); document inventories and Web sites of 18 organizations involved in HCP performance (for unpublished studies); and other sources to identify published and unpublished studies that tested strategies to improve HCP performance in LMICs.
The 15 electronic databases were:

- Campbell Collaboration
- Cumulative Index to Nursing & Allied Health Literature (CINAHL)
- Cochrane Library (which includes Database of Abstracts of Review of Effects [DARE] and the Cochrane Central Register of Controlled Trials [CENTRAL])
- Dissertation Abstracts (for theses and dissertations)
- EconLit
- Eldis
- Excerpta Medica database (EMBASE)
- The Effective Practice and Organization of Care (EPOC) specialized register
- Education Resources Information Center (ERIC)
- Global Health
- The Healthcare Management Information Consortium (HMIC)

- Medical Literature Analysis and Retrieval System Online (Medline)
- Science Citation Index (SCI)
- Sociological Abstracts
- Social Sciences Citation Index (SSCI).

The 18 organizations involved in HCP performance (searched to identify unpublished studies) were:

- Basic Support for Institutionalizing Child Survival (BASICS)
- Capacity Project
- CORE Project
- Danish International Development Agency (DANIDA)
- United Kingdom Department for International Development (DFID)
- Human Resources for Health (HRH) Global Resource Center
- International Conference on Social Health Insurance in Developing Countries 2005 proceedings,
- International Conferences on Improving Use of Medicines (ICIUM) 1997 and 2004 conference proceedings
- INRUD-Nepal
- Johns Hopkins International Education for Reproductive Health (JHPIEGO)
- Management Sciences for Health (MSH)
- Pan-American Health Organization (PAHO)
- Partners in Health
- Partners for Health Reformplus (PHRPlus)
- PRIME II (a USAID project to strengthen performance of primary care providers of family planning and reproductive health care services)
- Quality Assurance Project (QAP)
- United States Agency for International Development (USAID)
- World Bank.

Annex 3.2 Key Search Terms in a Medline Search

The following is an example of the search strategy (and number of citations found with each part of the search) used to search Medline:

S1   1543769 EDUCATION OR INSERVICE OR TRAINING OR AUDIT OR PRACTICE OR INTERVENTION? ? OR ASSURANCE OR KNOWLEDGE OR ATTITUDE? ? OR COVERAGE OR OCCUPATION? ? OR OCCUPATIONAL OR PLANNING OR VOCATION OR VOCATIONAL OR CAREER OR EMPLOYEE

S2   1825485 JOB( )SATISFACTION OR MENTORING OR WORK OR WORKING OR WAGE OR WAGES OR BENEFIT? ? OR SAFETY OR POPULATION OR DEMOGRAPHY OR INCENTIVES OR HUMAN( ) ADAPTIBILITY OR PREVENTION OR IMMUNIZATIONS OR IMMUNIZE OR VACCINATIONS OR VACCINATE

S3   4957568 VACCINE? ? OR DISEASE OR TREATMENT OR THERAPY OR PREVENTIVE OR SANITATION OR IMPROVEMENT OR ECONOMIC? ? OR INTEGRATION OR INITIATIVES OR STRATEGIC( ) PLANNING OR LEADERSHIP OR SECTOR( )WIDE OR DECENTRALIZATION OR DECONCENTRATION

S4   1259660 AUTONOMIZATION OR AUTHORITY OR FEE OR FEES OR PAYMENT OR RISK OR INSURANCE OR FINANCING OR COPAYMENT OR CASH OR VOUCHERS OR COST OR EFFICIENT OR EFFICIENCY OR SAVINGS( )ACCOUNT? ? OR MOBILIZATION OR EMPOWERMENT OR ENGAGEMENT

S5   1548180 COALITION? ? OR ORGANIZATION? ? OR CONSUMER OR PATIENT OR REPORT( )CARD? ? OR SCORECARDS OR PATIENT( ) SATISFACTION OR MARKETING OR FRANCHISING OR DEMAND

S6   7341918 S1 OR S2 OR S3 OR S4 OR S5

S7   1203296 CONTRACT OR CONTRACTING OR REGULATION OR ACCREDITATION OR LICENSING OR SERVICE( )AGREEMENT? ? OR PARTNERSHIP? ? OR STEWARDSHIP OR PERFORMANCE OR QUALITY OR BENCHMARK OR BENCHMARKING OR REORGANIZATION OR REDESIGN OR RE( )ENGINEERING OR TEAM

S8   731744 TEAMS OR GUIDELINE? ? OR SUPPLY( )CHAIN OR CERTIFICATE(1W)NEED OR ASSESSMENT OR MOTIVATION OR COMPETENCE OR STAFF OR STAFFING OR SKILL OR PRODUCTIVITY

S9   7986723 S6 OR S7 OR S8

S10   13335 AFGHANISTAN OR BANGLADESH OR BENIN OR BHUTAN OR BURKINA( )FASO OR BURUNDI OR CAMBODIA OR CAMEROON

S11   233582   CENTRAL( )AFRICAN( )REPUBLIC   OR   CHAD   OR COMOROS OR CONGO OR COTE( )D'IVOIRE OR ERITREA OR COTE( )D( )IVOIRE OR ETHIOPIA OR GAMBIA OR GHANA OR GUINEA OR HAITI OR INDIA OR KENYA OR KOREA—OR KYRGYSZSTAN OR LAO OR LAOS OR LESOTHO OR LIBERIA

S12   49258 MADAGASCAR OR MALAWI OR MALI OR MAURITANIA OR MOLDOVA OR MONGOLIA OR MOZAMBIQUE OR MYANMAR OR NEPAL OR NICARAGUA OR NIGER OR NIGERIA OR PAKISTAN OR RWANDA OR SAO( )TOME OR SENEGAL OR SIERRA( )LEONE OR SOLOMON( )ISLANDS OR SOMALIA OR SUDAN

S13 65091 TAJIKISTAN OR TANZANIA OR TIMOR OR TOGO OR UGANDA OR UZBEKISTAN OR VIETNAM OR YEMEN OR ZAIRE OR ZAMBIA OR ZIMBABWE OR ALBANIA OR ALGERIA OR ANGOLA OR ARMENIA OR AZERBAIJAN OR BELARUS OR BOLIVIA OR BOSNIA OR HERZEGOVINA OR BRAZIL

S14 93907 BULGARIA OR CAPE( )VERDE OR CHINA OR COLOMBIA OR CUBA OR DJIBOUTI OR DOMINICAN( )REPUBLIC OR ECUADOR OR EGYPT OR EL( )SALVADOR OR FIJI OR GEORGIA OR GUATEMALA OR GUYANA OR HONDURAS OR   INDONESIA OR IRAN OR IRAQ OR JAMAICA OR JORDAN

S15 28785 KAZAKHSTAN OR KIRIBATI OR MACEDONIA OR MALDIVES OR MARSHALL( )ISLANDS OR MICRONESIA OR MOROCCO OR NAMIBIA OR PARAGUAY OR PERU OR PHILIPPINES OR ROMANIA OR SAMOA OR SERBIA OR MONTENEGRO OR SRI( )LANKA OR SURINAME OR SWAZILAND OR SYRIA

S16 32076 THAILAND OR TONGA OR TUNISIA OR TURKMENISTAN OR UKRAINE OR VANUATU OR WEST( )BANK OR GAZA

S17 46899 ANTIGUA OR BARBUDA OR ARGENTINA OR BARBADOS OR BELIZE OR BOTSWANA OR CHILE OR COSTA( )RICA OR CROATIA OR CZECH( )REPUBLIC OR DOMINICA OR EQUATORIAL( )GUINEA OR ESTONIA OR GABON OR GRENADA OR HUNGARY OR LATVIA OR LEBANON OR LIBYA OR LITHUANIA

S18 88268 MALAYSIA OR MAURITIUS OR MAYOTTE OR MEXICO OR MARIANA( )ISLANDS OR OMAN OR PALAU OR PANAMA OR POLAND OR RUSSIAN( )FEDERATION OR SEYCHELLES OR SLOVAK( )REPUBLIC OR SOUTH( )AFRICA OR ST( )KITTS OR ST(1W)KITTS OR NEVIS OR ST( )LUCIA OR ST(1W)LUCIA

S19 23371 ST( )VINCENT OR GRENADINES OR TRINIDAD OR TOBAGO OR TURKEY OR URUGUAY OR VENEZUELA

S20 113013 ASIA OR WEST( )INDIES OR POLYNESIA OR MICRONESIA OR MIDDLE EAST OR AFRICA OR LATIN AMERICA OR CENTRAL AMERICA OR SOUTH AMERICA OR CARIBBEAN OR WEST INDIES REGION OR HISPA?OLA OR SOUTHEAST ASIA OR SUB( )SAHA-RAN( )AFRICA OR EASTERN( )EUROPE

S21 44 HISPANIOLA

S22 84172 BURMA OR EAST( )TIMOR OR CONGO OR GUIANA OR CZECHOSLOVAKIA OR LAOS OR NORTH( )KOREA OR IVORY( ) COAST OR REPUBLIC(1W)GEORGIA OR YEMEN OR ZAIRE OR SLOVAKIA OR SOVIET( )UNION OR SURINAM OR USSR OR SAMOA OR YUGOSLAVIA

S23 65946 DEVELOPING( )(NATION? ? OR COUNTRIES) OR LESS( ) DEVELOPED( )(NATION? ? OR COUNTRIES) OR THIRD( )

WORLD( )(NATION? ? OR COUNTRIES) OR UNDER( )DEVELOPED( )(NATION? ? OR COUNTRIES) OR POOR( )(NATION? ? OR COUNTRIES OR ECONOMIES)

S24 761381 S10 OR S11 OR S12 OR S13 OR S14 OR S15 OR S16 OR S17 OR S18 OR S19 OR S20 OR S21 OR S22 OR S23

S25 1624852 DOCTOR? ? OR PERSONNEL OR WORKER? ? OR STUDENT? ? OR PHYSICIAN? ? OR PROVIDER? ? OR PARAMEDICAL OR MIDWIFE OR MIDWIVES OR PROFESSIONAL? ? OR NURSE? ? OR PRACTITIONER? ? OR THERAPIST? ? OR ATTENDANT? ? OR HOSPITAL? ? OR POST? ?

S26 825622 CENTER? ? OR FACILITIES OR FACILITY OR SERVICE? ? OR COMMUNITY

S27 2087266 S25 OR S26

S28 188544 S27 AND S24

S29 154907 S9 AND S28

S30 73085 S29 AND (STUDY OR STUDIES)

S31 69232 S30/AB

S32 5865106 S9/TI,AB

S33 63989 S32 AND S31

S34 44508 S33/ENG,HUMAN

S35 91295 S24/TI,AB AND S27/TI,AB

S36 30610 S35 AND S34

S37 30610 S24/TI,AB AND S36

S38 2640315 S6/TI OR S7/TI OR S8/TI

S39 10541 S38 AND S37

S40 604079 S26/TI OR S27/TI

S41 2816 S39 AND S40

S42 2640315 S1/TI OR S2/TI OR S3/TI OR S4/TI OR S5/TI OR S7/TI OR S8/TI

S43 15518 S42 AND S34

S44 7555 S10/AB

S45 6014 S10/TI

S46 136210 S11/TI,AB

S47 33979 S12/TI,AB

S48 41149 S13/TI,AB

S49 53060 S14/TI,AB

S50 53060 S14/TI,AB

S51   15223 S15/TI,AB

S52   10079 S10/TI,AB

S53   13621 S16/TI,AB

S54   25662 S17/TI,AB

S55   39308 S18/TI,AB

S56   16152 S19/TI,AB

S57   48666 S20/TI,AB

S58   44 S21/TI,AB

S59   23652 S22/TI,AB

S60   20797 S23/TI,AB

S61   771237 60 OR S59 OR S58 OR S57 OR S56 OR S55 OR S54 OR S53 OR S52 OR S51 OR S50 OR S48 OR S47 OR S46

S62   406325 S60 OR S59 OR S58 OR S57 OR S56 OR S55 OR S54 OR S53 OR S52 OR S51 OR S50 OR S48 OR S47 OR S46

S63   72102 S62 AND S42

S64   11352 S34 AND S63

S65   10541 S64 AND (S25/TI,AB OR S26/TI,AB)

S66   721008   CHILDREN(2W)HOSPITAL? ?/TI   OR   COMMUNITY( ) HEALTH( )SERVICES/DE OR DOCTOR/TI,AB OR DOCTORS/TI,AB OR   HEALTH   PERSONNEL!   OR   HEALTH( )POSTS/TI,AB   OR HEALTH( )SERVICES( )RESEARCH/DE   OR   HEALTH( )WORKERS/ TI,AB OR HOSPITAL/TI,AB OR HOSPITALS/TI,AB

S67   153675 MEDICAL( )STUDENTS/TI OR OBSTETRIC( )CARE/TI OR PHARMACEUTICAL( )SERVICES/DE OR PHARMACY( )SERVICE( ) HOSPITAL/DE OR PHYSICIANS/TI,AB OR PRIMARY( )HEALTH( ) CARE/TI,AB   OR   PRIMARY( )HEALTH( )CENTRES/TI,AB   OR PROVIDERS/ TI,AB

S68   818451 S66 OR S67

S69   413517 AUDIT/TI OR EDUCATION, CONTINUING! OR HEALTH CARE COSTS! OR HEALTH EDUCATION! OR HEALTH KNOWL-EDGE, ATTITUDES, PRACTICE! OR IMPACT/TI OR INSERVICE TRAINING! OR INTERVENTION/TI,AB OR QUALITY ASSURANCE, HEALTHCARE! OR TRAINING/TI

S71   149104 QUALITY ASSURANCE, HEALTH CARE!

S72   539997 S71 OR S69

S73   11369 S72 AND S68 AND S24

S74   8890 S65 NOT S73

S75   6723 S74 AND EPIDEMIOLOGIC METHODS!

S76 6723 S75/ENG, HUMAN, AB
S77 6716 S76/1970:2006
S78 6705 S76/1975:2006
S79 6657 S76/1980:2006

Annex 3.3 Studies Included in the Review

The following lists 75 citations reviewed that related to the 56 studies of adequate design with a nonintervention control group included in the preliminary analysis:

Afenyadu, G.Y., I.A. Agyepong, G. Barnish, and S. Adjei. 2005. "Improving Access To Early Treatment of Malaria: A Trial with Primary School Teachers As Care Providers." *Tropical Medicine & International Health* 10(10): 1065–72.

Ali, B.S., M. H. Rahbar, S. Naeem, A. Gul, S. Mubeen, and A. Iqbal. 2003. "The Effectiveness of Counseling on Anxiety and Depression by Minimally Trained Counselors: A Randomized Controlled Trial." *American Journal of Psychotherapy* 57(3): 324–336.

Ali, B. S, H. Reza, M. M. Khan, and I. Jehan. 1996. "Development of an Indigenous Screening Instrument in Pakistan: The Aga Khan University Anxiety and Depression Scale." *The Journal of the Pakistan Medical Association* 48(9): 261–265.

Althabe, F, J. M. Belizan, J. Villar, S. Alexander, E. Bergel, S. Ramos, M. Romero, A. Donner, G. Lindmark, A. Langer, U. Farnot, J.G. Cecatti, G. Carroli, and E. Kestler. 2004. For the Latin American Caesarean Section Study Group. "Mandatory Second Opinion To Reduce Rates of Unnecessary Caesarean Sections in Latin America: A Cluster Randomised Controlled Trial." *Lancet* 363: 1934–40.

Angunawela, I. I., V. K. Diwan, and G. Tomson. 1991. "Experimental Evaluation of the Effects of Drug Information on Antibiotic Prescribing: A Study in Outpatient Care in an Area of Sri Lanka." *International Journal of Epidemiology* 20(2): 558–564.

Bailey, P.E., J.A. Szaszdi, and L. Glover. 2002. "Obstetric Complications: Does Training Traditional Birth Attendants Make a Difference?" *Pan American Journal of Public Health* 11(1): 15–23.

Belizán, J.M., F. Barros, A. Langer, U. Farnot, C. Victora, and J. Villar. 1995. "Impact of health education during pregnancy on behavior and utilization of health resources." Latin American Network for Perinatal and Reproductive Research. *American Journal of Obstetrics and Gynecology*.;173(3 Pt 1): 894–9.

Benitez, I., J. De la Cruz, A. Suplido, V. Oblepias, K. Kennedy, and C. Visness. 1992. "Extending lactational amenorrhea in Manila: a successful breast-feeding education programme." *Journal of Biosocial Science* 24(2): 211–231.

Bexell, A., E. Lwando, B. von Hofsten, S. Tembo, B. Eriksson, and V.K. Diwan. 1996. "Improving Drug Use Through Continuing Education: A Randomized Controlled Trial in Zambia." *The Journal of Clinical Epidemiology* 49(3): 355–357.

Bhandari, N., S. Mazumder, R. Bahl, J. Martines, R.E. Black, M.K. Bhan, and the Infant Feeding Study Group. 2004. "An Educational Intervention to Promote Appropriate Complementary Feeding Practices and Physical Growth in Infants and Young Children in Rural Haryana, India." *Journal of Nutrition*; 134: 2342–2348.

Carrier, J. 2006. "Educational Outreach Visits to Primary Care Nurses Improved Tuberculosis Detection and Treatment of Obstructive Lung Disease." *Evidence Based Nursing* 9(2): 58.

Clarke, M., J. Dick, and L. Bogg. 2006. "Cost-effectiveness Analysis of an Alternative Tuberculosis Management Strategy for Permanent Farm Dwellers in South Africa Amidst Health Service Contraction." *Scandinavian Journal of Public Health.*; 34(1): 83–91.

Clarke, M., J. Dick, M. Zwarenstein, C.J. Lombard, and V.K. Diwan. 2005. "Lay Health Worker Intervention with Choice of DOT Superior to Standard TB Care for Farm Dwellers in South Africa: A Cluster Randomised Control Trial." *The International Journal of Tuberculosis and Lung Disease* 9(6): 673–9.

F.M. Coeytaux, T. Kilani, and M. McEvoy. 1987. "The Role of Information, Education, and Communication in Family Planning Service Delivery in Tunisia." Studies in Family Planning 18(4): 229–234.

de Vries, T.P.G.M., R.H. Henning, H.V. Hogerzeil, J.S. Bapna, L. Bero, K.K. Kafle, A.F.B. Mabadeje, B. Santoso, and A.J. Smith. 1995. "Impact of a Short Course in Pharmacotherapy For Undergraduate Medical Students: An International Randomised Controlled Study." *Lancet* 346: 1454–5.

Delacollette, C., P. Van der Stuyft, and K. Molima. 1996. "Using Community Health Workers For Malaria Control: Experience in Zaire." *Bulletin of the World Health Organization* 74(4): 423–430.

Dick, J., S. Lewin, E. Rose, M. Zwarenstein, and H. van der Walt. 2004. "Changing Professional Practice in Tuberculosis Care: An Educational Intervention." *Journal of Advanced Nursing* 48(5): 434–442.

Diop, F., A. Yazbeck, and R. Bitran. 1995. "The Impact of Alternative Cost Recovery Schemes on Access and Equity in Niger." *Health Policy and Planning* 10(3): 223–240.

Dusitsin, N., S. Varakamin, P. Ningsanon, S. Chalapati, B. Boonsiri, and R. H. Gray. 1980. "Post-partum Tubal Ligation by Nurse-Midwives and Doctors in Thailand." *Lancet* 1(8169): 638–639.

Fairall, L.R., M. Zwarenstein, E.D. Bateman, et al. 2005. "Effect of Educational Outreach to Nurses on Tuberculosis Case Detection and Primary Care of

Respiratory Illness: Pragmatic Cluster Randomized Controlled Trial." *British Medical Journal* 331: 750–754.

Fauveau, V., K. Stewart, S.A. Khan, and J. Chakraborty. 1991. "Effect on Mortality of Community-based Maternity-care Programme in Rural Bangladesh." *Lancet.*; 338(8776): 1183–1186.

Fauveau, V., M.K. Stewart, J. Chakraborty, and S.A. Khan. 1992. "Impact on Mortality of a Community-based Programme to Control Acute Lower Respiratory Tract Infections." *Bulletin of the World Health Organization* 70(1): 109–116.

Flores, R., J. Robles, and B.R. Burkhalter. 2002. "Distance Education with Tutoring Improves Diarrhea Case Management in Guatemala." *International Journal for Quality in Health Care* 14(suppl. 1): 47–56.

Flores, R., J. Robles, and B.R. Burkhalter. 1998. "Implementation and Evaluation of a Distance Education Course on the Management of Cholera and Diarrheal Diseases." Published for INCAP, PAHO/WHO, and USAID by the BASICS Project, Arlington, VA. http://www.basics.org/publications/pubs/implementation/contents.htm

Gonzalez Ochoa, E., L. Armas Perez, J.R. Bravo Gonzalez, J. Cabrales Escobar, R. Rosales Corrales, and G. Abreu Suarez. 1996. "Prescription of Antibiotics for Mild Acute Respiratory Infections in Children." *Bulletin of the Pan American Health Organization* 30(2): 106–117.

Gul, A., and B.S. Ali. 2004. "The Onset and Duration of Benefit from Counselling by Minimally Trained Counsellors on Anxiety and Depression in Women." *Journal of the Pakistan Medical Association* 54(11): 549–552.

Gutierrez, G., H. Guiscafre, M. Bronfman, J. Walsh, H. Martinez, and O. Munoz. 1994. "Changing Physician Prescribing Patterns: Evaluation of an Educational Strategy For Acute Diarrhea in Mexico City." *Medical Care* 32(5): 436–446.

Hadiyono, J.E, S. Suryawati, S.S. Danu, Sunartono, and B. Santoso. 1996. "Interactional Group Discussion: Results of a Controlled Trial Using A Behavioral Intervention To Reduce The Use of Injections in Public Health Facilities." *Social Science and Medicine* 42(8): 1177–83.

Haider, R., A. Ashworth, I. Kabir, and S.R. Huttly. 2000. "Effect of Community-Based Peer Counselors on Exclusive Breastfeeding Practices in Dhaka, Bangladesh: A Randomized Controlled Trial." *Lancet* 356(9242): 1643–47.

Haider, R., I. Kabir, S.R. Huttly, and A. Ashworth. 2002. "Training Peer Counselors To Promote and Support Exclusive Breastfeeding in Bangladesh." *Journal or Human Lactation* 18(1): 7–12.

Harrison, A., S.A. Karim, K. Floyd, C. Lombard, M. Lurie, N. Ntuly, and D. Wilkinson. 2000. "Syndrome Packets and Health Worker Training Improve Sexually Transmitted Disease Case Management in Rural South Africa: Randomized Controlled Trial." *AIDS* 14(17): 2769–2779.

Hermida, J., and M.E. Robalino. 2002. "Increasing Compliance with Maternal and Child Care Quality Standards in Ecuador." *International Journal for Quality in Health Care* 14(suppl. 1): 25–34.

Hubacher, D., R. Vilchez, R. Gmach, C. Jarquin, J. Medrano, A. Gadea, T. Grey, and B. Pierre-Louis. 2006. "The Impact of Clinician Education on IUD Uptake, Knowledge and Attitudes: Results of a Randomized Trial." *Contraception* 73: 628–633.

Jintaganont, P., J. Stoeckel, and S. Butaras. 1988. "The Impact of an Oral Rehydration Therapy Program in Southern Thailand." *American Journal of Public Health* 78(10): 1302–1304.

Kafle, K.K., A.D. Shrestha, S.B. Karkee, B.P. Yadav, R.R. Prasad, N. Shrestha, P.L. Das, Y.M.S. Pradhan, T.N. Jha, S.S. Jha, and B.R. Bhatta. 1995. "Intervention Test of Training and Supervision on Dispensing Practices." Report submitted to USAID/RPM/JSI Nepal. Kathmandu, Nepal. August.

———. 1995. "Intervention Test of Training and Supervision on Prescribing Practices." Report submitted to USAID/RPM/JSI Nepal. Kathmandu, Nepal. August.

Kafle, K.K., Y.M.S. Pradhan, A.D. Shrestha, S.B. Karkee, P.L. Das, N. Shrestha, and R.R. Prasad. 1997. "Better Primary Health Care Delivery Through Strengthening The Existing Supervision/Monitoring." Poster presented at the International Conference on Improving Use of Medicines, Chiang Mai, Thailand.

Kafle, K.K., A.D. Shrestha, S.B. Karkee, P.L. Das, N. Shrestha, R.R. Prasad, Y.M.S. Pradhan, J.D. Quick, D. Ross-Degnan, B.R. Shrestha, R. Baniya, R. Adhikary, K.K. Singh, R. Bhandari, R. Lamichhane, A. Lamichhane, and S. Upadhyaya. 1998. "Impact of Action-oriented Training and/or Mailed Print Material on Retailer Practices: Safe Dispensing, Correct Advice, and Appropriate Referral For Diarrhoea, ARI, and Pregnancy." Unpublished report, Kathmandu, Nepal, 21 July.

Kafuko, J.M, C. Zirabamuzaale, and D. Bagenda. 1997. "Rational Drug Use in Rural Health Units of Uganda: Effect of National Standard Treatment Guidelines on Rational Drug Use." International Conferences on Improving Use of Medicines, Chiang Mai, Thailand, http://mednet3.who.int/icium/icium1997/posters/2f3_text.html, accessed July 20, 2006.

Khan, A.J., J.A. Khan, M. Akbar, and D.J. Addiss. 1990. "Acute Respiratory Infections in Children: A Case Management Intervention in Abbottabad District, Pakistan." *Bulletin of the World Health Organization* 68(5): 577–585.

Kielmann, A.A., A.B. Mobarak, M.T. Hammamy, A.I. Gomaa, S. Abou-El-Saad, R.K. Lotfi, I. Mazen, and A. Nagaty. 1985. "Control of Deaths from Diarrheal Disease in Rural Communities: I. Design of an Intervention Study and Effects on Child Mortality." *Tropical Medicine and Parasitology* 36: 191–198.

Kielmann, A.A., A. Nagaty, and C.A. Ajello. 1986. "Control of Deaths from Diarrheal Disease in Rural Communities: II. Motivating and Monitoring the Community." *Tropical Medicine and Parasitology* 37: 15–21.

Lewin, S., J. Dick, M. Zwarenstein, and CJ. Lombard. 2005. "Staff Training and Ambulatory Tuberculosis Treatment Outcomes: A Cluster Randomized Controlled Trial in South Africa." *Bulletin of the World Health Organization*83(4): 250–259.

Loevinsohn, B.P., E.T. Guerrero, and S.P. Gregorio. 1995. "Improving Primary Health Care through Systematic Supervision: A Controlled Field Trial." *Health Policy and Planning* 10(2): 144–153.

Maine, D., M.Z. Akalin, J. Chakraborty, A. de Francisco, and M. Strong. 1996. "Why Did Maternal Mortality Decline in Matlab?" *Studies in Family Planning* 27(4): 179–187.

Manandhar, D.S., D. Osrin, B.P. Shrestha, N. Mesko, J. Morrison, K.M. Tumbahangphe, S. Tamang, S. Thapa, D. Shrestha, B. Thapa, JR. Shrestha, A. Wade, J. Borghi, H. Standing, M. Manandhar, A.M. Costello, and Members of the MIRA Makwanpur Trial Team. 2004. "Effect of a Participatory Intervention with Women's Groups on Birth Outcomes in Nepal: Cluster-Randomised Controlled Trial." *Lancet.*; 364(9438): 970–9.

Miller, P., and N. Hirschhorn. 1995. "The Effect of a National Control of Diarrheal Diseases Program on Mortality: The Case of Egypt." *Social Science and Medicine* 40(10):S1-S30.

Mohagheghi, M.A., A. Mosavi-Jarrahi, M. Khatemi-Moghaddam, A. Afhami, S. Khodi, and O. Azemoodeh. 2005. "Community-based Outpatient Practice of Antibiotics Use in Tehran." *Pharmacoepidemiology and Drug Safety* 14: 135–38.

Moongtui, W., D.K. Gauthier, and J.G. Turner. 2000. "Using Peer Feedback to Improve Handwashing and Glove Usage among Thai Health Care Workers." *American Journal of Infection Control* 28: 365–9.

Moongtui, W. 1999. "Compliance with Components of Universal Precautions Guidelines: Using Peer Feedback Program as a Cue to Action among Health Care Workers in Thailand." DSN Dissertation, University of Alabama at Birmingham.

National Control of Diarrheal Diseases Project. 1988. "Impact of the National Control of Diarrhoeal Diseases Project on Infant and Child Mortality in Dakahlia, Egypt." *Lancet* 2(8603): 145–148.

Okonofua, F.E., P. Coplan, S. Collins, F. Oronsaye, D. Ogunsakin, J.T. Ogonor, J.A. Kaufman, and K. Heggenhougen. 2003. "Impact of an Intervention to Improve Treatment-seeking Behavior and Prevent Sexually Transmitted Diseases among Nigerian Youths." *International Journal of Infectious Diseases* 7: 61–73.

O'Rourke, K. 1995. "The Effect of Hospital Staff Training on Management of Obstetrical Patients Referred by Traditional Birth Attendants." *International Journal of Gynecology & Obstetrics* 48(suppl): S95-S102.

Penny, M.E, H.M. Creed-Kanashira, R.C. Robert, M.R. Narro, L.E. Caulfield, and R.E. Black. 2005. "Effectiveness of an Educational Intervention Delivered through the Health Services to Improve Nutrition in Young Children: A Cluster-randomised Controlled Trial." *Lancet* 365: 1863–1872.

Perez-Cuevas, R., H. Guiscafre, O. Munoz, H. Reyes, P. Tome, V. Libreros, and G. Gutierrez. 1996. "Improving Physician Prescribing Patterns to Treat Rhinopharyngitis: Intervention Strategies in Two Health Systems of Mexico." *Social Science and Medicine* 42(8): 1185–1194.

Podhipak, A., W. Varavithya, P. Punyaratabandhu, K. Vathanophas, and R. Sangchai. 1993. "Impact of an Educational Program on the Treatment Practices of Diarrheal Diseases among Pharmacists and Drugsellers." *Southeast Asian Journal of Tropical Medicine and Public Health* 24(1): 32–39.

Ratanajamit, C., V. Chongsuvivatwong, and A. F. Geater. 2002. "A Randomized Controlled Educational Intervention on Emergency Contraception among Drugstore Personnel in Southern Thailand." *Journal of the American Medical Women's Association.*; 57(4): 196–9, 207.

Reddaiah, V. P., and S. F. Kapoor. 1991. "Effectiveness of ARI Control Strategy on Under Five Mortality." *Indian Journal of Pediatrics* 58: 123–130.

Ross-Degnan, D., S.B. Soumerai, P.K. Goel, J. Bates, J. Makhulo, N. Dondi, Sutoto, D. Adi, L. Ferraz-Tabor, and R. Hogan. 1996. "The Impact of Face-to-face Educational Outreach on Diarrhea Treatment in Pharmacies." *Health Policy and Planning* 11(3): 308–318.

Ruangkanchanasetr, S. 1993. "Laboratory Investigation Utilization in Pediatric Out-patient Department Ramathibodi Hospital." *Journal of the Medical Association of Thailand* 76(suppl 2): 194–208.

Santoso, B., S. Suryawati, and J.E. Prawaitasari. 1996. "Small group intervention vs. formal seminar for improving appropriate use." *Social Science and Medicine* 42(8): 1163–1168.

Theron, G.B. 1999. "The Effect of the Maternal Care Manual of the Perinatal Education Programme on the Attitude of Midwives towards their Work." *Curationis* 22(4): 63–8.

———. 1999. "Effect of the Maternal Care Manual from the Perinatal Education Programme on the Quality of Antenatal and Intrapartum Care Rendered by Midwives." *South African Medical Journal* 89: 336–42.

———. 1999. "Effect of the Maternal Care Manual of the Perinatal Education Programme on the Abilitiy of Midwives to Interpret Antenatal Cards and Partograms." *Journal of Perinatology* 19(6): 432–435.

———. 1999. "Improved Cognitive Knowledge of Midwives Practising in the Eastern Cape Province of the Republic of South Africa through the Study of a Self-education Manual." *Midwifery* 15(2): 66–71.

————. 2000. "Improved Practical Skills of Midwives Practicing in the Eastern Cape Province of the Republic of South Africa through the Study of a Self-education Manual. *Journal of Perinatology.*" 20(3): 184–188.

Thuo, H.M., and S.F.A.M. Gelders. 1997 "Multi-feedback Approach to Rational Drug Use: Using Inpatient Drug Use Indicators as an Intervention Tool." Presented at International Conference on the Rational Use of Medicines (ICIUM).

Trap, B., C.H. Todd, H. Moore, and R. Laing. "The Impact of Supervision on Stock Management and Adherence to Treatment Guidelines: A Randomized Controlled Trial." *Health Policy and Planning,* 2001;16(3): 273–280.

Villar, J., U. Farnot, F. Barros, C. Victora, A. Langer, and J.M. Belizan. 1992. "A Randomized Trial of Psychosocial Support during High-risk Pregnancies. The Latin American Network for Perinatal and Reproductive Research." *The New England Journal of Medicine* 327(18): 1266–71.

Waters, H.R., M.E. Penny, H.M. Creed-Kanashiro, R.C. Robert, R. Narro, J. Willis, L.E. Caulfield, and R.E. Black. 2006. "The Cost-effectiveness of a Child Nutrition Education Programme in Peru." *Health Policy and Planning.*;21(4): 257–264.

Wesson, J., A. Olawo, V. Bukusi, M. Solomon, B. Pierre-Louis, J. Stanback, and B. Janowitz. 2008. "Reaching Providers is not Enough to Increase IUD Use: A Factorial Experiment of 'Academic Detailing' in Kenya." *Journal of Biosocial Science* 40(1): 69–82.

Widyastuti, S., I. Dwiprahasto, and Bakri Z. Andajaningsih. 1997. "The Impact of Problem-based Rational Drug Use Training on Prescribing Practices, Cost Reallocations and Savings in Primary Care Facilities." Poster presented at International Conferences on Improving Use of Medicines (ICIUM), Chiang Mai, Thailand. http://mednet3.who.int/icium/icium1997/posters/2b4_text.html, accessed July 20, 2006.

Winch, P.J., A. Bagayoko, A. Diawara, M. Kane, F. Thiero, K. Gilroy, Z. Daou, Z. Berthe, and E. Swedberg. 2003. "Increases in Correct Administration of Chloroquine in the Home and Referral of Sick Children to Health Facilities through a Community-based Intervention in Bougouni District, Mali." *Transactions of the Royal Society of Tropical Medicine and Hygiene* 97: 481–90.

Wu, Z., R. Detels, J. Zhang, V. Li, and J. Li. 2002. "Community-based Trial to Prevent Drug Use among Youths in Yunnan, China." *American Journal of Public Health.*; 92(12): 1952–7.

Yeager, B.A., S.R. Huttly, J. Diaz, R. Bartolini, M. Marin, and C.F. Lanata. 2002. "An Intervention for the Promotion of Hygienic Feces Disposal Behaviors in a Shanty Town of Lima, Peru." *Health Education Research* 17(6): 761–73.

The following lists the 25 citations reviewed that related to studies of adequate design that were excluded from the preliminary analysis either because they lacked nonintervention controls or because there were questions about their data:

Adamolekun, B., J.K. Mielke, and D.E. Ball. 1999. "An Evaluation of the Impact of Health Worker and Patient Education on the Care and Compliance of Patients with Epilepsy in Zimbabwe." *Epilepsia* 40(4): 507–511.

Bhushan, I., S. Keller, and B. Schwartz. 2002. "Achieving the Twin Objectives of Efficiency and Equity: Contracting Health Services in Cambodia." ERD Policy Brief Series, Number 6, Economics and Research Department, Asian Development Bank, Manila.

Chalker, J., and N.K. Phuong. 1997. "Combating the Growth of Resistance to Antibiotics. Antibiotic Dose as an Indicator for Rational Drug Use." In ICIUM Conference Proceedings. http://mednet3.who.int/icium/icium1997/posters/2E1_txtf.html.

Chalker, J. 2001. "Improving Antibiotic Prescribing in Hai Phong Province, Viet Nam: the 'Antibiotic-Dose' Indicator." *Bulletin of the World Health Organization*, 79(4): 313–320.

Chongsuvivatwong, V., L. Bujakorn, V. Kanpoy, and R. Treetrong. 1993. "Control of Neonatal Tetanus in Southern Thailand." *International Journal of Epidemiology.*; 22(5): 931–935.

Chowdhury, M.E., R. Botlero, M. Koblinsky, SK. Saha, G. Dieltiens, and C. Ronsmans. 2007. "Determinants of Reduction in Maternal Mortality in Matlab, Bangladesh: A 30-year Cohort Study." *Lancet* 370(9595): 1320–28.

el-Rafie, M., W.A. Hassouna, N. Hirschhorn, S. Loza, P. Miller, A. Nagaty, S. Nasser, and S. Riyad. 1990. "Effect of Diarrhoeal Disease Control on Infant and Childhood Mortality in Egypt." *Lancet* 335(8685): 334–38.

Fahdhy, M., and V. Chongsuvivatwong. 2005. "Evaluation of World Health Organization Partograph Implementation by Midwives for Maternity Home Birth in Medan, Indonesia." *Midwifery* 21(4): 301–10.

Gokcay, G., A. Bulut, and O. Neyzi. 1993. "Paraprofessional Women as Health Care Facilitators in Mother and Child Health." *Tropical Doctor* 23(2): 79–81.

Kohler, F., C. Schierbaum, W. Konertz, M. Schneider, H. Kern, E. Int, K. Tael, U. Siigur, K. Kleinfeld, K. Buhlmeyer, P. Fotuhi, and S.F. Winter. 2005. "Partnership for the heart German-Estonian health project for the treatment of congenital heart defects in Estonia." *Health Policy* 73: 151–159.

Mathur, H.N., Damodar, P.N. Sharma, and T.P. Jain. 1979. "The Impact of Training Traditional Birth Attendants on the Utilisation of Maternal Health Services." *Journal of Epidemiology and Community Health* 33(2): 142–4.

Miller, P., and N. Hirschhorn. 1995. "The Effect of a National Control of Diarrheal Diseases Program on Mortality: The Case of Egypt." *Social Science and Medicine* 40(10):S1-S30.

Mohan, P., S.D. Iyengar, J. Martines, S. Cousens, and K. Sen. 2004. "Impact of Counselling on Careseeking Behaviour in Families with Sick Children: Cluster Randomised Trial in Rural India." *British Medical Journal* 329(7460): 266–, originally published online 20 Jul 2004.

Mtango, F.D.E., and D. Neuvians. 1986. "Acute Respiratory Infections in Children under Five Years. Control Project in Bagamoyo District, Tanzania." *Transactions of the Royal Society of Tropical Medicine and Hygiene* 80: 851–858.

Rashad, H. 1989. "Oral Rehydration Therapy and its Effect on Child Mortality in Egypt." *Journal of Biosocial Science* 10(suppl.): 105–113.

Rattanavong, P., T. Thammavong, D. Louanvilayvong, L. Southammavong, V. Vioounalath, W. Laohasiriwong, S. Saowakontha, A. Merkle, and F.P. Schelp. 2000. "Reproductive Health in Selected Villages in Lao PDR." *The Southeast Asian Journal of Tropical Medicine and Public Health* 31(suppl. 2): 51–62.

Ronsmans, C., A.M. Vanneste, J. Chakraborty, and J. van Ginneken. 1997. "Decline in Maternal Mortality in Matlab, Bangladesh: A Cautionary Tale." *Lancet* 350: 1810–14.

Roter, D., J. Rosenbaum, B. de Negri, D. Renaud, L. DiPrete-Brown, and O. Hernandez. 1998. "The Effects of a Continuing Medical Education Programme in Interpersonal Communication Skills on Doctor Practice and Patient Satisfaction in Trinidad and Tobago." *Medical Education* 32: 181–189.

Schwartz, J.B., and I. Bhushan. 2004. "Cambodia: Using Contracting to Reduce Inequity in Primary Health Care Delivery." Health, Nutrition, and Population Family (HNP) Dicussion Paper. Reaching the Poor Program Paper No. 3, World Bank, Washington, DC.

———. 2004. "Improving Immunization Equity through a Public-private Partnership in Cambodia." *Bulletin of the World Health Organization* 82(9): 661–667.

———. 2004. "Reducing Inequity in the Provision of Primary Health Care Services: Contracting in Cambodia." Prepared for Conference on Reaching the Poor with Effective Health, Nutrition and Population Services: What Works, What Doesn't, and Why, February 18–20. Washington, DC. http://wbln0018.worldbank.org/HDNet/hddocs.nsf/vtlw/BE2F3B5B9E4D1 64385256E00006863DC?OpenDocument, accessed January 10, 2006.

———. 2005. "Cambodia: Using Contracting to Reduce Inequity in Primary Health Care Delivery." In *Reaching the Poor with Health, Nutrition, and Population Services: What Works, What Doesn't, and Why*, ed. D.R. Gwatkin, A. Wagstaff, and A. Yazbeck, 137–161. Washington, DC: World Bank.

Singhal, N., D.D. McMillan, F.L. Cristobal, R.S. Arciaga, W. Hocson, J. Franco, R. Farrales, and L. Famor. 2001. "Problem-based Teaching of Birth Attendants in the Phillippines." *Health Care for Women International* 22: 569–583.

Suwanrath-Kengpol, C., S. Pinjaroen, O. Krisanapan, and P. Petmanee. 2004. "Effect of a Clinical Practice Guideline on Physician Compliance." *International Journal of Quality in Health Care* 16(4): 327–332.

Van der Hoek, W. "Prescription Audit for Antibiotics in a District Hospital." 1994. *Tropical Doctor* April: 85–86.

CHAPTER 4

Review of Community Empowerment Strategies for Health

Bahie Rassekh and Nathanial Segaren

Summary

Objective: To evaluate the published literature on community empowerment strategies with respect to health outcomes in LMICs.

Methods: A systematic literature search was conducted on strategies to empower communities for health, through a comprehensive set of databases using standardized search strategies. The results of primary outcomes were assessed for each type of study. Odds ratios were used to compare different strategies.

Key messages:

- Many different types of community empowerment approaches have worked to improve health services and health outcomes. About 90 percent of all studies using community empowerment approaches had a positive primary outcome.

(continued)

- The most successful approaches included: providing training opportunities for local health workers; promoting communication and collective action by communities; supporting community ownership and management of services; and holding service providers, officials, and private organizations accountable.
- The manner in which community empowerment strategies are implemented matters. Partnerships between communities, policy makers, and experts have been more successful than approaches that do not create such partnerships. Providing feedback through sharing results with communities, using systems for local adaptive learning, harnessing community resources to support programs, and promoting equity are particularly successful.
- Initial conditions, such as the presence of strong leadership and previous community empowerment strategies, are important contributors to successful results.
- It is too simplistic to believe that certain factors may be generalizable to empowerment strategies as a whole.

Reasons for Conducting the Review

Community engagement—or empowerment—in health systems gained momentum after the Alma Ata Declaration in 1978, as it was seen as an integral aspect of primary health care. However, the challenges of involving communities in health planning and resource allocation, although large then, remain significant today. This is due, in part, to the lack of consensus as to whether community empowerment has tangible health benefits in LMICs. The ability of such empowerment approaches to make a difference beyond the provincial or national level has also been questioned, since many empowerment strategies have been implemented on a small scale. The sustainability and impact of these strategies on a larger scale is not well known.

Objectives of the Review

This review was conducted in order to examine the available evidence on community empowerment interventions on health outcomes in LMICs. From this, the aim was to examine the relative health outcomes of different approaches and to identify factors that facilitated or hindered their implementation. This systematic review synthesizes the literature on this broad topic and provides evidence of measured results in terms of health services, empowerment, or health status outcomes.

The World Bank (2002) defines community empowerment as "the process of enhancing the capacity of individuals or groups to make choices and to transform those choices into desired actions and outcomes." In practical terms, this means that a community has the autonomy to mobilize resources and its members have sufficient education to make informed decisions and sufficient power to transform those decisions into desired outcomes.

Many empowerment strategies exist. For this review they have been categorized into four broad themes and one set of financial empowerment approaches that cover several of these themes:

- *Information and education* aims to equip citizens sufficiently so that they can take advantage of opportunities, access services, exercise rights, negotiate effectively, and hold state and nonstate actors accountable to make appropriate choices and meaningful actions.
- *Inclusion and participation* aim to promote the participation of service users in providing care, and extend care to marginalized groups.
- *Accountability* allows citizens to hold public officials, private employers, or other service providers accountable.
- *Local organizational capacity* refers to citizens' capacity to collaborate, organize themselves, and mobilize resources to identify and resolve issues.
- *Financial empowerment* refers to a set of approaches that use financing mechanisms either to raise funds for households and community groups or to turn over control of financing of health services to citizen's groups and households.

Methods Used

On the basis of the methods described for the systematic reviews in the *Overview*, a comprehensive literature search was conducted using a list of health and empowerment intervention terminologies from a variety of databases (annex 4.1) and key search terms. Of the 26,985 studies included after the initial term search, only 282 studies met the criteria (annex 4.2) for inclusion in the final review, including a sufficient study design, namely RCTs, NRCTs, uncontrolled BATs including uncontrolled time-series studies, and case-control studies. (These represent study designs D1 through D4 in table 4 in the *Overview*.) The initial stage of analysis in this chapter incorporates all these studies, but for analysis concerning potential determinants of positive outcomes, the focus was on studies with the strongest designs (D1 and D2 of that table).

The various study designs and measurements of outcomes meant than comparison between the papers was not straightforward, given multiple outcomes, comparison groups, and measures. A primary outcome was identified by the paper, and reviewed independently by two abstractors, on the basis of the outcome most central to the objective of the paper or for which there was the most data. If the outcome produced a beneficial effect it was labeled a "positive outcome"; a negative effect was labeled a "negative outcome." Each strategy was assessed on the likelihood of producing a positive result, with each type of study design taken separately.

To see which strategy was more likely to produce a positive effect, comparisons were made across all the community empowerment studies. This was done on the assumption that the comprehensive search was a fair representation (given the time and resources available for this search) of the published literature on community empowerment approaches in health. The analysis involved making comparisons of different strategies to empower communities in health using an odds ratio (OR), which was defined as the ratio of odds of an event occurring in one group (for example, empowerment studies where the strategy was implemented) to the odds of it occurring in another group (for example, empowerment studies where the strategy was not used). An OR greater than 1 suggested that the strategy was correlated with a positive health outcome, whereas an OR less than 1 suggested that it was correlated with a negative or unchanged health outcome.

Main Findings

Of the 282 studies analyzed, 243 (86 percent) were peer-reviewed articles, 5 were books (2 percent), 29 were project reports (10 percent), 3 were World Bank papers (1 percent), and 2 were unpublished papers (1 percent). An increasing number of studies were published each decade or period: 2 (1 percent) in 1975–79; 30 (10 percent) in the 1980s; 93 (33 percent) in the 1990s; and the majority 157 (56 percent) after 2000 (two high-quality studies were published in 2007 and are included in the review).

Studies were included from 66 countries and the following regions: South Asia (35 percent), Sub-Saharan Africa (32 percent), Latin America and the Caribbean (17 percent), East Asia and the Pacific (12 percent), Middle East and North Africa (2 percent), and Europe and Central Asia (1 percent).

A broad array of community empowerment strategies was pursued (table 4.1). Of the different types of empowerment strategies used in the included studies, nearly all (89 percent) involved some kind of education strategy, with educating health workers at the community level the most common (studies may involve more than one type of community empowerment strategy). Over 60 percent of the studies involved training community health workers or other local cadres in preventive or curative roles, whereas over 40 percent of the studies involved training of women in the community. Some kind of community organizational activity was found in almost half the studies, with organizing community groups or taking community collective action found in nearly a third of them. About one-quarter of the studies involved community managing or partnering in the delivery of services. One-quarter of the studies involved some kind of financing mechanism, with community financing of services the most common (9 percent). Less than one-fifth of the studies involved some kind of mechanism to improve accountability, with the most common approach involving joint monitoring of services (9 percent of studies).

The scale of implementation of strategies examined in the studies is shown in table 4.2, which shows that about 40 percent of the strategies were implemented at the village or subdistrict level, and about one-third at one or more district levels. Yet many strategies were implemented at provincial to national levels (18 percent). Of the studies reviewed, 225 reported the estimated population potentially affected by the intervention(s), with a median value of 171,000, ranging from 206 people to over 1 billion; 86 studies reported over 1 million of the population potentially affected; 24 studies reported over 10 million; and 1 reported over 1 billion. Most studies were conducted in rural areas (63.9 percent), with just 9.1 percent in urban areas. Peri-urban areas and slums were represented by just under 5 percent of the studies. However, analysis showed no clear relationship between the scale of the strategy and the likelihood of a positive outcome.

In terms of outcomes, of the 282 studies reviewed, nearly 90 percent of the strategies had a positive effect on the primary outcome (table 4.3). There was no real difference between the type of study design and

Table 4.1 Types of Community Empowerment Strategies Used

Method of community empowerment	Type of study design (number and % in parentheses)				
	Randomized controlled trial	Nonrandomized controlled trial	Before-after trial (uncontrolled)	Case-control study	Total studies
Information and education	56 (90.3)	79 (84.0)	82 (89.1)	34 (100.0)	251 (89.0)
Training of community health workers, traditional birth attendants, informal health cadres	38 (61.3)	55 (58.5)	58 (63.0)	22 (64.7)	173 (61.3)
Community education—Group meetings	19 (30.6)	14 (14.9)	26 (28.3)	20 (58.8)	79 (28.0)
Training of women and mothers	25 (40.3)	38 (40.4)	31 (33.7)	17 (50.0)	111 (39.4)
Community education—Home visits	6 (9.7)	4 (4.3)	8 (8.7)	5 (14.7)	23 (8.2)
Community education—Media/printed	12 (19.4)	13 (13.8)	19 (20.7)	6 (17.6)	50 (17.7)
In person teacher at facility	24 (38.7)	24 (25.5)	32 (34.8)	15 (44.1)	95 (33.7)
Community education—Arts	27 (43.5)	35 (37.2)	30 (32.6)	16 (47.1)	108 (38.3)
Training of youth/young people	29 (46.8)	33 (35.1)	43 (46.7)	18 (52.9)	123 (43.6)
Inclusion and participation	18 (29.0)	35 (37.2)	35 (38.0)	14 (41.2)	102 (36.2)
Community-managed services	17 (27.4)	27 (28.7)	21 (22.8)	6 (17.6)	71 (25.2)
Community partnership	12 (19.4)	18 (19.1)	28 (30.4)	12 (35.3)	70 (24.8)
Community-owned services	10 (16.1)	15 (16.0)	10 (10.9)	6 (17.6)	41 (14.5)
Community comanagement of drugs	6 (9.7)	10 (10.6)	3 (3.3)	1 (2.9)	20 (7.1)
Accountability	9 (14.5)	20 (21.3)	21 (22.8)	3 (8.8)	53 (18.8)
Joint monitoring of access and quality	6 (9.7)	9 (9.6)	8 (8.7)	2 (5.9)	25 (8.9)
Providers held accountable	6 (9.7)	11 (11.7)	6 (6.5)	1 (2.9)	24 (8.5)

Provider performance bonus decided by community	1 (1.6)	4 (4.3)	8 (8.7)	0 (0.0)	13 (4.6)
Community score cards	0 (0.0)	1 (1.1)	3 (3.3)	0 (0.0)	4 (1.4)
Complaints bureau	0 (0.0)	1 (1.1)	1 (1.1)	0 (0.0)	2 (.07)
Access to courts/legal advice	0 (0.0)	0 (0.0)	1 (1.1)	0 (0.0)	1 (0.4)
Complaints lines	0 (0.0)	0 (0.0)	0 (0.0)	0 (0.0)	0 (0.0)
Local organizational capacity	32 (51.6)	42 (44.7)	43 (46.7)	15 (44.1)	132 (46.8)
Community mobilization	19 (30.6)	35 (37.2)	25 (27.2)	13 (37.2)	92 (32.6)
Community collective action	24 (38.7)	29 (30.9)	26 (28.3)	8 (23.5)	87 (30.9)
Community meetings	18 (29.0)	14 (14.9)	21 (22.8)	5 (14.7)	58 (20.6)
Community boards	5 (8.1)	9 (9.6)	8 (8.7)	1 (2.9)	23 (8.2)
Revolving drug funds	2 (3.2)	3 (3.2)	5 (5.4)	0 (0.0)	10 (3.5)
Financial empowerment	15 (24.2)	24 (25.5)	25 (27.2)	8 (23.5)	72 (25.5)
Community financing	6 (9.7)	3 (3.2)	13 (14.1)	3 (8.8)	25 (8.9)
In-kind subsidies for health services	2 (3.2)	7 (7.4)	4 (4.3)	3 (8.8)	16 (5.7)
Community participatory budgeting	3 (4.8)	4 (4.3)	6 (6.5)	1 (2.9)	14 (5.0)
Vouchers for health services	3 (4.8)	3 (3.2)	5 (5.4)	1 (2.9)	12 (4.3)
Income generation schemes	0 (0.0)	4 (4.3)	5 (5.4)	2 (5.9)	11 (3.9)
Conditional cash transfers	2 (3.2)	4 (4.3)	3 (3.3)	0 (0.0)	9 (3.2)
Microcredit	2 (3.2)	0 (0.0)	3 (3.3)	0 (0.0)	5 (1.8)

Source: Authors.

Note: Studies may involve more than one type of community empowerment strategy. Parentheses indicate percentage of total number of studies of that study design using that strategy.

Table 4.2   Scale of Community Empowerment Studies

Scale of study	Number of studies	% of total
One village/town	39	13.8
Two or more villages/towns	79	28.0
One district/administrative unit	61	21.6
Two or more districts/administrative units	36	12.8
One province/state	16	5.7
Two or more provinces/states	12	4.2
Nationwide	22	7.8
Not specified	17	6.0
Total	282	100.0

Source: Authors.

Table 4.3   Study Design and Positive Outcomes

	Positive outcome		
	(number)	(%)	Total (number)
Randomized controlled trial	57	91.9	62
Nonrandomized controlled trial	85	90.4	94
Before-after trial (uncontrolled)	88	95.7	92
Case-control study	30	88.2	34
Total	260	89.8	282

Source: Authors.

whether the outcome was positive. We also examined whether some types of outcomes were more likely to be positive (for example, measures of mortality, morbidity, health service, health financing, or type of empowerment), and found no differences in the likelihood of a positive outcome.

For the remainder of this chapter, we restricted the analysis to the stronger studies (RCTs and NRCTs), which have more comparable outcome measures (both using comparison groups and at least two measures in time). Table 4.4 shows the likelihood of specific types of community empowerment strategies producing a positive effect. Every type of strategy used had a high likelihood of a positive outcome, as shown by the "Positive outcome with strategy" column, which ranges from 83.3 percent (for vouchers and conditional cash transfers) to 100 percent (for holding providers accountable, community boards, community managed drug revolving funds, community financing, in-kind subsidies, income generation, and microcredit schemes).

To try to find out which type of community empowerment strategy worked better, we compared the positive outcomes in those using a

Table 4.4 Specific Community Empowerment Strategies and Their Effects on Outcomes (RCT and NRCT Studies)

Community empowerment strategy	Positive outcome with strategy (%)	Positive outcome without strategy (%)	Odds ratio	Lower 95% CI	Upper 95% CI	Studies with strategy (number)
Information and education	93.3	76.2	4.375	1.304	14.681	135
Training of community health workers, traditional birth attendants, informal health cadres	93.5	87.3	2.109	.694	6.406	93
Community education—Group meetings	84.8	92.7	0.442	0.137	1.423	33
Training of women and mothers	90.5	91.4	0.894	0.295	2.714	63
Community education —Home visits	90.0	91.1	0.880	0.103	7.500	10
Community education—Media/printed	92.0	90.8	1.160	0.243	5.530	25
In person teacher at facility	93.8	89.8	1.701	0.452	6.397	48
Community education—Arts	91.9	90.4	1.207	0.385	3.788	62
Training of youth/young people	91.9	90.4	1.207	0.385	3.788	62
Inclusion and participation	94.3	89.3	1.993	0.531	7.476	53
Community-managed services	95.5	89.3	2.520	0.540	11.751	44
Community partnership	90.0	91.3	0.861	0.225	3.300	30
Community-owned services	96.0	90.1	2.644	0.330	21.180	25
Community comanagement of drugs	93.8	90.7	1.535	0.187	12.578	16
Accountability	93.1	90.6	1.409	0.298	6.667	29
Joint monitoring of access and quality	86.7	91.5	0.605	0.122	3.001	15
Providers held accountable	100	89.9	n.a.	n.a.	n.a.	17

(continued)

Table 4.4   Specific Community Empowerment Strategies and Their Effects on Outcomes (RCT and NRCT Studies) *(Continued)*

Community empowerment strategy	Positive outcome with strategy (%)	Positive outcome without strategy (%)	Odds ratio	Lower 95% CI	Upper 95% CI	Studies with strategy (number)
Local organizational capacity	94.6	87.8	2.431	0.728	8.113	74
Community mobilization	94.4	89.2	2.055	0.548	7.707	54
Community collective action	96.2	88.3	3.363	0.724	15.618	53
Community meetings	96.9	89.5	3.631	0.457	28.846	32
Community boards	100	90.1	n.a.	n.a.	n.a.	14
Revolving drug funds	100	90.7	n.a.	n.a.	n.a.	5
Financial empowerment	92.3	90.4	1.245	0.329	4.715	39
Community financing	100	90.5	n.a.	n.a.	n.a.	9
In-kind subsidies for health services	100	90.5	n.a.	n.a.	n.a.	9
Community participatory budgeting	85.7	91.3	0.574	0.064	5.136	7
Vouchers for health services	83.3	91.3	0.474	0.051	4.373	6
Income generation schemes	100	90.8	n.a.	n.a.	n.a.	4
Conditional cash transfers	83.3	91.3	0.474	0.051	4.373	6
Microcredit	100	90.9	n.a.	n.a.	n.a.	2

Source: Authors.

Note: Reference group for each strategy is the absence of the strategy; multiple strategies are possible.
n.a. = not applicable (odds ratio undefined).

particular strategy with other strategies that did not use the strategy in question (shown in the "Odds ratio" column in table 4.4). In this analysis, the highest OR was for use of any type of education approach (OR 4.4; 95 percent confidence interval [CI] 1.3–14.7). Although none of the other strategies achieved statistical significance at p value <0.05, use of any of the other main strategies also had a positive effect, with strategies involving local capacity building having the next highest OR (of 2.4), followed by inclusion strategies (OR 1.8), accountability (OR 1.4), and financing mechanisms (OR 1.2). The specific strategies with the highest ORs were strategies involving community meetings (OR 3.6), community collective action (OR 3.4), and community-owned services (OR 2.6). However, ORs could not be calculated for some strategies where 100 percent of the studies had a positive outcome, usually when there were only few studies. Most notably, 17 studies showed the strategy involved holding providers accountable to the community, all of which were successful. Other specific strategies that had 100 percent positive outcomes involved fewer than 10 studies.

Those strategies that appeared relatively less correlated with positive health outcomes included community group education (OR 0.4), voucher schemes (OR 0.5), and conditional cash transfers (OR 0.5). However, none of these reached a level of statistical significance of p value <0.05, which in part is due to the small number of studies within each of these categories.

In addition to analyzing the thematic approaches to community empowerment, we also examined other key characteristics concerning their context and how they were implemented. Figure 4.1 demonstrates that contextual factors (the top two horizontal bars), such as strong local leadership, was strongly associated with a positive outcome (OR 8.2; 95 percent CI 1.04–64.6). Having a pre-existing strategy probably helped (OR 2.0), though this did not reach statistical significance. Involvement of nonstate providers (organizations comprise the bottom four horizontal bars) may have had a positive effect (OR 2.5), whereas involvement of government providers may have decreased the odds of having a positive effect (OR 0.4). Involvement of political parties was uncommon (only 17 studies), and the use of government funding had a statistically lower chance of success than its nonuse (OR 0.3; 95 percent CI 0.08–0.9).

The way in which community empowerment strategies were implemented may also matter (figure 4.2). Although none of the approaches to implementing community empowerment strategies reached statistical significance in comparison to empowerment strategies that did not use them, in all cases, they were associated with a very high probability of

success (>90 percent) (annex table 4.3.1). (The 22 studies that involved empowerment approaches where results are shared with communities had a 100 percent success rate, reinforcing the importance of feedback to the community. Those approaches that forge partnerships between the community and policy makers or technical experts also had relatively high odds of success (OR 2.5). When communities are expected to contribute to an intervention, a sense of ownership is conveyed, and the outcomes may have a greater chance of success (OR 2.3). Other approaches to empowerment that had relatively higher odds of success were those that promote equity (OR 2.2) and those that use systems for local adaptive learning (OR 1.8). Further analysis on factors associated with positive outcomes is detailed in the annex tables.

Main Limitations

The review has several limitations, some common to all literature reviews and some specific to this study. First, a systematic review tends to show what has worked for a common set of interventions rather than how or why more complex strategies have worked (see the *Overview*). The majority of published work on community empowerment is not designed with rigorous scientific methodology to produce probability inferences, and the types of intervention are often not suited to randomized trials. The review also focuses on articles that are in the published literature, only in English or with English abstracts, and in scientific journals, which may have introduced a publication bias toward positive outcomes. (Publication bias is discussed in more detail in the section "Main limitations" in chapter 2.) The analysis of a binary outcome (positive or not) as the measure of success of each study also represents an oversimplification, but was also one way of dealing with very different outcomes in each study.

Just as the strategies are quite different in each context, so are the outcomes. Many of the papers presented multiple outcomes, yet they were not accounted for in this analysis, nor was the magnitude of change conveyed. However, this approach is a very conservative indication as to the success of a strategy compared to other attempts to empower communities that do not use the same strategy. (Further analysis of the data is ongoing to better account for the different types of outcomes and the magnitude of the measured effects.)

This review's premise that certain factors may be generalizable to empowerment strategies as a whole is overly simplistic. The interventions compared were from 66 different countries, targeting different sectors of the population; were managed in different ways; and had a diverse set of aims, inputs, and outcomes. Still, this review should stimulate further research into empowerment for health, and provides some encouragement and useful insights for decision makers, communities, and organizations interested in pursuing such approaches.

Implications for Decision Makers

This systematic review brings together the research on strategies that can empower communities and that can lead to improved health outcomes. Many types of community empowerment approaches have been successful in LMICs across all of the main thematic approaches: access to information; inclusion and participation; accountability; local organizational capacity; and financial empowerment. Although there were more studies conducted on small populations, success was commonly found in both small-scale interventions on the one hand, and national and other large-scale community empowerment strategies on the other. This suggests that the scale of operations does not need to be a constraint to pursuing community empowerment approaches, although the specific requirements of a strategy may still limit the size of the population covered.

It was also found that the context within which a strategy was implemented was important. In particular, the presence of strong local leadership was strongly correlated with improved outcomes, and the experience of using previous community empowerment strategies also appeared helpful. But in places where these conditions did not exist, the success rate with community empowerment approaches was also very high, so these should not be limitations to initiating these strategies. The finding that government financing, the involvement of public health providers, and the involvement of political parties appear relatively less likely to be successful than alternative approaches, particularly those involving nongovernmental providers, does not mean that governments should not be involved in community empowerment approaches. But it does suggest that there is an important role for other civil society organizations, and that governments need to carefully consider their roles. Communities that entered into partnerships with policy makers and technical experts tended to achieve better results than those that did not, suggesting that governments may want to play a more collaborative role.

Governments, civil society organizations, and technical experts can also play a role by promoting good practice in community empowerment strategies. Interventions that appear particularly promising as part of community empowerment strategies include: promoting community communication and action; promoting community ownership and management of services; and providing training opportunities for health workers. Practices that are relatively promising and should be considered in the design and implementation of strategies include: providing feedback by sharing results with communities; using systems for local adaptive learning; using community resources to support programs; and promoting equity.

There is also an important need to better understand how different strategies work. There is relatively limited experience with strategies that involve changing accountability relationships or incorporating financial empowerment in studies that measure health outcomes. Even if the initial findings are encouraging, it is important to test these approaches more systematically in various settings.

It is clear from this analysis that there is a large variation in the contexts, actors, approaches to implementation, and results obtained in community empowerment strategies. More robust research on community empowerment strategies is needed. In addition to strengthening the evidence on strategies that can provide lessons across countries, such research could facilitate the learning and testing of approaches within a country.

Reference

World Bank. 2002. *Empowerment and Poverty Reduction: A Sourcebook.* http://siteresources.worldbank.org/INTEMPOWERMENT/Resources/48631 2-1095094954594/draft.pdf.

Annex 4.1 Electronic Databases Searched

Studies were required to present the following information for initial inclusion in the review:

- health outcome data before and after the empowering strategy was implemented, either through a pre-post design with controls, or with multiple study arms;
- health outcomes specifically related to health, including: morbidity, mortality, service utilization or coverage, empowerment outcomes, financial protection and health financing outcomes; and
- health outcomes recorded in a quantitative manner, that is, enabling a numerical calculation of the effect of intervention.

All articles were in English, and those that could not be found through the Internet (open domain), Johns Hopkins University, and World Bank libraries (virtual and physical) were not included.

The databases used include: Medline, the Cochrane Library, Social Sciences Citation Index, Popline, and the World Bank database. Over 40,000 articles were highlighted from the initial search and went on to title screening. Those articles progressing through the title screen went on for abstract screening. A total of 1,067 papers were selected for detailed, full paper analysis for inclusion into the review. These papers were searched for by graduate students at the Johns Hopkins School of Public Health. Of these, 113 had insufficient data to be tracked, or were not contained in the resources mentioned. Full papers were analyzed by a team trained in the review inclusion criteria. Accepted articles were sent for data abstraction. Review articles were not included in the review, but their constituent individual papers were screened for inclusion.

Annex 4.2 Studies Reviewed

Abatemarco, D.J., B. West, et al. 2004. "Project Northland in Croatia: A Community-based Adolescent Alcohol Prevention Intervention." *Journal of Drug Education* 34(2): 167–78.

Abdu, Z., Z. Mohammed, et al. 2004. "The Impact of User Fee Exemption on Service Utilization and Treatment-seeking Behaviour: The Case of Malaria in Sudan." *The International Journal of Health Planning and Management* 19(suppl. 1): S95–106.

Abdulla, S., et al. 2001. "Impact on Malaria Morbidity of a Programme Supplying Insecticide-treated Nets in Children Aged Under 2 Years in Tanzania: Community Cross-sectional Study." *British Medical Journal* 322 (7281): 270–3.

Adatu, F., et al. 2003. "Implementation of the DOTS Strategy for Tuberculosis Control in Rural Kiboga District, Uganda, Offering Patients the Option of Treatment Supervision in the Community, 1998–1999." *The International Journal of Tuberculosis and Lung Disease* 7(9):S63-S71.

Afari, E.A., F.K. Nkrumah, et al. 1995. "Impact of Primary Health Care on Child Morbidity and Mortality in Rural Ghana: The Gomoa Experience." *The Central African Journal of Medicine* 41(5): 148–53.

Agboatwalla, M. 1997. "Impact of Health Education on Mothers' Knowledge of Preventive Health Practices." *Tropical Doctor* 27: 199–202.

Ahluwalia, I.B., T. Schmid, et al. 2003. "An Evaluation of a Community-Based Approach to Safe Motherhood in Northern Tanzania." *International Journal of Gynaecology and Obstetrics* 82(2): 231–40.

Ahmed, N.U., M.F. Zeitlin, et al. 1993. "A Longitudinal Study of the Impact of Behavioural Change Intervention on Cleanliness, Diarrhoeal Morbidity and Growth of Children in Rural Bangladesh." *Social Science & Medicine* 37(2): 159–71.

Akashi, H., T. Yamada, E. Huot, and K. Kanal. 2003. "User Fees at a Public Hospital in Cambodia: Effects on Hospital Perfomnance and Provider Attitudes." *Social Science & Medicine.*

Akram, D.S., and M. Agboatwalla. 1992. "A Model for Health Intervention." *Journal of Tropical Pediatrics* 38(2): 85–7.

Akram, D.S., M. Agboatwalla, et al. 1997. "Effect of Intervention on Promotion of Exclusive Breast Feeding." *The Journal of the Pakistan Medical Association* 47(2): 46–8.

Al Quds University, Center for Development in Primary Health Care. 2003. "Improving Postpartum Care among Low-parity Mothers in Palestine." Frontiers in Reproductive Health. Population Council, Washington, DC, May.

Ali, M., C. Miyoshi, et al. 2006. "Emergency Medical Services in Islamabad, Pakistan: A Public-Private Partnership." *Public Health* 120(1): 50–7.

Ali, M., M. Emch, et al. 2001. "Implications of Health Care Provision on Acute Lower Respiratory Infection Mortality in Bangladeshi Children." *Social Science & Medicine* 52(2): 267–77.

Ali, M., T. Asefaw, et al. 2005. "Helping Northern Ethiopian Communities Reduce Childhood Mortality: Population-based Intervention Trial." *Bulletin of the World Health Organization* 83(1): 27–33.

Alisjahbana, A., C. Williams, et al. 1995. "An Integrated Village Maternity Service to Improve Referral Patterns in a Rural Area in West-Java." *International Journal of Gynaecology and Obstetrics* 48(suppl.): S83–94.

Allen, C.W., and H. Jeffery. 2006. "Implementation and Evaluation of a Neonatal Educational Program in Rural Nepal." *Journal of Tropical Pediatrics* 52(3): 218–22.

Amaral, J., A.J.M. Leite, et al. 2005. "Impact of IMCI Health Worker Training on Routinely Collected Child Health Indicators in Northeast Brazil." *Health Policy and Planning* 20: 142–148.

Ande, O., O. Oladepo, et al. 2004. "Comparison of Knowledge on Diarrheal Disease Management between Two Types of Community-based Distributors in Oyo State, Nigeria." *Health Education Research* 19(1): 110–3.

Anderson, J.D., and C.C. Bentley. 1986. "Role of Community Health Workers in Trachoma Control. Case Study from a Somali Refugee Camp." *Tropical Doctor* 16(2): 66–9.

Arole, M., and R. Arole. 1994. *Jamkhed: A Comprehensive Rural Health Project.* London: Macmillan Press, Ltd.

Asamoah-Adu, A., et al. 1994. "Evaluation of a Targeted AIDS Prevention Intervention to Increase Condom Use among Prostitutes in Ghana." *AIDS* 8: 239–246.

Attanasio, O., E. Fitzsimons, et al. 2006. "Child Education and Work Choices in the Presence of a Conditional Cash Transfer Programme in Rural Colombia." SSRN.

Aubel, J., I. Toure, et al. 2004. "Senegalese Grandmothers Promote Improved Maternal and Child Nutrition Practices: The Guardians of Tradition Are Not Averse to Change." *Social Science & Medicine* 59(5): 945–59.

Awasthi, S., M. Nichter, et al. 2000. "Developing an Interactive STI-prevention Program for Young Men: Lessons from a North Indian Slum." *Studies in Family Planning* 31 (2): 138–50.

Aziz, K.M., B.A. Hoque, et al. 1990. "Reduction in Diarrhoeal Diseases in Children in Rural Bangladesh by Environmental and Behavioural Modifications." *Transactions of the Royal Society of Tropical Medicine and Hygiene* 84(3): 433–8.

Bairagi, R., M.M. Islam, and M.K. Barua. 2000. "Contraceptive Failure: Levels, Trends and Determinants in Matlab, Bangladesh." *Journal of Biosocial Science* 32(1): 107–23.

Bairagi, R., and M. Rahman. 1996. "Contraceptive Failure in Matlab, Bangladesh." *International Family Planning Perspectives* 22(1): 21–5.

Bajracharya, D. 2003. "Myanmar Experiences in Sanitation and Hygiene Promotion: Lessons Learned and Future Directions." *International Journal of Environmental Health Research* 13(suppl. 1): S141–52.

Bang, A.T., H.M. Reddy, et al. 2005. "Neonatal and Infant Mortality in the Ten Years (1993 to 2003) of the Gadchiroli Field Trial: Effect of Home-based Neonatal Care." *Journal of Perinatology* 25(suppl. 1): S92–107.

Bang, A.T., R.A. Bang, et al. 1990. "Reduction in Pneumonia Mortality and Total Childhood Mortality by Means of Community-based Intervention Trial in Gadchiroli, India." *Lancet* 336(8709): 201–6.

Bang, A.T., R.A. Bang, et al. 1993. "Pneumonia in Neonates: Can it be Managed in the Community?" *Archives of Disease in Childhood* 68(5 Spec No.): 550–6.

Bang, A.T., R.A. Bang, et al. 1994. "Management of Childhood Pneumonia by Traditional Birth Attendants." The SEARCH Team. *Bulletin of the World Health Organization* 72(6): 897–905.

Bang, A.T., R.A. Bang, et al. 1999. "Effect of Home-based Neonatal Care and Management of Sepsis on Neonatal Mortality: Field Trial in Rural India." *Lancet* 354(9194): 1955–61.

Bang, A.T., R.A. Bang, et al. 2005. "Management of Birth Asphyxia in Home Deliveries in Rural Gadchiroli: The Effect of Two Types of Birth Attendants and of Resuscitating with Mouth-to-Mouth, Tube-Mask or Bag-Mask." *Journal of Perinatology* 25(suppl. 1): S8.

Bang, A.T., R.A. Bang, et al. 2005. "Methods and the Baseline Situation in the Field Trial of Home-based Neonatal care in Gadchiroli, India." *Journal of Perinatology* 25(suppl. 1): S11–7.

Bang, A.T., R.A. Bang, et al. 2005. "Home-based Neonatal Care: Summary and Applications of the Field Trial in Rural Gadchiroli, India (1993 to 2003)." *Journal of Perinatology* 25(suppl. 1): S108–22.

Bang, A.T., R.A. Bang, et al. 2005. "Reduced Incidence of Neonatal Morbidities: Effect of Home-based Neonatal Care in Rural Gadchiroli, India." *Journal of Perinatology* 25(suppl. 1): S51–61.

Bang, A.T., S.B. Baitule, et al. 2005. "Low Birth Weight and Preterm Neonates: Can They Be Managed at Home by Mother and a Trained Village Health Worker?" *Journal of Perinatology* 25(suppl. 1): S72–81.

Baqui, A.H., R.E. Black, et al. 2004. "Zinc Therapy for Diarrhoea Increased the Use of Oral Rehydration Therapy and Reduced the Use of Antibiotics in Bangladeshi Children." *Journal of Health, Population, and Nutrition* 22(4): 440–2.

Behrman, J.R., and E. Skoufias. 2006. "Mitigating Myths about Policy Effectiveness: Evaluation of Mexico's Antipoverty and Human Resource Investment Program." *Annals of the American Academy of Political and Social Science* 606: 244–275.

Bell, D., R. Go, et al. 2005. "Unequal Treatment Access and Malaria Risk in a Community-based Intervention Program in the Philippines." *The Southeast Asian Journal of Tropical Medicine and Public Health* 36(3): 578–86.

Berggren, G.G. 1985. Comparison of Haitian Children in a Nutrition Intervention Programme with Children in the Haitian National Nutrition Survey. *Bulletin of the World Health Organization* 63(6): 1141–1153.

Berggren, W.L., D.C. Ewbank, et al. 1981. "Reduction of Mortality in Rural Haiti Through a Primary-health-care Program." *The New England Journal of Medicine* 304(22): 1324–30.

Berman, P.A. 1984. "Village Health Workers in Java, Indonesia: Coverage and Equity." *Social Science & Medicine* 19(4): 411–22.

Bhandari, N., R. Bahl, et al. 2003. "Effect of Community-based Promotion of Exclusive Breastfeeding on Diarrhoeal Illness and Growth: A Cluster Randomised Controlled Trial." *Lancet* 361(9367): 1418–23.

Bhandari, N., S. Mazumder, et al. 2004. "An Educational Intervention to Promote Appropriate Complementary Feeding Practices and Physical Growth in Infants and Young Children in Rural Haryana, India." *Journal of Nutrition* 134(9): 2342–8.

Bhandari, N., S. Mazumder, et al. 2005. "Use of Multiple Opportunities for Improving Feeding Practices in Under-twos within Child Health Programmes." *Health Policy and Planning* 20(5): 328–36.

Björkman, M., Svensson, J. 2007. "Power to the People: Evidence from a Randomized Field Experiment of a Community-Based Monitoring Project in Uganda." World Bank Policy Research Working Paper 4268. June.

Bian, J.Y., B.X. Zhang, et al. 1995. "Evaluating the Social Impact and Effectiveness of Four-year 'Love Teeth Day' Campaign in China." *Advances in Dental Research* 9: 130–133.

Billig, P., E. Gurzau, et al. 1999. "Innovative Intersectoral Approach Reduces Blood Lead Levels of Children and Workers in Romania." *International Journal of Occupational and Environmental Health* 5(1): 50–6.

Blas, E., and M. Limbambala. 2001. "User-payment, Decentralization and Utilization in Zambia." *Health Policy and Planning* 16(suppl. 2): 19–28.

Boelee, E., and H. Laamrani. 2004. "Environmental Control of Schistosomiasis through Community Participation in a Moroccan Oasis." *Tropical Medicine & International Health* 9(9): 997–1004.

Borghi, J., A. Gorter, et al. 2005. "The Cost-effectiveness of a Competitive Voucher Scheme to Reduce Sexually Transmitted Infections in High-risk Groups in Nicaragua." *Health Policy and Planning* 20(4): 222–31.

Borghi, J., B. Thapa, et al. 2005. "Economic Assessment of a Women's Group Intervention to Improve Birth Outcomes in Rural Nepal." *Lancet* 366(9500): 1882–4.

Brieger, W.R., G.E. Delano, et al. 2001. "West African Youth Initiative: Outcome of a Reproductive Health Education Program." *Journal of Adolescent Health* 29(6): 436–46.

Broadhead, R.S., V.L. Volkanevsky, et al. 2006. "Peer-driven HIV Interventions for Drug Injectors in Russia: First Year Impact Results of a Field Experiment." *International Journal of Drug Policy* 17(5): 379–392.

Brugha, R.F., and J.P. Kevany. 1996. "Maximizing Immunization Coverage through Home Visits: A Controlled Trial in an Urban Area of Ghana." *Bulletin of the World Health Organization* 74(5): 517–24.

Burnham, G.M., G. Pariyo, et al. 2004. "Discontinuation of Cost Sharing in Uganda." *Bulletin of the World Health Organization* 82(3): 187–95.

Chaiken, M.S., H. Deconinck, et al. 2006. "The Promise of a Community-based Approach to Managing Severe Malnutrition: A Case Study from Ethiopia." *Food and Nutrition Bulletin* 27(2): 95–104.

Chakraborty, S., S.A. D'Souza, et al. 2000. "Improving Private Practitioner Care of Sick Children: Testing New Approaches in Rural Bihar." *Health Policy and Planning* 15(4): 400–7.

Chand, A.D. 1987. "Community Financing for Primary Health Care. Report of a study." *Economic and Political Weekly* 22(24): 951–6.

Chandler, Rudolph, Kaytie Decker, and Bernard Nziyige. 2004. "Estimating the Cost of Providing Home-based Care for HIV/AIDS in Rwanda." The

Partners for Health Reform*plus* Project, Abt Associates Inc., Bethesda, Maryland. June.

Chaoniyom, W., N. Suwannapong, et al. 2005. "Strengthening the Capability of Family Health Leaders for Sustainable Community-based Health Promotion." *The Southeast Asian Journal of Tropical Medicine and Public Health* 36(4): 1039–47.

Chatterjee, S., V. Patel, et al. 2003. "Evaluation of a Community-based Rehabilitation Model for Chronic Schizophrenia in Rural India." *The British Journal of Psychiatry* 182: 57–62.

Chaudhuri, S.N. 1988. "Growth monitoring in the Evolution of Clinic based Health Care through a Community-based Action Program." *Indian Journal of Pediatrics* 55(suppl. 1): S84–7.

Chaudhury, N., and D. Parajuli. 2006. "Conditional Cash Transfers and Female Schooling: The Impact of the Female School Stipend Program on Public School Enrollments in Punjab, Pakistan." SSRN.

Chen, L.C., M. Rahman, et al. 1983. "Mortality Impact of an MCH-FP Program in Matlab, Bangladesh." *Studies in Family Planning* 14(8–9): 199–209.

Chopra, Micky, and David Wilkinson. 1997. "Vaccination Coverage is Higher in Children Living in Areas with Community Health Workers in Rural South Africa." *Journal of Tropical Pediatrics* 43(6): 372–4.

Chowdhury, A.M., et al. 1988. "Teaching ORT to Women: Individually or in Groups?" *Journal of Tropical Medicine and Hygiene*, 91, 283–287.

Chowdhury, A.M., F. Karim, et al. 1997. "The Status of ORT (oral rehydration therapy) in Bangladesh: How Widely is it Used?" *Health Policy and Planning* 12(1): 58–66.

Chowdhury, A.M., J.P. Vaughan, et al. 1988a. "Mothers Learn How to Save the Lives of Children." *World Health Forum* 9(2): 239–44.

Chowdhury, A.M., J.P. Vaughan, et al. 1988b. "Use and Safety of Home-made Oral Rehydration Solutions: An Epidemiological Evaluation from Bangladesh." *International Journal of Epidemiology* 17(3): 655–65.

Chowdhury, A.M., et al. 1999. *Hope Not Complacency: State of Primary Education in Bangladesh*. Dhaka: Bangladesh University Press.

Clay, R.M. 1985. "The Health Guide Scheme. The Mysore District, India: The Community's Perspective." *Medical Anthropology* 9(1): 49–56.

Community Health Waiver Scheme (CHEWS). 2006. Kafue District Team. "Zambia Community Health Waiver Scheme: Final Evaluation." Abt Associates, Partners for Health Reform*plus*, Bethesda, Maryland. February.

Cooper, P.J., M. Landman, et al. 2002. "Impact of a Mother-infant Intervention in an Indigent Peri-urban South African Context. Pilot Study." *British Journal of Psychiatry* 180: 76–81.

Corbett, E.L., E. Dauya, R. Matambo, Y.B. Cheung, et al. 2006. "Uptake of Workplace HIV Counselling and Testing: A Cluster-randomised Trial in Zimbabwe." *PloS Medicine* 3(7): e238.

Coutinho, S.B., P.I. de Lira, et al. 2005. "Comparison of the Effect of Two Systems for the Promotion of Exclusive Breastfeeding." *Lancet* 366(9491): 1094–100.

Cropley, L. 2004. "The Effect of Health Education Interventions on Child Malaria Treatment-seeking Practices among Mothers in Rural Refugee Villages in Belize, Central America." *Health Promotion International* 19(4).

Curtale, F., and B. Siwakoti. 1995. "Improving Skills and Utilization of Community Health Volunteers in Nepal." *Social Science Medicine* 40(8): 1117–25.

Darmstadt, G. L., V. Kumar, et al. 2006. "Introduction of Community-based Skin-to-skin Care in Rural Uttar Pradesh, India." *Journal of Perinatology* 26(10): 597–604.

Datta, N., et al. 1987. "Application of Case Management to the Control of Acute Respiratory Infections in Low-birth-weight Infants: A Feasibility Study." *Bulletin of the World Health Organization* 65(1): 77–82.

Davies-Adetugbo, A.A. 1996. "Promotion of Breast Feeding in the Community: Impact of Health Education Programme in Rural Communities in Nigeria." *Journal of Diarrhoeal Diseases Research* 14(1): 5–11.

Debpuur, C., J.F. Phillips, et al. 2002. "The Impact of the Navrongo Project on Contraceptive Knowledge and Use, Reproductive Preferences, and Fertility." *Studies in Family Planning* 33(2): 141–64.

Delacollette, C., P. Van der Stuyft, and K. Molima. 1996. "Using Community Health Workers for Malaria Control: experience in Zaire." *Bulletin of the World Health Organization* (4): 423–430.

Diallo, D.A., S.N. Cousens, et al. 2004. "Child Mortality in a West African Population Protected with Insecticide-treated Curtains for a Period of up to 6 Years." *Bulletin of the World Health Organization* 82(2): 85–91.

Douthwaite, M., and P. Ward. 2005. "Increasing Contraceptive Use in Rural Pakistan: An Evaluation of the Lady Health Worker Programme." *Health Policy and Planning* 20(2): 117–23.

Dow, W.H., and K.K. Schmeer. 2003. "Health Insurance and Child Mortality in Costa Rica." *Social Science & Medicine* 57(6): 975–86.

Dror, D.M., E.S. Soriano, et al. 2005. "Field-based Evidence of Enhanced Healthcare Utilization among Persons Insured by Micro Health Insurance Units in Philippines." *Health Policy* 73(3): 263–271.

Dubois, D. 2004. "Uganda Family Planning Programs: Lessons from the Field. Partnering with Communities and District Health Teams." Minnesota International Health Volunteers/CORE.

Dunston, C., D. McAfee, et al. 2001. "Collaboration, Cholera, and Cyclones: A Project to Improve Point-of-use Water Quality in Madagascar." *American Journal of Public Health* 91(10): 1574–6.

Duresamin, A., and A. Mubina. 1992. "Gastroenteritis: A Grass Root Approach." *Community Development Journal* 27(1): 42–49.

Dutt, D., and D.K. Srinivasa. 1997. "Impact of Maternal and Child Health Strategy on Child Survival in a Rural Community of Pondicherry." *Indian Pediatrics* 34(9): 785–92.

Elder, J.P., T. Louis, O. Sutisnaputra, N.S. Sulaeiman, L. Ware, W. Shaw, C. de Moor, and J. Graeff. 1992. "The Use of Diarrhoeal Management Counselling Cards for Community Health Volunteer Training in Indonesia: The Healthcom Project." *Journal of Tropical Medicine and Hygiene* 95(5): 301–8.

Eng, E., J. Briscoe, et al. 1990. "Participation Effect from Water Projects on EPI." *Social Science & Medicine* 30(12): 1349–58.

Esu-Williams, E., K.D. Schenk, et al. 2006. "We are No Longer Called Club Members but Caregivers: Involving Youth in HIV and AIDS Caregiving in Rural Zambia." *AIDS Care* 18(8): 888–94.

Ethiraj, T., P. Antony, et al. 1995. "A Study on the Effect of Patient and Community Education in Prevention of Disability Programme." *Indian Journal of Leprosy* 67(4): 435–45.

Dudley, L., V. Azevedo, R. Grant, J. H. Schoeman, L. Dikweni, and D. Maher. 2003. "Evaluation of Community Contribution to Tuberculosis Control in Cape Town, South Africa." *International Journal of Tuberculosis and Lung Disease* 7(9 suppl. 1): S48–55.

Farmer, P., S. Robin, et al. 1991. "Tuberculosis, Poverty, and Compliance: Lessons from Rural Haiti." *Seminars in Respiratory Infections* 6(4): 254–60.

Fauveau, V., et al. 1992. "Impact on Mortality of a Community-based Programme to Control Acure Lower Respiratory Tract Infections." *Bulletin of the World Health Organization* 70(1): 109–116.

Fauveau, V., B. Wojtyniak, et al. 1990. "The Effect of Maternal and Child Health and Family Planning Services on Mortality: Is Prevention Enough?" *British Medical Journal* 301(6743): 103–7.

Fauveau, V., B. Wojtyniak, et al. 1990. "Perinatal Mortality in Matlab, Bangladesh: A Community-based Study." *International Journal of Epidemiology* 19(3): 606–12.

Fofana, P., O. Samai, et al. 1997. "Promoting the Use of Obstetric Services through Community Loan Funds, Bo, Sierra Leone. The Bo PMM Team." *International Journal of Gynaecology and Obstetrics* 59(suppl. 2): S225–30.

Foongming Moy, Atiya A. B. Sallam, and Meelan Wong. 2006. "The Results of a Worksite Health Promotion Programme in Kaula Lumpur, Malaysia." *Health Promotion International* 21(4).

Fullerton, J. T., R. Killian, et al. 2005. "Outcomes of a Community- and Home-based Intervention for Safe Motherhood and Newborn Care." *Health Care for Women International* 26(7): 561–76.

Ghosh, S.K., R.R. Patil, et al. 2006. "A Community-based Health Education Programme for Bio-environmental Control of Malaria through Folk Theatre (Kalajatha) in Rural India." *Malaria Journal* 5: 123.

Goodman, C.A., W.M. Mutemi, et al. 2006. "The Cost-effectiveness of Improving Malaria Home Management: Shopkeeper Training in Rural Kenya." *Health Policy and Planning* 21(4): 275–88.

Greenwood, B.M., A.K. Bradley, et al. 1990. "Evaluation of a Primary Health Care Programme in The Gambia. II. Its Impact on Mortality and Morbidity in Young Children." *Journal of Tropical Medicine and Hygiene* 93(2): 87–97.

Hadi, A. 2003. "Management of Acute Respiratory Infections by Community Health Volunteers: Experience of Bangladesh Rural Advancement Committee (BRAC)." *Bulletin of the World Health Organization* 81(3): 183–9.

Haggerty, P.A., K. Muladi, et al. 1994. "Community-based Hygiene Education to Reduce Diarrhoeal Disease in Rural Zaire: Impact of the Intervention on Diarrhoeal Morbidity." *International Journal of Epidemiology* 23(5): 1050–9.

Hammett, T.M., R. Kling, et al. 2006. "Patterns of HIV Prevalence and HIV Risk Behaviors among Injection Drug Users Prior to and 24 Months Following Implementation of Cross-border HIV Prevention Interventions in Northern Vietnam and Southern China." *AIDS Education and Prevention* 18(2): 97–115.

Hardeman, W., W. Van Damme, et al. 2004. "Access to Health Care for All? User Fees Plus a Health Equity Fund in Sotnikum, Cambodia." *Health Policy and Planning* 19(1): 22–32.

Hartman, A.F., M.D. Hartman, et al. 1984. "Impact of a Community-based Intervention of Health and Nutrition Status in the Central Amazon of Brazil." *Journal of Tropical Pediatrics* 30(1): 30–6.

Herrel, N. 2004. "Improving Malaria Case Management in Ugandan Communities: Lessons from the Field." Minnesota International Health Volunteers/CORE.

Hii, J.L., K.C. Chee, et al. 1996. "Sustainability of a Successful Malaria Surveillance and Treatment Program in a Runggus Community in Sabah, East Malaysia." *The Southeast Asian Journal of Tropical Medicine and Public Health* 27(3): 512–21.

Holanda, F., Jr., A. Castelo, et al. 2006. "Primary Screening for Cervical Cancer through Self Sampling." *International Journal of Gynaecology and Obstetrics* 95(2): 179–84.

Hollander, D. 2002. "As Desired Fertility Falls, Contraceptive Services Help Women Avoid Abortions." *International Family Planning Perspectives* 28(2): 130.

Hossain, J., and S.R. Ross. 2006. "The Effect of Addressing Demand for as Well as Supply of Emergency Obstetric Care in Dinajpur, Bangladesh." *International Journal of Gynaecology and Obstetrics* 92(3): 320–8.

Hossain, S.M., A. Duffield, et al. 2005. "An Evaluation of the Impact of a US$60 million Nutrition Programme in Bangladesh." *Health Policy and Planning* 20(1): 35–40.

Howard-Grabman, L., G. Seoane, et al. 2002. "The Warmi Project: A Participatory Approach to Improve Maternal and Neonatal Health. An Implementor's Manual." Westport, CT, John Snow International, MotherCare Project, Save the Children.

Huerta, M.C. 2006. "Child Health in Rural Mexico: Has Progresa Reduced Children's Morbidity Risks?" *Social Policy & Administration* 40(6): 652–677.

Huicho, L., M. Davila, et al. 2005. "Implementation of the Integrated Management of Childhood Illness Strategy in Peru and its Association with Health Indicators: An Ecological Analysis." *Health Policy and Planning* 20(suppl. 1): i32–i41.

Interchurch Medical Assistance. 2006. "SANRU III Final Evaluation." New Windsor, Maryland.

Islam, M.A., E. Biswas, et al. 1994. "Factors Associated with Safe Preparation and Home-use of Sugar-salt Solution." *Public Health* 108(1): 55–59.

Jacobs, B., N. Price. 2005. "Improving Access for the Poorest to Public Sector Health Services: Insights from Kirivong Operational Health District in Cambodia." Advance Publication. November 17.

Jacobson, M.L., M.H. Labbok, et al. 1985. "Individual and Group Supervision of Community Health Workers in Kenya: A Comparison." *J Health Admin Educ* 5: 83–94.

Jacobson, M.L., M.H. Labbok, et al. 1989. "A Case Study of the Tenwek Hospital Community Health Programme in Kenya." *Social Science & Medicine* 28(10): 1059–62.

Jahanfar, S., Z. Ghodsy, et al. 2005. "Community-based Distribution and Contraception Usage in Iran." *The Journal of Family Planning and Reproductive Health Care* 31(3): 194–7.

Jana, S., and S. Singh. 1995. "Beyond Medical Model of STD Intervention: Lessons from Sonagachi." *Indian Journal of Public Health* 39(3): 125–31.

Jokhio, A.H., H.R. Winter, et al. 2005. "An Intervention Involving Traditional Birth Attendants and Perinatal and Maternal Mortality in Pakistan." *The New England Journal of Medicine* 352(20): 2091–9.

Joseph, A., S. Abraham, et al. 1988. "Improving Immunization Coverage." *World Health Forum* 9(3): 336–40.

Jutting, J.P. 2004. "Do Community-based Health Insurance Schemes Improve Poor People's Access to Health Care? Evidence from Rural Senegal." *World Development* 32(2): 273–288.

Kachur, S.P., P.A. Phillips-Howard, A.M. Odhacha, T.K. Ruebush, A.J. Oloo, and B.L. Nahlen. 1999. "Maintenance and Sustained Use of Insecticide-treated Bednets and Curtains Three Years after a Controlled Trial in Western Kenya." *Tropical Medicine & International Health* 4(11): 72.

Kassaye, M., et al. 1994. "A Randomized Community Trial of Prepackaged and Homemade Oral Rehydration Therapies." *Archives of Pediatrics & Adolescent Medicine* 148.

Kay, B.H., V.S. Nam, et al. 2002. "Control of Aedes Vectors of Dengue in Three Provinces of Vietnam by Use of Mesocyclops (Copepoda) and Community-based Methods Validated by Entomologic, Clinical, and Serological Surveillance." *The American Journal of Tropical Medicine and Hygiene* 66(1): 40–8.

Khan, M.A., J.D. Walley, S.N. Witter, A. Imran, and N. Safdar. 2002. "Costs and Cost-effectiveness of Different DOT Strategies for the Treatment of Tuberculosis in Pakistan." *Health Policy and Planning* 17(2): 178–86.

Khan, A.J., J.A. Khan, et al. 1990. "Acute Respiratory Infections in Children: A Case Management Intervention in Abbottabad District, Pakistan." *Bulletin of the World Health Organization* 68(5): 577–85.

Khan, M.U. 1982. "Interruption of Shigellosis by Hand Washing." *Transactions of the Royal Society of Tropical Medicine and Hygiene* 76(2): 164–8.

Khan, N.C., H.T. Thanh, et al. 2005. "Community Mobilization and Social Marketing to Promote Weekly Iron-folic Acid Supplementation: A New Approach toward Controlling Anemia among Women of Reproductive Age in Vietnam." *Nutrition Reviews* 63(12 Pt 2): S87.

Khandekar, R., T. Khim Thana, and Phi Do Thi. 2006. "Impact of Face Washing and Environmental Improvement on Education of Active Trachoma in Vietnam: A Public Health Intervention Study." *Ophthalmic Epidemiology* 13(1): 43–52.

Khatun, M., H. Stenlund, et al. 2004. "BRAC Initiative towards Promoting Gender and Social Equity in Health: A Longitudinal Study of Child Growth in Matlab, Bangladesh." *Public Health Nutrition* 7(8): 1071–9.

Kidane, G., and R.H Morrow. 2000. "Teaching Mother to Provide Home Treatment of Malaria in Tigray, Ethiopa: A Randomised Trial." *Lancet* 356(9229): 550–5.

Kielmann, A.A., A.B. Mobarak, M.T. Hammamy, A.I. Gomaa, S. Abou-el-Saad, R.K. Lotfi, I. Mazen, and A. Nagaty. 1985. "Control of Deaths from Diarrheal Disease in Rural Communities. I. Design of an Intervention Study and Effects on Child Mortality." *Tropical Medicine and Parasitology* 36(4):191–8.

Kilaru, A., P.L. Griffiths, et al. 2005. "Community-based Nutrition Education for Improving Infant Growth in Rural Karnataka." *Indian Pediatrics* 42(5): 425–32.

King, M. 1983. *An Iranian Experiment in Primary Health Care. The West Azerbaijan Project.* Oxford University Press, New York, NY.

Kittayapong, P., U. Chansang, et al. 2006. "Community Participation and Appropriate Technologies for Dengue Vector Control at Transmission Foci in Thailand." *Journal of the American Mosquito Control Association* 22(3): 538–46.

Koum, K., J. Busch-Hallen, T. Cavalli-Sforza, B. Crape, and S. Smitasiri. "Weekly Iron-Folic Acid Supplementation to Prevent Anemia among Cambodian Women in Three Settings: Process and Outcomes of Social Marketing and Community Mobilization." *Nutrition Reviews* 63(S2) S126–S133.

Kowli, S.S., R.R. Kumar, M.J. Trivedi, and V.R. Bhalerao. 1984. "Experience with Under-five Clinic in Malavani, A Slum Area near Bombay." *Journal of Postgraduate Medicine* 30(1): 13–9.

Kroeger, A., R. Meyer, et al. 1996. "Health Education for Community-based Malaria Control: An Intervention Study in Ecuador, Colombia and Nicaragua." *Tropical Medicine & International Health* 1(6): 836–46.

Kumar, R., A. Raizada, et al. 2002. "A Community-based Rheumatic Fever/Rheumatic Heart Disease Cohort: Twelve-year Experience." *Indian Heart Journal* 54(1): 54–8.

Kwast, B.E. 1995. "Building a Community-based Maternity Program." *International Journal of Gynecology & Obstetrics* 48(suppl.): S67-S82.

Lagerkvist, B. 1992. "Community-based Rehabilitation: Outcome for the Disabled in the Philippines and Zimbabwe." *Disability and Rehabilitation* 14(1): 44–50.

Landry, E.G., R. Louisy, et al. 1987. "Distribution of Contraceptives in Factories in St. Lucia." *Journal of Health Administration Education* 5(1): 105–17.

Landry, E., et al. 1991. "Information and Education Strategies to Increase Knowledge and Improve Attitudes toward Vasectomy in Chogoria, Kenya." Presented at the 19th Annual Meeting of the American Public Health Association (APHA), Atlanta, Georgia. November 11–14.

Leite, A.J., R.F. Puccini, et al. 2005. "Effectiveness of Home-based Peer Counselling to Promote Breastfeeding in the Northeast of Brazil: A Randomized Clinical Trial." *Acta Paediatrica* 94(6): 741–6.

Leon, F.R., R. Hurtado, et al. 1992. "Provider Knowledge Concerning Depo-Provera and Other Contraceptives before and after Training: A Study in Rural Peru."

Leontsini, E., E. Gil, et al. 1993. "Effect of a Community-based *Aedes Aegypti* Control Programme on Mosquito Larval Production Sites in El Progreso, Honduras." *Transactions of the Royal Society of Tropical Medicine and Hygiene* 87(3): 267–71.

Levy-Bruhl, D., A. Soucat, et al. 1997. "The Bamako Initiative in Benin and Guinea: Improving the Effectiveness of Primary Health Care." *The International Journal of Health Planning and Management* 12(suppl. 1): S49–79.

Litvack, J.I., and C. Bodart. 1993. "User Fees Plus Quality Equals Improved Access To Health-Care. Results of a Field Experiment in Cameroon." *Social Science & Medicine* 37(3): 369–383.

Lloyd, L.S, Winch, P., et al. 1992."Results of a Community-based *Aedes Aegypti* Control Program in Merida, Yucatan, Mexico." *The American Journal of Tropical Medicine and Hygiene* 46(6): 635–642.

Lou, C.H., B. Wang, et al. 2004. "Effects of a Community-based Sex Education and Reproductive Health Service Program on Contraceptive Use of Unmarried Youths in Shanghai." *Journal of Adolescent Health* 34(5): 433–40.

Lovell, C.H. 1992. "Breaking the Cycle of Poverty: The BRAC Case." Kumarian Press, Boulder, Colorado.

Luby, S.P., M. Agboatwalla, et al. 2005. "Effect of Handwashing on Child Health: A Randomised Controlled Trial." *Lancet* 366(9481): 225–33.

Luby, S.P., M. Agboatwalla, et al. 2006. "Combining Drinking Water Treatment and Hand Washing for Diarrhoea Prevention: A Cluster Randomised Controlled Trial." *Tropical Medicine & International Health* 11(4): 479–89.

Lucumi, D.I., O.L. Sarmiento, et al. 2006. "Community Intervention to Promote Consumption of Fruits and Vegetables, Smoke-free Homes, and Physical Activity among Home Caregivers in Bogota, Colombia." *Preventing Chronic Disease* 3(4): A120.

Lwilla, F., D. Schellenberg, et al. 2003. "Evaluation of Efficacy of Community-based vs. Institutional-based Direct Observed Short-course Treatment for the Control of Tuberculosis in Kilombero District, Tanzania." *Tropical Medicine & International Health* 8(3): 204.

Lynch, M., S.K. West, et al. 2003. "Azithromycin Treatment Coverage in Tanzanian Children using Community Volunteers." *Ophthalmic Epidemiology* 10(3): 167–175.

Lynch, M., S.K. West, et al. 1994. "Testing a Participatory Strategy to Change Hygiene Behaviour: Face Washing in Central Tanzania." *Transactions of the Royal Society of Tropical Medicine and Hygiene* 88(5): 513–7.

Manandhar, D.S., D. Osrin, et al. 2004. "Effect of a Participatory Intervention with Women's Groups on Birth Outcomes in Nepal: Cluster-randomised Controlled Trial." *Lancet* 364(9438): 970–9.

Manikutty, S. 1997. "Community Participation: So What? Evidence from a Comparative Study of Two Rural Water Supply and Sanitation Projects in India." *Development Policy Review* 15(2): 115. V140.

Marsh, V.M., W.M. Mutemi, J. Muturi, A. Haaland, W.M. Watkins, G. Otieno, and K. Marsh. 1999. "Changing Home Treatment of Childhood Fevers by Training Shop Keepers in Rural Kenya." *Tropical Medicine & International Health* 4(5): 383–9.

Marsh, V.M., W.M. Mutemi, A. Willetts, K. Bayah, S. Were, A. Ross, and K. Marsh. 2004. "Improving Malaria Home Treatment by Training Drug Retailers in Rural Kenya." *Tropical Medicine & International Health* 9(4): 451–60.

Maru, R.M. 1983. "The Community Health Volunteer Scheme in India: An Evaluation." *Social Science & Medicine* 17(19): 1477–83.

Massow, F., et al. 1998. "Financially Independent Primary Health Care Drug Supply System in Cameroun." *Tropical Medicine & International Health* 3(10): 788–801.

Mathur, S.S., V.R. Bhalerao, et al. 1992. "An Integrated Community based Approach in Undergraduate Medical Teaching of Maternal and Child Health: An Experiment." *Journal of Postgraduate Medicine* 38(1): 16–8.

Mbugua, J.K., G.H. Bloom, et al. 1995. "Impact of User Charges on Vulnerable Groups: The Case of Ibwezi in Rural Kenya." *Social Science & Medicine* 41(6): 829–835.

Mburu, F.M., H.C. Spencer, et al. 1987. "Changes in Sources of Treatment Occurring after Inception of a Community-based Malaria Control Programme in Saradidi, Kenya." *Annals of Tropical Medicine and Parasitology* 81(suppl. 1): 105–10.

McCord, C., et al. 2001. "Efficient and Effective Obstetric Care in a Rural Indian Community where Most Deliveries are at Home." *International Journal of Gynecology and Obstetrics* 75: 297–307.

McQuestion, M.J., and A. Velasquez. 2006. "Evaluating Program Effects on Institutional Delivery in Peru." *Health Policy* 77(2): 221–32.

Meegan, M., D.C. Morley, et al. 1994. "Child Weighing by the Unschooled: A Report of a Controlled Study of Growth Monitoring over 12 Months of Maasai Children Using Direct Recording Scales." *Transactions of the Royal Society of Tropical Medicine and Hygiene* 88(6): 635–7.

Melville, B., T. Fidler, et al. 1995. "Growth Monitoring: The Role of Community Health Volunteers." *Public Health* 109(2): 111–6.

Meuwissen, L.E., A.C. Gorter, et al. 2006. "Does a Competitive Voucher Program for Adolescents Improve the Quality of Reproductive Health Care? A Simulated Patient Study in Nicaragua." *BMC Public Health* 6: 9.

Meuwissen, L.E., A.C. Gorter, et al. 2006. "Impact of Accessible Sexual and Reproductive Health Care on Poor and Underserved Adolescents in Managua, Nicaragua: A Quasi-experimental Intervention Study." *Journal of Adolescent Health* 38(1): 56.

Meuwissen, L.E., A.C. Gorter, Z. Segura, A.D.M. Kester, and J.A. Knottnerus. 2006. "Uncovering and Responding to Needs for Sexual and Reproductive Health Care among Poor Urban Female Adolescents in Nicaragua." *Tropical Medicine & International Health* 11(12): 1858–1867.

Middelkoop, K., L. Myer, et al. 2006. "Design and Evaluation of a Drama-based Intervention to Promote Voluntary Counseling and HIV Testing in a South African Community." *Sexually Transmitted Diseases* 33(8): 524–6.

Miti, S., Mfungwe, V., et al. 2003. "Integration of Tuberculosis Treatment in a Community-based Home Care Programme for Persons Living with HIV/AIDS in Ndola, Zambia." *The International Journal of Tuberculosis and Lung Disease* 7(9): 592–598.

Moens, F. 1990. "Design, Implementation, and Evaluation of a Community Financing Scheme for Hospital Care in Developing Countries: A Pre-paid Health Plan in the Bwamanda Health Zone, Zaire." *Social Science & Medicine* 30(12): 1319–27.

Mohan, C.I., D. Bishai, et al. 2005. "Changes in Utilization of TB health services in Nepal." *The International Journal of Tuberculosis and Lung Disease* 9(9): 1054–6.

Morisky, D.E., C. Nguyen, et al. 2005. "HIV/AIDS Prevention among the Male Population: Results of a Peer Education Program for Taxicab and Tricycle Drivers in the Philippines." *Health Education & Behavior* 32(1): 57–68.

Morisky, D.E., A. Ang, A. Coly, and T.V. Tiglao. 2004. "A Model HIV/AIDS Risk Reduction Program in the Philippines: A Comprehensive Community-based Approach through Participatory Action Research." *Health Promotion International* (19)1.

Morris, S.S., P. Olinto, et al. 2004. "Conditional Cash Transfers are Associated with a Small Reduction in the Rate of Weight Gain of Preschool Children in Northeast Brazil." *Journal of Nutrition* 134: 2336–2341.

Moses, S., F. Manji, et al. 1992. "Impact of User Fees on Attendance at a Referral Centre for Sexually Transmitted Diseases in Kenya." *Lancet* 340(8817): 463–6.

Mtango, F.D., and D. Neuvians. 1986. "Acute Respiratory Infections in Children under Five Years. Control Project in Bagamoyo District, Tanzania." *Transactions of the Royal Society of Tropical Medicine and Hygiene* 80(6): 851–8.

Mushi, A.K., J.R. Schellenberg, et al. 2003. "Targeted Subsidy for Malaria Control with Treated Nets Using a Discount Voucher System in Tanzania." *Health Policy and Planning* 18(2): 163–71.

Mushtaque, A., R. Chowdhury, Fazlul Karim, Jalaluddin Ahmad. 1988. "Teaching ORT to Women: Individually or in Groups." *Journal of Tropical Medicine and Hygiene* 283–287.

Mustaphi, P., and M. Dobe. 2005. "Positive Deviance: The West Bengal Experience." *Indian Journal of Public Health* 49(4): 207–13.

Nag, M. 1992. "Family Planning Success Stories in Bangladesh and India." WPS 1041. Policy Research Dissemination Center, p. 3. World Bank, Washington, DC.

Naimoli, J.F., A. Gbekley, et al. 1994. "Working with Communities to Increase the Use of Health Services: An Experience from Togo, West Africa." *International Quarterly of Community Health Education* 14(3): 257–71.

Nam, V.S., et al. 2005. "Elimination of Dengue by Community Programs Using Mesocyclops (Copepoda) against *Aedes Aegypti* in Central Vietnam." *The American Journal of Tropical Medicine and Hygiene* 72(1): 67–73.

Norr, K.F., J.L. Norr, et al. 2004. "Impact of Peer Group Education on HIV Prevention among Women in Botswana." *Health Care for Women International* 25(3): 210–26.

O'Rourke, K., L. Howard-Grabman, et al. 1998. "Impact of Community Organization of Women on Perinatal Outcomes in Rural Bolivia." *Revista panamericana de salud pública (Pan American Journal of Public Health)* 3(1): 9–14.

O'Toole, B. 1988. "A Community-based Rehabilitation Programme for Pre-school Disabled Children in Guyana." *International Journal of Rehabilitation Research* 11(4): 323–34.

Ohnishi, M., K. Nakamura, and T. Takano. 2005. "Improvement in Maternal Health Literacy among Pregnant Women Who Did Not Complete Compulsory Education: Policy Implications for Community Care Services." *Health Policy* 72(2): 157–64.

Ojofeitimi, E.O., M.K. Jinadu, and I. Elegbe. 1988. "Increasing the Productivity of Community Health Workers in Rural Nigeria through Supervision." *Socio-economic Planning Sciences* 22(1): 29–37.

Okello, D., K. Floyd, F. Adatu, R. Odeke, and G. Gargioni. 2003. "Cost and Cost-effectiveness of Community-based Care for Tuberculosis Patients in Rural Uganda." *The International Journal of Tuberculosis and Lung Disease* 7(9 suppl. 1): S72–9.

Olaniran, N., S. Offiong, et al. 1997. "Mobilizing the Community to Utilize Obstetric Services, Cross River State, Nigeria." *International Journal of Gynecology and Obstetrics* 59(suppl. 2): S181–9.

Olukoya, A.A., M.A. Ogunyemi, et al. 1997. "Upgrading Obstetric Care at a Secondary Referral Hospital, Ogun State, Nigeria." *International Journal of Gynecology and Obstetrics* 59(suppl. 2): S67–74.

Onwujekwe, O., N. Dike, et al. 2006. "Consumers' Stated and Revealed Preferences for Community Health Workers and Other Strategies for the Provision of Timely and Appropriate Treatment of Malaria in Southeast Nigeria." *Malaria Journal* 5: 117.

Pagnoni, F., N. Convelbo, et al. 1997. "A Community-based Programme to Provide Prompt and Adequate Treatment of Presumptive Malaria in Children." *Transactions of the Royal Society of Tropical Medicine and Hygiene* 91(5): 512–7.

Pandey, M.R., N.M. Daulaire, et al. 1991. "Reduction in Total Under-five Mortality in Western Nepal through Community-based Antimicrobial Treatment of Pneumonia." *Lancet* 338(8773): 993–7.

Pandey, M.R., P.R. Sharma, et al. 1989. "Impact of a Pilot Acute Respiratory Infection (ARI) Control Programme in a Rural Community of the Hill Region of Nepal." *Annals of Tropical Paediatrics* 9: 212–220.

Pandey, P., Sehgal, A.R.,Riboud, M., Levine, D., Goyal, M. 2007. "Informing Resource-Poor Populations and the Delivery of Entitled Health and Social Services in Rural India: A Cluster Randomized Controlled Trial." *Journal of the American Medical Association* 298(16):1867–1875.

Partnership for Child Health Care. 2004. "Basic Support for Institutionalizing Child Survival [BASICS]. Improving Family Health using an Integrated, Community-based Approach. Madagascar case study." Technical report. Arlington, Virginia, BASICS. February.

———. 2004. "Basic Support for Institutionalizing Child Survival [BASICS]. CHWs in Senegal Can Appropriately Treat Pneumonia with Cotrimoxazole." Senegal. Ministère de la Santé, de l'Hygiène et de la Prévention. Arlington, Virginia, BASICS. September.

Parvanta, C.F., P. Gottert, et al. 1997. "Nutrition Promotion in Mali: Highlights of a Rural Integrated Nutrition Communication Program (1989–1995)." *Journal of Nutrition Education* 29(5): 274–280.

Pasha, O., J. Del Rosso, et al. 2003. "The Effect of Providing Fansidar (sulfadox-ine-pyrimethamine) in Schools on Mortality in School-age Children in Malawi." *Lancet* 361(9357): 577–8.

Pattussi, M.P., R. Hardy, et al. 2006. "The Potential Impact of Neighborhood Empowerment on Dental Caries among Adolescents." *Community Dentistry and Oral Epidemiology* 34(5): 344–50.

Paxman, J.M., A. Sayeed, et al. 2005. "The India Local Initiatives Program: A Model for Expanding Reproductive and Child Health Services." *Studies in Family Planning* 36(3): 203–20.

Peer Morris, S.S., R. Flores, et al. 2004. "Monetary Incentives in Primary Health Care and Effects on Use and Coverage of Preventive Health Care Interventions in Rural Honduras: Cluster Randomised Trial." *Lancet* 364(9450): 2030–7.

Pence, B.W., P. Nyarko, et al. 2007. "The Effect of Community Nurses and Health Volunteers on Child Mortality: The Navrongo Community Health and Family Planning Project." *Scandinavian Journal of Public Health* 35 (6): 599–608.

Peng, B., P.E. Petersen, et al. 1997. "Changes in Oral Health Knowledge and Behaviour 1987–95 among Inhabitants of Wuhan City, PR China." *International Dental Journal* 47(3): 142–7.

Perez-Cuevas, R., H. Reyes, et al. 1999. "Immunization Promotion Activities: Are They Effective in Encouraging Mothers to Immunize their Children?" *Social Science & Medicine* 49(7): 921–32.

Perry, H.B., D.S. Shanklin, et al. 2003. "Impact of a Community-based Comprehensive Primary Healthcare Programme on Infant and Child Mortality in Bolivia." *Journal of Health, Population, and Nutrition* 21(4): 383–95.

Perry, H., M. Cayemittes, et al. 2006. "Reducing Under-five Mortality through Hospital Albert Schweitzer's Integrated System in Haiti." *Health Policy and Planning* 21(3): 217–30.

Pineda, M.A., J.T. Bertrand, et al. 1983. "Increasing the Effectiveness of Community Workers through Training of Spouses: A Family Planning Experiment in Guatemala." *Public Health Reports* 98(3): 273–7.

Pinfold, J.V., and N.J. Horan. 1996. "Measuring the Effect of a Hygiene Behaviour Intervention by Indicators of Behaviour and Diarrhoeal Disease." *Transactions of the Royal Society of Tropical Medicine and Hygiene* 90(4): 366–71.

Pongpaew, P., et al. 1990. "Aspects of Community-based Nutritional Intervention." *Journal of the Medical Association of Thailand* 73(4): 223–7.

Population Council. 2005. "Female Genital Cutting. Community Education Program Scaled-up in Burkina Faso." Frontiers in Reproductive Health or Summary No. 55. Population Council, Washington, DC.

———. 2005. "India Community Involvement. Broad Representation Supports Credibility of Village Committees. Frontiers in Reproductive Health or Summary No. 52. Population Council, Washington, DC.

Quigley, P., and G.J. Ebrahim. 1994. "Can Women's Organizations Bring about Health Development?" *Journal of Tropical Pediatrics* 40(5): 294–8.

Quinn, V.J., A.B. Guyon, et al. 2005. "Improving Breastfeeding Practices on a Broad Scale at the Community Level: Success Stories from Africa and Latin America." *Journal of Human Lactation* 21(3): 345–54.

Rahaman, M.M., K.M. Aziz, et al. 1979. "Diarrhoeal Mortality in Two Bangladeshi Villages with and Without Community-based Oral Rehydration Therapy." *Lancet* 2 (8147): 809.

Rao, V., and A.M. Ibanez. 2005. "The Social Impact of Social Funds in Jamaica: A 'Participatory Econometric' Analysis of Targeting, Collective Action, and Participation in Community-driven Development." *Journal of Development Studies* 41(5): 788.

Rodriguez-Garcia R., K., J. Aumack, and A. Ramos. 1990. "A Community-based Approach to the Promotion of Breastfeeding in Mexico." *Journal of Obstetric, Gynecologic, and Neonatal Nursing* 19(5): 431–8.

Ronsmans, C., A.M. Vanneste, et al. 1997. "Decline in Maternal Mortality in Matlab, Bangladesh: A Cautionary Tale." *Lancet* 350(9094): 1810–4.

Safe Motherhood Newsletter. "Bangladesh: Village Midwives Save Lives" 8: 8.

Sakondhavat, C., et al. 2000. "AIDS Prevention Strategies for Rural Families in Northeastern Thailand." *Journal of the Medical Association of Thailand* 83: 1175–1186.

Saowakontha, S., P. Pongpaew, et al. 2000. "Promotion of the Health of Rural Women Towards Safe Motherhood: An Intervention Project in Northeast Thailand." *The Southeast Asian Journal of Tropical Medicine and Public Health* 31(suppl. 2): 5–21.

Save-Guinea. 2006. "Child Survival 18-Guinea. Final Evaluation Report, Save the Children.

Schmeller W. 1998. "Community Health Workers Reduce Skin Diseases in East African Children." *International Journal of Dermatology* 37(5): 370–7.

Schmeller, W., S. Baumgartner, et al. 1997. "Dermatophytomycoses in Children in Rural Kenya: The Impact of Primary Health Care." *Mycoses* 40(1–2): 55–63.

Schuler S.R., and S.M. Hashemi. 1994. "Credit Programs, Women's Empowerment, and Contraceptive Use in Rural Bangladesh." *Studies in Family Planning* 25(2): 65–76.

Sennun, P., N. Suwannapong, N. Howteerakul, and O. Pacheun. 2006. "Participatory Supervision Model: Building Health Promotion Capacity among Health Officers and the Community." *Rural and Remote Health* 6(2): 440. Epub 2006 Apr 3.

Shah, P., and A. Junnarkar. 1976. "Communitywide Surveillance of 'At Risk' Under-fives in Need of Special Care." *Journal of tropical pediatrics and environmental child health* 22(3): 103–7.

Shahid, N.S., W.B. Greenough 3rd, et al. 1996. "Hand Washing with Soap Reduces Diarrhoea and Spread of Bacterial Pathogens in a Bangladesh Village." *Journal of Diarrhoeal Diseases Research* 14(2): 85–9.

Sharma, V.P., and R.C. Sharma. 1989. "Community-based Bioenvironmental Control of Malaria in Kheda District, Gujarat, India." *Journal of the American Mosquito Control Association* 5(4): 514–21.

Stalker, L., G.V. Abhyankar, and P. Iyer. 2002. "Why Some Village Water and Sanitation Committees Are Better than Others: A Study of Karnataka and Uttar Pradesh (India)." New Delhi Water and Sanitation Program, South Asia.

Steen, R., V. Mogasale, et al. 2006. "Pursuing Scale and Quality in STI Interventions with Sex Workers: Initial Results from Avahan India AIDS Initiative." *Sexually Transmitted Infections* 82(5): 381–5.

Steyn, K., et al. 1993. "The Intervention Effects of a Community-based Hypertension Control Programme in Two Rural South African Towns: The CORIS Study." *South African Medical Journal* 83: 885–891.

Sultan, M., J.G. Cleland, et al. 2002. "Assessment of a New Approach to Family Planning Services in Rural Pakistan." *American Journal of Public Health* 92(7): 1168–72.

Sur, D., D.R. Saha, et al. 2005. "Periodic Deworming with Albendazole and its Impact on Growth Status and Diarrhoeal Incidence among Children in an Urban Slum of India." *Transactions of the Royal Society of Tropical Medicine and Hygiene* 99(4): 261–7.

Sutter, E., and S. Maphorogo. 1996. "Integration of Community-based Trachoma Control in Primary Health Care in South Africa." *Revue internationale du trachome et de pathologie oculaire tropicale et subtropicale et de santé publique* 73: 19–50.

Swaddiwudhipong, W., et al. 1992. "Effect of Health Education on Community Participation in Control of Dengue Hemorrhagic Fever in an Urban Area of Thailand." *The Southeast Asian Journal of Tropical Medicine and Public Health* 23(2).

Sweat, M., et al. 2006. "Cost-effectiveness of Environmental-structural Communication Interventions for HIV Prevention in the Female Sex Industry in the Dominican Republic." *Journal of Health Communication* 11(1): 123–142.

Tate, R.B., N. Fernandez, et al. 2003. "Change in Health Risk Perception Following Community Intervention in Central Havana, Cuba." *Health Promotion International* 18(4): 279–86.

Tawye, Y., F. Jotie, et al. 2005. "The Potential Impact of Community-based Distribution Programmes on Contraceptive Uptake in Resource-poor Settings: Evidence from Ethiopia." *African Journal of Reproductive Health* 9(3): 15–26.

Therawiwat, M., et al. 2005. "Community-based Approach for Prevention and Control of Dengue Hemorrhagic Fever in Kanchanaburi Province, Thailand." *The Southeast Asian Journal of Tropical Medicine and Public Health* 36(6).

Thim, S., Sath, S., et al. 2004. "Research Letter: A Community-based Tuberculosis Program in Cambodia." *JAMA* 292 (5).

Thomesn, S.C., W. Ombidi, et al. 2006. "A Prospective Study Assessing the Effects of Introducing the Female Condom in a Sex Worker Population in Mombasa, Kenya." *Sexually Transmitted Infections* 82(5): 397–402.

Trujillo, A.J., J.E. Portillo, et al. 2005. "The Impact of Subsidized Health Insurance for the Poor: Evaluating the Colombian Experience Using Propensity Score Matching." *International Journal of Health Care Finance and Economics* 5(3): 211–39.

Turan, J.M., and L. Say. 2003. "Community-based Antenatal Education in Istanbul, Turkey: Effects on Health Behaviours." *Health Policy and Planning* 18(4): 391–8.

Uchoa, E., Barreto, S.M, et al. 2000. "The Control of Schistosomiasis in Brazil: An Ethno-epidemiological Study of the Effectiveness of a Community

Mobilization Program for Health Education." *Social Science & Medicine* 51: 1529–1541.

Vernon, R., G. Ojeda, and R. Murad. 1990. "Incorporating AIDS Prevention Activities into a Family Planning Organization in Colombia." *Studies in Family Planning* 21(6): 335–343.

Vijayakumar, V., et al. 2004. "Quality of Life after Community-Based Rehabilitation for Blind Persons in a Rural Population of South India." *Indian Journal of Ophthalmology* 52: 331–35.

Walton, D.A., P.E. Farmer, et al. 2004. "Integrated HIV Prevention and Care Strengthens Primary Health Care: Lessons from Rural Haiti." *Journal of Public Health Policy* 25(2): 137–58.

Wang'Ombe, J.K. 1984. "Economic Evaluation in Primary Health Care: The Case of Western Kenya Community-based Health Care Project." *Social Science & Medicine* 18(5): 375–385.

Waterkeyn, J., et al. 2005. "Creating Demand for Sanitation and Hygiene through Community Health Clubs: A Cost-effective Intervention in Two Districts in Zimbabwe." *Social Science and Medicine* 61: 1958–1970.

Weeden, D., A. Bennett, et al. 1986. "Community-based Incentives: Increasing Contraceptive Prevalence and Economic Opportunity." *Asia-Pacific Population Journal/United Nations* 1(3): 31–46.

Wilkinson, D. 1999. "Eight Years of Tuberculosis Research in Hlabisa: What Have We Learned?" *South African Medical Journal* 89(2): 155–9.

Wilkinson, D., and G.R. Davies. 1997. "Coping with Africa's Increasing Tuberculosis Burden: Are Community Supervisors an Essential Component of the DOT Strategy?" *Tropical Medicine & International Health* 2(7): 700–704.

———. 1998. "Pediatric Tuberculosis in Rural South Africa: Value of Directly Observed Therapy." *Journal of Tropical Pediatrics* 44(5): 266–269.

Wilson, J.M., G.N. Chandler, Muslihatun, and Jamiluddin. 1991. "Hand-washing Reduces Diarrhoea Episodes: A Study in Lombok, Indonesia." *Transactions of the Royal Society of Tropical Medicine and Hygiene* 85:819–21.

Wilson, J.M., and G.N. Chandler. 1993. "Sustained Improvements in Hygiene Behaviour amongst Village Women in Lombok, Indonesia." *Transactions of the Royal Society of Tropical Medicine and Hygiene* 87(6): 615–6.

Winch, P.J., et al. 2003. "Increases in Correct Administration of Chloroquine in the Home and Referral of Sick Children to Health Facilities through a Community-based Intervention in Bougouni District, Mali." *Transactions of the Royal Society of Tropical Medicine and Hygiene* 97(5): 481–90.

Wouters, A., and A. Kouzis. 1994. "Quality of Health Care and its Role in Cost Recovery in Africa: Cost Recovery and Improved Drug Availability in Niger: Implications for Total Patient Treatment Costs. Phases 2 and 3: Field Work,

Research Research Results, and Policy Recommendations." Abt Associates, Health Financing and Sustainability Project, Bethesda, Maryland.

Wright, J., et al. 2004. "Direct Observation of Treatment for TB: A Randomized Controlled Trial of Community Health Workers versus Family Members." *Tropical Medicine & International Health* 9(5): 559–565.

Wu, Z., R. Detels, J. Zhang, V. Li, and J. Li. 2002. "Community-based Trial to Prevent Drug Use Among Youths in Yunan, China." *American Journal of Public Health* 92(12).

Yassi, A., N. Fernandez, et al. 2003. "Community Participation in a Multisectoral Intervention to Address Health Determinants in an Inner-city Community in Central Havana." *Journal of Urban Health* 80(1): 61–80.

Yeudall, F., Gibson, R.S., et al. 2005. "Efficacy of a Community-based Dietary Intervention to Enhance Micronutrient Adequacy of High-phytate Maize-based Diets of Rural Malawian Children." *Public Health Nutrition*: 8(7): 826–836.

Zhan, S., L. Wang, et al. 2004. "Revenue-driven in TB Control: Three Cases in China." *The International Journal of Health Planning and Management* 19(suppl. 1): S63–78.

Zimmerman, M.A., J. Ramirez-Valles, et al. 1997. "An HIV/AIDS Prevention Project for Mexican Homosexual Men: An Empowerment Approach." *Health Education & Behavior* 24(2): 177–90.

Annex Table 4.3.1   Effect of Approaches Used in Community Empowerment Strategies

Factor (number of studies)	Randomized controlled trial				Nonrandomized controlled trial				Total			
	Positive (%)	Odds ratio	95% CI, lower	95% CI, upper	Positive (prop)	Odds ratio	95% CI, lower	95% CI, upper	Positive (prop)	Odds ratio	95% CI, lower	95% CI, upper
"Bottom-up" approach used (88)	90.6	.690	.107	4.449	87.9	0.71	0.14	3.89	90.5	0.95	0.27	3.52
"Top-down" approach used (63)	93.3				91.1				90.9			
Partnerships between community and policy makers/ technical experts (75)	97.0	5.120	.538	48.718	92.9	1.696	.398	7.229	94.7	2.500	.749	8.344
Not specified (81)	86.2				88.5				87.7			
Systems for local adaptive learning (64)	92.6	1.172	.182	7.559	94.6	2.450	.480	12.501	93.8	1.829	.547	6.112
Not specified (92)	91.4				87.7				89.1			
Local community resources used for program support (85)	93.9	1.788	.277	11.530	94.2	2.722	.638	11.618	94.1	2.323	.741	7.280
Not specified (71)	89.7				85.7				87.3			

Category												
Results shared with community (22)	100.0	n.a.			100.0	n.a.			100.0	n.a.		
Not specified (134)	90.4				89.0				89.6			
Community part of decision making (47)	82.4	.217	.033	1.434	100.0	n.a.			93.6	1.646	.437	6.195
Not specified (109)	95.6				85.9				89.9			
Holistic and iterative action (10)	100.0	n.a.			100.0	n.a.			100.0	n.a.		
Not specified (146)	91.2				89.9				90.4			
Equity promoted (56)	100.0	n.a.			91.9	1.333	.312	5.697	94.6	2.184	.583	8.183
No promotion of equity (100)	88.4				89.5				89.0			
Poor engaged (74)	96.8	4.444	.467	42.258	88.4	.647	.162	2.578	91.9	1.225	.404	3.712
Not specified (82)	87.1				92.2				90.2			
Scaling up promoted (53)	86.4	.333	.051	2.167	96.8	4.364	.521	-36.570	92.5	1.317	.393	4.417
Not specified (103)	95.0				87.3				90.3			

Source: Authors.

n.a. = not applicable (odds ratio undefined).

Annex Table 4.3.2 Scale of Study and Association with Positive Outcomes

Factor (number of studies)	Randomized controlled trial				Nonrandomized controlled trial				Total			
	Positive (%)	Odds ratio	95% CI, lower	95% CI, upper	Positive (%)	Odds ratio	95% CI, lower	95% CI, upper	Positive (%)	Odds ratio	95% CI, lower	95% CI, upper
Scale of the study												
Village level to 1 district												
(N=102)	92.1	1.94	0.03	29.01	92.2	1.31	0.02	13.86	92.2	1.57	0.15	8.95
≥2 districtts to 1 province												
(N=25)	87.5	1.17	0.01	104.5	82.4	0.52	0.01	7.87	84.0	0.70	0.06	5.69
≥2 provinces or larger												
(N=17)	85.7				90.0				88.2			

Source: Authors.

Note: Odds ratios calculated by comparison with the largest scale group (≥2 provinces).

Annex Table 4.3.3   Influence of the Type of Community Empowerment Strategy

Factor (number of studies)	Randomized controlled trial				Nonrandomized controlled trial				Total			
	Positive (%)	Odds ratio	95% CI, lower	95% CI, upper	Positive (%)	Odds ratio	95% CI, lower	95% CI, upper	Positive (%)	Odds ratio	95% CI, lower	95% CI, upper
Access to education (135)	92.9	2.600	0.242	27.972	93.7	5.382	1.251	23.160	93.3	4.375	1.304	14.681
Not part of strategy (21)	83.3				73.3				76.2			
Inclusion and participation (53)	100.0	n.a.			91.4	1.208	.282	5.167	94.3	1.993	.531	7.476
Not part of strategy (103)	88.6				89.8				89.3			
Accountability (29)	88.9	.653	.064	6.614	95.0	2.303	.271	19.586	93.1	1.409	.298	6.667
Not part of strategy (127)	92.5				89.2				90.6			
Local organizational capacity (74)	93.8	1.667	.259	10.741	95.2	3.111	.611	15.850	94.6	2.431	.728	8.113
Not part of strategy (82)	90.0				86.5				87.8			
Financial empowerment (39)	100.0	n.a.			87.5	.656	.151	2.857	92.3	1.245	.329	4.715
Not part of strategy (117)	89.4				91.4				90.6			

Source: Authors.

n.a. = not applicable (odds ratio undefined).

Annex Table 4.3.4   Influence of Organizations Involved in Community Empowerment Strategies

Factor (number of studies)	Randomized controlled trial				Nonrandomized controlled trial				Total			
	Positive (%)	Odds ratio	95% CI, lower	95% CI, upper	Positive (%)	Odds ratio	95% CI, lower	95% CI, upper	Positive (%)	Odds ratio	95% CI, lower	95% CI, upper
Government providers involved (97)	90.5	.500	.052	4.789	87.3	.371	.073	1.890	88.7	.419	.112	1.568
No government providers involved (59)	95.0				94.9				94.9			
Government financing of intervention (68)	90.0	.600	.093	3.867	81.6	.164	.032	.839	85.3	.276	.083	.923
No government financing (88)	93.8				96.4				95.5			
Political parties involved (17)	88.9	.653	.064	6.614	87.5	.718	.078	6.597	88.2	.700	.145	3.474
No political party involved (139)	92.5				90.7				91.4			
Nonstate providers involved (125)	90.0	n.a.			94.7	6.339	1.511	26.604	92.8	2.479	.767	8.010
No nonstate providers involved (31)	100.0				73.7				83.9			

Source: Authors.
n.a. = not applicable (odds ratio undefined).

Annex Table 4.3.5　Influence of Women's Involvement in Community Empowerment

Factor (number of studies)	Randomized controlled trial				Nonrandomized controlled trial				Total			
	Positive (%)	Odds ratio	95% CI, lower	95% CI, upper	Positive (%)	Odds ratio	95% CI, lower	95% CI, upper	Positive (%)	Odds ratio	95% CI, lower	95% CI, upper
Women actively engaged in intervention (79)	96.4	3.600	.379	34.229	88.2	.562	.132	2.398	91.1	1.029	.343	3.084
Not specified (77)	88.2				93.0				90.9			
Training of mothers/women in the community (63)	92.0	1.015	.157	6.556	89.5	.833	.209	3.328	90.5	.894	.295	2.714
Not specified (93)	91.9				91.1				91.4			
Women's empowerment promoted (76)	96.6	3.862	.406	36.715	91.5	1.280	.321	5.096	93.4	1.800	.575	5.637
Not specified (80)	87.9				89.4				88.8			

Source: Authors.

Annex Table 4.3.6 Community Health Worker Factors and Association with Positive Outcomes

Factor (number of studies)	Randomized controlled trial				Nonrandomized controlled trial				Total			
	Positive (%)	Odds ratio	95% CI, lower	95% CI, upper	Positive (%)	Odds ratio	95% CI, lower	95% CI, upper	Positive (%)	Odds ratio	95% CI, lower	95% CI, upper
Remuneration of CHWs												
Any remuneration (N=31)	90.0	.900	.049	16.594	85.7	.462	.043	4.952	87.1	.587	.098	3.502
No remuneration (N=25)	90.9				92.9				92.0			
CHWs supervised												
≥12 visits/year (N=25)	100.0	n.a.			92.3	n.a.			96.0	4.800	.255	90.298
<12 visits/year (N=6)	75.0				100.0				83.3			
Population covered per CHW												
(≥1000 people) (N=14)	100.0	n.a.			100.0	n.a.			100.0	n.a.		
(<1000 people) (N=20)	88.9				100.0				95.0			

Source: Authors.

n.a. = not applicable (odds ratio undefined).

Annex Table 4.3.7   Influence of Contextual Factors on Outcomes of Community Empowerment Strategies

Factor (number of studies)	Randomized controlled trial				Nonrandomized controlled trial				Total			
	Positive (%)	Odds ratio	95% CI, lower	95% CI, upper	Positive (prop)	Odds ratio	95% CI, lower	95% CI, upper	Positive (prop)	Odds ratio	95% CI, lower	95% CI, upper
Pre-existing strategy present (55)	100.0	n.a.	n.a.	n.a.	92.7	1.407	.316	6.277	94.5	2.016	.530	7.662
No pre-existing strategy (96)	89.1				90.0				89.6			
Presence of strong local leadership (56)	95.8	2.706	.284	25.783	100	n.a.			98.2	8.218	1.046	64.596
No presence of strong local leadership (100)	89.5				85.5				87.0			

Source: Authors.

n.a. = not applicable (odds ratio undefined).

CHAPTER 5

Analysis of Cross-country Changes in Health Services

Toru Matsubayashi, David H. Peters,
and Hafiz Rahman

Summary

Objectives: Identify the levels of sustainable changes in priority health services that LMICs can reasonably expect to achieve, as well as how changes in one priority health service are associated with changes in a different type of health service at a national level.

Methods: Longitudinal analyses using multilevel random intercept and coefficient models were used to test national panel data from international databases of key health services (1990–2004) for 162 countries.

Key messages:

- Less than two-thirds of LMICs are projected to reach international and Millennium Development Goal targets for health services by the target date of 2015, but identifying negative or slow rates of change in a country is probably a more important strategy than setting universal targets for health attainment.

(continued)

- Individual country differences (in delivery of health services, health status, and macro context) may be more important than international averages imply, undermining the relevance of targets set without reference to country-specific experience.
- Rather than showing a common pattern of progress for health services, countries tend to follow their own pathways.
- Countries' very different starting points affect their prospects of achieving the targets and their rate of change.
- Improvements in health services are usually not associated with changes in other health services.
- Since changes in national governance are significantly associated with heath status improvements, health programs should be planned within a broader framework.

Reasons for Conducting the Study

Recent years have seen increased attention, new global health initiatives, and more funding related to the provision of health services in developing countries, often focused on achieving the Millennium Development Goals (MDGs) (Gottret and Schieber 2006). Many initiatives have been organized around categorical disease-control programs or for specific health interventions, notably the Global Fund to Fight AIDS, TB, and Malaria; the GAVI Alliance; and the U.S. President's Emergency Plan for AIDS Relief. The "priority health services" in this chapter relate to child and maternal mortality, immunization, tuberculosis (TB), and skilled birth attendance, both because they are leading causes of mortality and morbidity, and because data were hard to come by for some other conditions. International agencies have set ambitious targets, not only for the MDGs related to reducing child and maternal mortality, but also for specific health services that address conditions representing a high burden of disease.

Annual data are available for only a few of these indicators across LMICs, including: proportion of one-year-old children immunized against measles (MDG indicator 15); proportion of births attended by skilled personnel (MDG indicator 17); and proportion of tuberculosis cases detected and proportion of TB cases cured under directly observed treatment, short-course (DOTS) (MDG indicator 24). This study analyzes trends in these indicators, as well as the proportion of one-year-old children immunized with three doses of diphtheria, pertussis, and tetanus vaccine (DPT3) (or its equivalent that may also include hepatitis B or hemophilus influenza B antigens), which is a longstanding indicator for the Expanded Programme on Immunization (EPI), and is a good indicator of how well the routine immunizations are delivered (annual data for this are also available in most LMICs).

International targets set for immunization coverage, tuberculosis treatment, and safe delivery include the following: 90 percent coverage for DPT3 immunization, 70 percent case detection rate for TB, 85 percent TB treatment completion rate, and 80 percent skilled birth attendance (UN 2007). These targets were set for LMICs without recourse to country-based plans, experiences, or expectations, and without a thorough assessment of what improvements are feasible and sustainable. However, since national governments are responsible for overall health sector policy, planning, and oversight of health financing and delivery in their own countries, it is useful to identify what levels of changes in health services delivery have been achieved in order to provide a yardstick for expectations globally. This may be useful for national ministries of health and program managers in setting appropriate benchmarks in health services delivery.

In addition to determining what has been feasible in scaling up individual health services, it is also important to understand whether the efforts that increase coverage of a specific health service have an effect on raising coverage of other health services in the country, or whether there is any correlation between changes across different health services. Disease-specific initiatives are vulnerable to criticism that they create poorly coordinated undertakings that can distort public health priorities in recipient countries as well as duplicate or fragment global health assistance (for example, Travis et al. 2004; Garrett 2007). This would suggest that improvements in targeted health services may occur at the expense of other health services. Yet there is little systematic evidence as to whether disease-specific programs, broad-based approaches, or combinations of them are the more effective in bringing changes to health services and outcomes on a large scale in different contexts (see chapter 1).

Using existing country-level data on health services, this study will help identify the actual changes that have been achieved in specific health services in LMICs, in order to provide more practical benchmarks for improving them further. It is hoped that such benchmarks will also be useful to decision makers in setting targets in formulating national strategies to improve essential health services. This study will also demonstrate how priority health services affect each other at a national level, and identify which country characteristics most influence changes in health services delivery at that level. Based on the conceptual framework outlined in the *Overview*, some of the macro-environment characteristics of a country are incorporated into the analysis, including national economic, political, and social factors, and measures of governance and development assistance.

Objectives of the Study

In general terms the study sought to:

- identify the levels of sustainable changes in priority health services (child immunization coverage, TB case detection and treatment completion, and skilled birth attendance) that LMICs can reasonably expect to achieve;
- identify how changes in one priority health service are associated with changes in a different type of health service at a national level;
- examine the relationships between changes in the selected health service outputs over time at the national level in LMICs in order to identify economic, political, and social characteristics that enhance or inhibit health services delivery nationally.

No high-quality prospective studies with time-series data collection are readily available to conduct a longitudinal analysis that could be used to answer the questions of interest. However, to capture changes over time in health services, a longitudinally collected dataset is necessary. Therefore, we used data sources, largely from United Nations (UN) and World Bank sources, which report annual levels of health outcomes, health services, and other contextual data of LMICs nationally from 1990 to 2004, and limited our enquiry to questions that the data would be able to inform.

Addressing the first objective provides us with estimates of feasible rates of improvements in priority health services in LMICs in areas where sufficient data are available. The second objective addresses the hypothesis that change in one type of health service is not necessarily associated with changes in other health services. Information obtained through this analysis will provide some insight as to whether a categorical program targeting a specific disease or intervention would have positive (synergistic) or negative (antagonistic) effects on other services in a national health system. It will also help identify which country characteristics most affect changes in health services delivery.

Methods Used

This study involved national panel data of selected health services between 1990 and 2004 on all 162 countries considered LMICs in 1990, according to World Bank definitions. Annual data on relevant economic, demographic, and social information from sources that allow standardized comparisons at a country level were also incorporated (World Bank, Demographic and Health Surveys, World Health Organization, UNICEF, and other UN organizations). The health services variables of interest are five indicators reflecting three distinct health service areas: immunization (DPT3 immunization rate, measles immunization rate), tuberculosis control (TB case detection rate, TB successful treatment rate), and skilled birth attendance rate. Several variables indicative of social, economic, and health sector characteristics were included in the longitudinal analysis, since they are likely to influence the trends in health services (for example, Lu et al. 2006; Mohan et al. 2006; Reidpath and Allotey 2006). Actual variables included in the analyses are: national population, gross national income (GNI) per capita, official development assistance (ODA) per capita, health expenditure per capita, governance ratings, adult literacy rate, and the number of people affected by disasters.

The key feature of the dataset is that most variables for each country were measured repeatedly over time rather than taken from single measures for each country, as in cross-sectional studies. Such repeated measuring violates the usual regression model assumption of independent observations. Since successive measures for the same country are correlated, they require special statistical methods to account for the correlation. A longitudinal analysis taking account of a country-level correlation was conducted, with two different models. One was a marginal model with generalized estimating equations (described in Ballinger 2004; Diggle 2002; Zeger et al. 1988), treating countries as clusters and using robust variance estimation. This model provides estimates of change for an "average" country beginning at an average starting point. The other model was a multilevel analysis, which allowed for a country-specific random intercept, representing its starting point in 1990, and a country-specific random slope in the annual trend of essential health services (outlined in Rabe-Hesketh and Skrondal 2005). As demonstrated below, there are large heterogeneities in the baseline values (intercepts) and trends (slopes) in each of the health service indicators among LMICs, leading us to use the multilevel models in our final analyses.

Main Findings

Historical Rates of Change for Health Services

Figure 5.1 shows how average national levels of five health services have changed in LMICs over a 15-year period, compared to the target figure for each indicator. With the exception of two years for skilled birth attendance (1998 and 2002), none of the targets was reached during this period, suggesting that on average, improvements in health services coverage take longer than expected to achieve the targets. Immunization coverage, TB case detection, and TB treatment completion rates tend to show slow but steady increases in levels, but with results significantly below the targets set for them. Coverage of skilled birth attendance is more variable, but with coverage in most years being significantly below its target.

In figure 5.2, we use the multilevel (random effects) models to estimate the country-specific effects for two of the health services indicators: DPT3 coverage and skilled birth attendance. Each line represents the experience for an individual country over the same 15-year period.[1] The first impression is one of much more variation than is illustrated in the "average" country models shown in figure 5.1. Relatively few countries actually experience a change in DPT3 coverage or skilled birth attendance shown in the "average" models (but the multilevel TB and measles estimates are similar in this respect). Figure 5.2 also demonstrates that quite a few countries are clearly falling behind in these essential health services (having negative or flat slopes), whereas other countries have much steeper positive slopes (indicating more rapid progress). Countries have very different starting points, which also affect their prospects of achieving the targets and their rate of change. Countries that have higher initial coverage tend to show lower rates of change than countries with lower starting points, and should not be expected to improve at the same rates. The observation reinforces the conclusion that achieving the highest levels of coverage may be the most difficult.

Applying the linear estimates produced from the multilevel models for the key health services, we projected how many countries would be expected to achieve the international and MDG targets by 2010 and 2015 for each health service (table 5.1). Based on trends over the 15 years from 1990 to 2004, about two-thirds of all countries would be projected

Figure 5.1   Trends in Selected Health Service Indicators in LMICs between 1990 and 2004

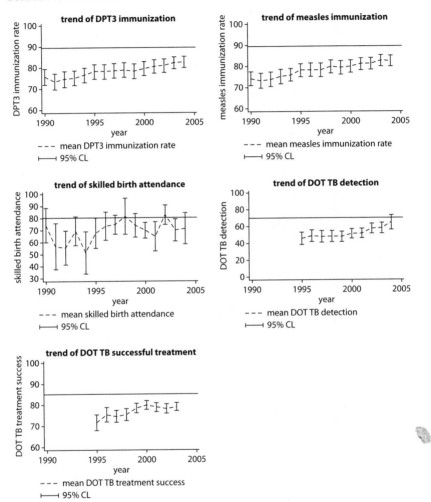

Source: Authors.
Note: 95% CI: mean value of indicator ± 2SD/   (n is the number of countries). Horizontal lines indicate the targets set in the MDGs (and the EPI for DPT3). Targets for DPT3 immunization coverage, measles immunization coverage, skilled birth attendance, TB detection, and TB treatment completion rate are 90 percent, 90 percent, 80 percent, 70 percent, and 85 percent, respectively.

to achieve the target levels of health services by 2015, when the MDG targets also expect these countries to have achieved dramatic reductions in child and maternal mortality. The health services with the fewest LMICs achieving the international and MDG targets are DPT3 immunization (55 percent), measles immunization (56 percent), and TB detection

Figure 5.2 Country-specific Estimates of DPT3 Immunization Coverage and Skilled Birth Attendance from 1990 to 2004 Using Multilevel Models

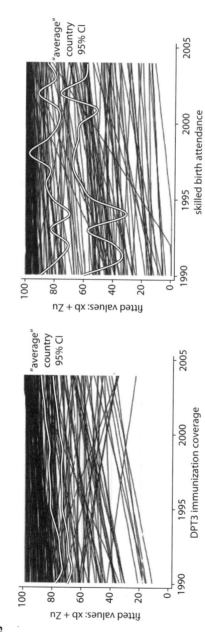

Source: Authors.

Note: Each line represents the data for one country.

Table 5.1   Number of Countries Estimated to Achieve the International and MDG Targets for Key Health Services

Health service	Target level %	1990 % (#/N)	2000 % (#/N)	2010[a] % (#/N)	2015[a] % (#/N)
DPT3 immunization rate	90	28 (37/130)	41 (63/155)	51 (79/156)	55 (86/156)
Measles immunization rate	90	15 (20/130)	37 (58/155)	50 (78/156)	56 (88/156)
TB detection rate	70	—	28 (35/127)	52 (80/153)	57 (87/153)
TB treatment completion rate	85	—	34 (42/123)	67 (102/152)	74 (113/152)
Skilled birth attendance	80	54 (6/11)	49 (38/77)	61 (96/158)	66 (104/158)

Source: Authors.
Note: N is the number of countries where data are available. # is the number of countries that meet the target. DPT3 target is based on the EPI.
— = data not available.
a. Projections based on models shown in table 5.2.

(57 percent), whereas the highest number of LMICs achieving the targets are for TB treatment completion (74 percent) and skilled birth attendance (66 percent).

These findings highlight not only the challenges of achieving international and MDG targets, but also that implementation experience for coverage of these key health services is very different across LMICs. In addition, the findings of large heterogeneity in starting points and annual changes clearly indicate that setting a cross-country target in health services and health outcomes might not serve as an achievable and practicable benchmark for many countries. Identifying negative or slow rates of change in a country is probably a more important programmatic strategy than setting universal targets.

Table 5.2 shows the multilevel analysis of change for each of the health services, health status, and country macro-environment characteristics that take into account the different starting points and rates of change for each country. The mean values of average annual changes and starting points are shown in the "fixed" part of the model, while the "random" part incorporates the different intercepts and slopes for each country. The selected health services show statistically significant improvements between 1990 and 2004, ranging from 0.56 percent coverage a year for DPT3 (95 percent CI 0.37–0.76) to 3.0 percent a year for TB case detection rate (95 percent

Table 5.2 Average Annual Changes in Health Services and Country Characteristics, Based on Multilevel (Random-Effects) Models for Each Variable

Variables	Fixed effect: Slope (95% CI)	Fixed effect: Intercept (95% CI)	Random effect: Slope (95% CI)	Random effect: Intercept (95% CI)
Health services				
DPT3 immunization rate change (%)	0.56 (0.37–0.76)	73.89 (70.42–77.36)	1.13 (0.99–1.29)	21.69 (19.32–24.36)
Measles immunization rate change (%)	0.65 (0.47–0.82)	73.50 (70.39–76.60)	0.99 (0.86–1.14)	19.29 (17.14–21.70)
TB detection rate change (%)[a]	3.03 (1.79–4.27)	35.14 (27.60–42.69)	7.36 (6.46–8.38)	44.18 (38.57–50.62)
TB treatment completion rate change (%)[a]	0.86 (0.49–1.24)	72.94 (70.11–75.77)	1.82 (1.47–2.26)	15.54 (13.31–18.14)
Skilled birth attendance change (%)	0.71 (0.46–0.97)	66.97 (61.79–72.16)	1.26 (1.05–1.52)	31.69 (28.05–35.81)
Health status				
Under-five mortality rate change (per 1,000 live births)	−1.20 (−1.54–0.86)	88.93 (77.81–100.04)	2.12 (1.89–2.38)	70.34 (62.90–78.66)
Infant mortality rate change (per 1,000 live births)	−0.81 (−1.04–0.57)	60.79 (54.25–67.34)	1.46 (1.30–1.64)	41.41 (37.03–46.31)
Maternal mortality ratio change (per 100,000 live births)	−7.89 (−12.80–2.98)	−458.93 (378.60–539.27)	19.73[c]	453.94[c]
Total fertility rate change (number of children)	−0.06 (−0.07–0.05)	4.09 (3.78–4.40)	0.04 (0.03–0.05)	2.00 (1.79–2.23)
TB mortality rate (per 100,000 pop.)	91.09 (−41.61–223.78)	9,923.32 (3,371.76–16,474.89)	825.36 (733.51–928.72)	42,226.86 (37,833.84–47,129.96)

Country characteristics

Population (× 10^6)	0.45	27.50	0.16	113.00
	(0.20–0.70)	(10.10–44.90)	(0.15–0.18)	(101.00–126.00)
GNI per capita ($)	66.85	1,617.96	108.07	1,837.43
	(49.20–84.50)	(1,324.97–1,910.96)	(95.94–121.74)	(1,640.49–2,058.23)
Governance[b]	−0.005	−0.242	0.051	0.851
	(−0.014–0.004)	(−0.385–0.100)	(0.044–0.058)	(0.749–0.967)
Literacy rate (%)	0.92	63.42	0.56[c]	29.50[c]
	(0.78–1.06)	(58.30–68.54)		
Official development assistance inflows ($ per capita)	0.25	74.25	9.40	100.91
	(−1.31–1.80)	(57.89–90.62)	(8.17–10.82)	(87.86–115.91)
Health expenditure ($ per capita)	6.01	81.59	18.79	197.32
	(2.88–9.15)	(48.61–114.57)	(16.58–21.29)	(174.06–223.68)
Disaster-affected people (number per 10^5 pop)	18.71	1,851.97	289.90	3,497.44
	(0.00–103.48)	(1,032.54–2,671.40)	(194.59–431.89)	(2,719.37–4,498.15)

Source: Authors.

Note: All the values were estimated by multilevel (random effects) models using the variable in question, and the country and year.

a. TB service indicators are available between 1995 and 2004, whereas other variables are available between 1990 and 2004.

b. Governance indicators are available between 1996 and 2004.

c. Convergence was not achieved due to the small sample size.

CI 1.8–4.3). The mean numbers and 95 percent CIs are a good reflection of the average rate of change that can be expected in LMICs on the basis of their past experience.

The other notable finding from table 5.2 is the large heterogeneity of annual change in health service indicators across countries. In every case, both the country-specific initial coverage (random intercept) and change in coverage (random slope) are statistically significant. For example, the table shows that the overall average DPT3 immunization coverage in 1990 was 73.9 percent (fixed effect intercept), and the overall average annual increase in coverage since then has been about 0.6 percent per year (fixed effect slope). However, the standard deviation for their initial coverage (random intercept) was 21.7 percent, demonstrating that there was a very large amount of variation in DPT3 coverage among different countries in 1990. In addition, the standard deviation for the annual increase in the DPT3 coverage was 1.13 percent per year, indicating that DPT3 coverage increase per year ranged from –1.61 percent to 2.81 percent per year (0.6 percent ± 1.96 × 1.13) in 95 percent of LMICs. This large variation and statistically significant differences in annual change is observed not only for health services, but also for health status indicators and variables related to the macro context for each country. This suggests that the individual country differences in delivery of health services, health status, and macro context may be a larger part of the story than that told by international averages. This has important programmatic implications for country-level implementation, as well as for the relevance of targets set without consideration of country-specific experience.

The mean annual changes shown in the fixed part of the model in table 5.2, which are based on the actual experiences by the studied countries, could serve as potential benchmarks for other countries when their decision makers set targets for national programs. For setting feasible targets for individual countries, a starting point could be based on the actual rate of change in that country. Annex 5.1 provides a table for each of these health services indicating each country's starting point in 1990 and the annual rate of change.

But more customized benchmarks could be developed by using each country's starting point and rate of change. This involves borrowing information from other countries to refine the projections for an individual country (the statistical model uses empirical Bayes estimates to incorporate information from other countries (as explained in Rabe-Hesketh and Skrondal 2005).

Correlations of Change in Coverage of Health Services

To examine the associations between different health services, we began by examining the simple correlations between changes in health services and country contextual factors. Table 5.3 shows that there is a strong correlation between changes in measles immunization coverage and DPT3 coverage (.899), and that all other correlations between changes in health services are relatively weak, but in the positive direction. DPT3 and measles immunization coverage are expected to be closely correlated because they are often part of the same program, even if measles immunization may also be supplemented by campaigns that do not include DPT vaccination. Because changes in DPT3 and measles immunization coverage are highly correlated, subsequent models only include one indicator—DPT3 coverage. The relatively low level of correlation between the other health services suggests that on average there is neither much synergy nor antagonism between changes in one type of health service and another—excluding DPT3 and measles immunization coverage, which involve similar if not identical service delivery mechanisms.

Determinants of Changes in Health Services Coverage

Having demonstrated that the "average" experience with health services represents the experience of very few countries (figures 5.1 and 5.2, and table 5.2), we thus turned to multilevel models to further investigate the associations between changes in health services delivery across health services, adjusting for changes in country characteristics and accounting for the heterogeneity of country experiences (table 5.4). The table describes four models showing the relationship between changes in health services and country contexts, changing one of four health services as the dependent variable. Marginal statistical models that estimate country averages produced similar coefficients as the fixed effects component shown at the top of each model. In the multilevel models, the coefficients for the country context variables were similar in each model, irrespective of whether the other health services were included or excluded. These factors suggest that the models are fairly stable, and that influence from the potential endogeneity of the health services variables may not be strong.

A major finding in this analysis is that improvements in selected health services are usually not associated with changes in other health services. The exception appears to be increases in skilled birth attendance, which was associated with increases in DPT3 coverage and in the TB detection

Table 5.3 Correlations between Annual Changes in Key Health Services and Country Context Variables

	DPT3	Measles	TB detection	TB treatment	Skilled birth attendance	Governance	Literacy	Population	Fertility	GNI per capita ($)	ODA ($ per capita)
DPT3	1										
Measles	0.8987	1									
TB detection	0.2533	0.1271	1								
TB treatment	0.2932	0.3921	0.2092	1							
Skilled birth attendance	0.6040	0.6568	0.2355	0.0866	1						
Governance	0.0165	0.0008	0.2869	-0.0955	0.1054	1					
Literacy	0.5528	0.6662	-0.0087	0.1950	0.7601	-0.0426	1				
Population	-0.1952	-0.2832	-0.2425	0.1139	-0.2353	0.1025	-0.2305	1			
Fertility	-0.6471	-0.7339	-0.1944	-0.5502	-0.6811	0.0106	-0.6508	-0.0459	1		
GNI per capita ($)	0.2298	0.3097	0.4285	-0.0076	0.4830	0.4068	0.2589	-0.1325	-0.3257	1	
ODA ($ per capita)	-0.0145	-0.0917	0.1762	0.0207	0.1900	0.1027	0.2342	-0.2139	-0.0918	-0.1197	1

Source: Authors.

Note: Pearson correlation coefficients.

Table 5.4 Determinants of Health Services Changes in LMICs: Multivariable Analyses, Multilevel (Random-Effects) Models

Predictors	DPT3 Coefficient (95% CI)	P value	TB detection Coefficient (95% CI)	P value	TB treatment completion rate Coefficient (95% CI)	P value	Skilled birth attendance Coefficient (95% CI)	P value
Health services								
DPT3 coverage			0.050 (−0.230, 0.331)	0.73	0.017 (−0.084, 0.117)	0.75	0.031 (−0.072, 0.134)	0.56
TB case detection	−0.004 (−0.070, 0.062)	0.91			0.032 (−0.017, 0.081)	0.21	0.031 (−0.022, 0.084)	0.25
TB treatment completion rate	0.072 (−0.109, 0.253)	0.78	0.286 (−0.092, 0.664)	0.14			−0.025 (−0.177, 0.127)	0.75
Skilled birth attendance	**0.157 (0.019, 0.294)**	**0.03**	**0.316 (0.032, 0.600)**	**0.03**	−0.031 (−0.139, 0.077)	0.57		
Country characteristics								
Governance rating	**4.882 (0.526, 9.239)**	0.03	**15.590 (6.652, 24.528)**	**0.001**	−2.113 (−5.530, 1.305)	0.23	−0.501 (−4.774, 3.772)	0.82
Literacy (baseline value)	−0.008 (−0.156, 0.140)	0.91	−0.221 (−0.526, 0.084)	0.16	−0.083 (−0.202, 0.036)	0.17	**0.447 (0.280, 0.614)**	**<0.001**
Population (baseline per 10⁶)	−0.005 (−0.020, 0.010)	0.53	**−0.032 (−0.063, −0.018)**	**0.04**	0.006 (−0.005, 0.019)	0.30	−0.004 (−0.022, 0.014)	0.70
Total fertility rate	**−4.586 (−7.335, −1.836)**	**0.001**	−0.015 (−5.789, 5.758)	0.99	**−3.445 (−5.618, −1.273)**	**0.002**	**−5.378 (−8.532, −2.224)**	**0.001**

(continued)

Table 5.4 Determinants of Health Services Changes in LMICs: Multivariable Analyses, Multilevel (Random-Effects) Models (Continued)

Predictors	DPT3 Coefficient (95% CI)	P value	TB detection Coefficient (95% CI)	P value	TB treatment completion rate Coefficient (95% CI)	P value	Skilled birth attendance Coefficient (95% CI)	P value
GNI per capita	-0.001 (-0.002, 0.001)	0.31	-0.002 (-0.004, 0.001)	0.23	-0.0001 (-0.001, 0.001)	0.90	0.002 (0.001, 0.003)	**0.02**
Year	**0.947 (0.183, 1.711)**	**0.02**	**1.993 (0.094, 3.891)**	**0.04**	-0.020 (-0.665, 0.626)	0.95	0.349 (-0.363, 1.061)	0.34
ODA inflows per capita								
$0–10	Reference		Reference		Reference		Reference	
$10–30	2.233 (-0.163, 6.286)	0.25	0.542 (-7.105, 8.189)	0.14	1.003 (-1.705, 3.712)	0.45	-<None>10.156 (-2.603, 2.293)	0.90
$31–100	5.303 (0.592, 10.013)	0.03	2.738 (-6.757, 12.234)	0.57	0.821 (-2.596, 4.239)	0.64	-2.716 (-6.132, 0.701)	0.20
>$101	4.785 (-1.463, 11.034)	0.13	0.254 (-12.572, 13.080)	0.97	4.119 (-0.492, 8.730)	0.08	-1.657 (-6.411, 3.098)	0.50
Random effects parameters								
SD for intercept (95% CI)	**21.93 (13.25 36.31)**		**63.07 (42.73 93.09)**		**20.04 (13.08 30.71)**		**29.17 (22.11 38.49)**	
SD for slope on year (95% CI)	**1.31 (0.50 3.44)**		**5.25 (3.34 8.26)**		**1.64 (1.02 2.64)**		**2.04 (1.48 2.84)**	

Source: Authors.

Note: All the values were estimated by using multilevel (random effects) models with each of the variables included in the model. Other models incorporating one, two, or three health services at one time show similar effects. Statistically significant relationships are in bold.

SD = standard deviation.

rate (p<0.05) in both multivariate models, whereas changes in TB indicators and DPT3 immunization coverage showed no association with each other. Of the 12 coefficients showing the relationships between changes in health services, nine are in a positive direction, suggesting that even if the relationships between changes in health services are weak, they tend at least to be positive.

As might be expected from the above analysis, the random components of each of the models are highly statistically significant (none of the 95 percent CIs for random intercepts or random slopes includes 0), suggesting that both where countries start and how they progress are highly heterogeneous. Rather than showing a common pattern of progress for health services, countries tend to follow their own pathways.

Five country characteristics were also associated with changes in specific health services (table 5.4). For example, changes in per capita national income and literacy rates were significantly associated with improvements in skilled birth attendance. More specifically, a $1 increase in per capita national income was associated with 0.002 percent increase (95 percent CI 0.001–0.003) in skilled birth attendance. Changes in national governance were significantly associated with DPT3 coverage and TB case detection. Furthermore, a decrease in the total fertility rate was associated with improvement in DPT3 coverage, TB successful treatment, and skilled birth attendance. Given these findings, it makes sense that health programs should be planned and assessed within a broader framework that also includes a more complete range of health services and country contextual factors. Country characteristics, especially governance index, literacy rate, and economic indicators have been identified in this study as key factors associated with changes in health services delivery, even after the heterogeneity of experience in health services across countries is accounted for.

Main Limitations

Several limitations need to be pointed out. First, some important health services are excluded from the analysis due to data limitations. These services include contraceptive prevalence, acute respiratory tract infection treatment at an appropriate facility, diarrhea treatment with oral rehydration salts, use of insecticide-treated bednets for malaria, or use of voluntary counseling and testing for HIV or treatment with anti-retroviral drugs. These services were originally intended to be included in the study, but since they are available in less than 20 percent of the countries on an annual basis, they could not be. Data that are more directly relevant to service delivery for the newer global programs on HIV/AIDS and malaria are the least available, and particularly since these programs have taken up much of the funding and have a large potential to influence the delivery of other services, this lack of data is unfortunate. Even for health services that have been more commonly measured, data for multiple time points are limited; the skilled birth attendance rate, for example, had fewer data available than others. The sample size in multivariate models is reduced from 162 to 101 when the skilled birth attendance rate is included in the models.

The second limitation relates to the reliability and validity of the national data themselves. The validity of officially reported data on vaccine coverage rates in low-income countries has been questioned in recent years (Murray et al. 2003), and there is no reason that the officially reported data on other types of health service indicators should be more valid than those for vaccine coverage. Tuberculosis case detection estimates are particularly vulnerable to assumptions made about the incidence of tuberculosis, which may not be as predictable as previously thought (van Leth et al. 2008). Wide and implausible changes in year-to-year levels of TB case detection are also seen, including some levels of over 100 percent, suggesting that this indicator may be less robust than others. We do not know how the problem with the validity of officially reported data affected the statistical results in this study. While this problem is likely to have increased "noise," making it more difficult to statistically detect relationships, systematic biases in the change in these indicators are not obvious. Despite this uncertainty, the results remain the best estimates that can be drawn from the currently available information.

Another limitation is that our statistical models could not assess a potential endogeneity problem, though this type of problem is more commonly encountered in cross-sectional data (Lozano et al. 2006). That is, an independent variable can be a predictor of the outcome of interest, while the same variable can also be predicted by the outcome measured on earlier occasions (Diggle 2002). To avoid this problem, we checked correlations between all the variables in order to exclude highly correlated variables (correlation coefficient >0.80) in the multivariate models such as DPT3 and measles immunization coverage, and tested the multivariate models with and without the other health services variables. However, there does not seem to be an established method to assess a potential endogeneity problem in the type of longitudinal data used in our study.

It should be made clear that the associations found throughout this analysis do not necessarily imply causality. Although a longitudinal design provides stronger evidence about the potential causal relationships between variables than cross-sectional studies, the study is based on national estimates and subject to an ecologic fallacy—that is, changes at the cross-country level do not necessarily imply there will be similar changes within countries or at the individual level, particularly as information about how individual programs were implemented within each country are not available (Morgenstern 1995; Blakely and Woodward 2000). The models that we used highlight the need to examine individual country experience rather than rely on the "average" experience of LMICs.

Implications for Decision Makers

After years of emphasis on specific disease-control programs, there is a growing interest in how these programs influence health systems. The multilevel analysis conducted here may serve as groundwork to examine the impact of specific programs, since it allows us to investigate effects occurring over time at different levels, such as individual effects on countries or on subnational levels. But this requires data to be collected over time on how health services and health outcomes are changing.

There is clearly a need for more data of higher quality to better address how the new global initiatives are affecting health services and outcomes, both within and across countries. In particular, more consistent reporting of services related to HIV/AIDS, malaria, and general curative care, both of outpatient and hospitalizations, are needed if countries are to better assess how their programs and health services are working. It also makes little sense for national decision makers to look at just one health service or outcome when assessing how well programs are working, since it is clear that improvements in one program area can be associated with positive or negative (or insignificant) changes in other health services in their country—improvements in one area do not in themselves produce improvements in other areas of health services. This means that health programs should be purposely planned and monitored in a broader framework of health systems to secure improvements across the full range of health services, rather than simply one area at a time (which, as said, may have deleterious effects elsewhere).

Despite the limitations, this study provides a reasonable alternative to the benchmarks of health services based on what LMICs actually achieve over time. Figure 5.1 above suggests that most of the service delivery targets may be achieved within a few years for the "average" country— but figure 5.2 above demonstrates that few countries are, in fact, average. The range of improvements that have been made for each health service and outcome have been calculated (table 5.2 above), and may provide a more appropriate set of benchmarks for individual countries.

Note

1. These models use empirical Bayes predictors and random intercepts and random slopes for each country.

References

Ballinger, G.A. 2004. "Using Generalized Estimating Equations for Longitudinal Data Analysis." *Organizational Research Methods* 7(127).

Blakely, T.A., and A.J. Woodward. 2000. "Ecological Effects in Multi-level Studies." *Journal of Epidemiology and Community Health* 54(5): 367–374.

Diggle, P. 2002. *Analysis of Longitudinal Data.* (2nd ed.) Oxford and New York: Oxford University Press.

Garrett, L. 2007. "The Challenge of Global Health." *Foreign Affairs* 2007. January/February.

Gottret, P.E., and G. Schieber. 2006. *Health Financing Revisited: A Practitioner's Guide.* Washington, DC: World Bank.

Lozano, R., P. Soliz, E. Gakidou, J. Abbott-Klafter, D.M. Feehan, C. Vidal, et al. 2006. "Benchmarking of Performance of Mexican States with Effective Coverage." *Lancet* 368(9548): 1729–1741.

Lu, C., C.M. Michaud, E. Gakidou, K. Khan, and C.J. Murray. 2006. "Effect of the Global Alliance for Vaccines and Immunisation on Diphtheria, Tetanus, and Pertussis Vaccine Coverage: An Independent Assessment." *Lancet* 368(9541): 1088–1095.

Mohan, A., M.V. Murhekar, N.S. Wairgkar, Y.J. Hutin, and M.D. Gupte. 2006. "Measles Transmission Following the Tsunami in a Population with a High One-dose Vaccination Coverage, Tamil Nadu, India 2004–2005." *BMC Infectious Diseases* 6: 143.

Morgenstern, H. 1995. "Ecologic Studies in Epidemiology: Concepts, Principles, and Methods." *Annual Review of Public Health* 16: 61–81.

Murray, C.J., B. Shengelia, N. Gupta, S. Moussavi, A. Tandon, and M. Thieren. 2003. "Validity of Reported Vaccination Coverage in 45 Countries." *Lancet* 362(9389): 1022–1027.

Rabe-Hesketh, S., and A. Skrondal. 2005. "Multilevel and Longitudinal Modeling Using Stata." College Station, Texas: A Stata Press Publication.

Reidpath, D.D., and P. Allotey. 2006. "Structure, (Governance) and Health: An Unsolicited Response." *BMC International Health and Human Rights* 6, 12.

Travis, P., S. Bennett, A. Haines, T. Pang, Z. Bhutta, A.A. Hyder, et al. 2004. "Overcoming Health-systems Constraints to Achieve the Millennium Development Goals." *Lancet* 364(9437): 900–906.

United Nations (UN). 2007. UN Millennium Development Goals. http://www.un.org/millenniumgoals/index.html, accessed March 17, 2008.

van Leth, F., M.J. van der Werf, and M.W. Borgdorff. 2008. "Prevalence of Tuberculous Infection and Incidence of Tuberculosis: A Re-Assessment of the Styblo Rule." *Bulletin of the World Health Organization* 86(1): 20–6.

Zeger, S. L., K.Y. Liang, and P.S. Albert. 1988. "Models for Longitudinal Data: A Generalized Estimating Equation Approach." *Biometrics* 44(4): 1049–1060.

Annex 5.1 Country-level Annual Changes in Key Health Services

Country or territory	DPT3 coverage 1990	DPT3 coverage projected 2015	DPT3 annual change	SBA rate 1990	SBA projected 2015	SBA annual change	TB case detection rate 1995	TB case detection projected 2015	TB case detection annual change	TB successful DOTS treatment 1995	TB successful DOTS treatment projected 2015	TB successful DOTS treatment annual change
Afghanistan	25	81.4	2.6		25.8	0.9		46.6	2.4		100.0	5.3
Albania	94	100.0	0.5		100.0	0.4		47.3	1.3		98.4	0.6
Algeria	89	88.9	0.0		100.0	1.7		100.0	0.0		93.3	0.5
American Samoa					100.0	0.6		0.0	-4.5	100	100.0	1.4
Angola	24	68.9	1.9		92.0	3.4		100.0	8.6		100.0	4.6
Antigua and Barbuda	99	98.1	0.0		100.0	0.1		40.8	-1.8		100.0	5.8
Argentina	86	87.0	0.3		100.0	0.3		100.0	9.9		83.8	1.6
Armenia		100.0	0.6		100.0	0.4	13	62.7	1.6	83	85.1	0.2
Aruba					100.0	0.6						
Azerbaijan		100.0	0.7		73.7	-1.1	5	90.9	4.6		61.7	-1.3
Bahrain	94	100.0	0.2		100.0	0.2		69.6	3.6		100.0	6.3
Bangladesh	69	98.3	1.1		20.7	0.6	7	79.7	3.4	71	100.0	1.5
Barbados	91	94.0	0.2		99.2	0.1		100.0	20.0		100.0	1.5
Belarus					100.0	0.3		50.6	0.8		83.2	0.7
Belize	91	98.4	0.5		94.7	0.7		100.0	1.6		92.8	0.8
Benin	74	88.8	0.8		79.3	1.0	81	85.6	0.3	73	93.7	1.1
Bhutan	96	90.8	0.1		58.4	2.1	29	49.8	1.3	97	81.1	-0.5
Bolivia	41	100.0	2.9		83.9	1.5	39	95.9	1.6	62	100.0	2.0

Country												
Bosnia and Herzegovina		100.0	2.6		100.0	0.3		100.0	4.5		100.0	0.6
Botswana	92	100.0	0.4		100.0	1.1	72	51.1	-1.5	67	93.0	1.4
Brazil	66	100.0	2.1		100.0	2.0		85.4	5.0		67.4	-0.8
Bulgaria	84	95.8	0.2		100.0	0.6		100.0	17.4		100.0	1.1
Burkina	66	92.2	2.2		33.3	-0.2	12	22.1	0.3	25	100.0	4.0
Burundi	86				42.5	1.1	20	44.5	1.0	45	100.0	3.1
Cambodia	38	94.7	2.6		44.9	0.7	40	91.1	2.7	91	90.9	0.0
Cameroon	48	87.9	2.1		64.3	0.3		100.0	11.7		65.1	-0.6
Cape Verde	88				100.0	4.4		71.2	2.1			
Central African Republic	82				49.9	0.3	37	0.0	-6.0	37	96.8	2.7
Chad	20	63.7	2.1		19.1	0.2		6.8	-1.2	47	100.0	2.9
Chile	99	99.3	0.3		100.0	0.1	71	100.0	4.3	79	94.3	0.8
China	97			81.8	100.0	4.2	15	83.0	3.2	96	89.2	-0.3
Colombia	88	82.6	0.1		96.3	0.6		0.0	-7.2		98.0	1.2
Comoros	94	87.6	1.1		84.8	1.6	54	15.2	-2.1	90	100.0	0.6
Congo, Dem. Rep. of	35	65.1	1.9		72.1	0.8	42	94.0	2.6	80	100.0	2.0
Congo, Rep. of	79						67	84.7	1.0		86.6	1.3
Costa Rica	95	89.3	0.0		98.8	0.1		100.0	15.1		100.0	1.8
Côte d'Ivoire	54	68.4	0.8		89.4	2.1	52	6.6	-2.1	68	88.0	1.4
Croatia		100.0	0.9	99.8	100.0	0.0		100.0		90	94.0	0.2
Cuba	92				100.0	0.1	82	100.0	0.7			

(continued)

Annex 5.1 Country-level Annual Changes in Key Health Services (*Continued*)

Country or territory	DPT3 coverage 1990	DPT3 coverage projected 2015	DPT3 annual change	SBA rate 1990	SBA projected 2015	SBA annual change	TB case detection rate 1995	TB case detection projected 2015	TB case detection annual change	TB successful DOTS treatment 1995	TB successful DOTS treatment projected 2015	TB successful DOTS treatment annual change
Czech Rep.		99.0	0.1		100.0	0.2	45	75.3	1.1	60	97.5	1.7
Djibouti	85	53.4	0.3		69.8	0.7		0.0	-6.7	76	77.1	0.1
Dominica	92	100.0	0.2		100.0	0.3		0.0	-5.9		89.0	-0.4
Dominican Rep.	69				100.0	0.5		100.0	12.4		87.3	0.5
Ecuador	68	100.0	1.4		84.9	1.0		100.0	5.8		94.8	0.9
Egypt, Arab Rep. of	87	100.0	1.4		98.8	2.5	43	100.0	5.2		87.1	0.2
El Salvador	80	100.0	1.3		100.0	3.0		71.8	1.2		100.0	1.7
Equatorial Guinea	77				100.0	6.8	83	86.2	0.5	89	34.8	-2.4
Eritrea		100.0	4.3		43.7	1.1		38.8	1.7		100.0	1.7
Estonia		100.0	0.7		100.0	0.6		100.0	3.3		82.7	1.1
Ethiopia	49	95.6	2.6		25.5	1.2	15	66.7	2.5	61	89.4	1.0
Fiji	97				100.0	0.2	47	87.4	2.1	86	78.8	-0.5
Gabon	78				94.8	0.6		100.0	1.8		43.0	-0.4
Gambia, The	92	94.0	0.2	44.1	70.8	1.1	75	64.8	-0.4	76	74.7	0.0
Georgia		100.0	1.7		100.0	0.5	18	100.0	5.3	58	77.2	0.7
Ghana	58	99.3	1.5		52.8	0.5	16	75.0	2.7	54	81.9	1.6
Greece	54	100.0	0.8									

Grenada	80	100.0	0.6		100.0	0.3		44.2	-0.4	61	100.0	2.1
Guatemala	66	100.0	1.4		56.2	1.1	42	59.9	0.6	78	73.0	-0.1
Guinea	17	90.1	2.1		73.6	2.0	43	100.0	5.2		100.0	3.9
Guinea-Bissau	61				58.8	1.6		100.0	2.9		51.6	-2.2
Guyana	83	95.1	0.5		83.9	-0.5		58.7	6.3		86.8	0.8
Haiti	41	50.3	0.5		41.0	1.1		100.0	14.1		84.1	-0.2
Honduras	84	96.4	0.2		72.3	1.1		100.0	2.6		28.8	-2.3
Hungary	99	99.5	0.0		100.0	0.6		73.3	6.9	79	96.0	0.8
India	70	65.1	0.1		61.3	1.2		100.0	5.1	91	97.6	1.4
Indonesia	60	83.6	0.8		100.0	3.2	1	100.0				
Iran, Islamic Rep. of	91	100.0	0.5		100.0	0.8	46	100.0	3.7		85.3	0.1
Iraq	83	86.4	0.5		83.1	0.7		58.6	2.9		96.0	0.6
Jamaica	86				100.0	0.5		64.4	-1.6	67	40.1	-1.8
Jordan	92	100.0	0.3	87.2	100.0	1.0	114	47.9	-2.1		86.4	-0.1
Kazakhstan		100.0	1.0		100.0	0.1		100.0	8.1		79.3	0.1
Kenya	84				41.5	-0.1	56	33.4	-1.2		91.9	0.9
Kiribati	97	83.8	0.0		100.0	1.8		100.0	0.0	75	99.3	0.8
Korea, Dem. People's Rep. of	98				100.0	0.4		100.0	17.6		86.3	-0.2
Korea, Rep. of	74	100.0	0.9	98	100.0	0.0	34	0.0	-3.4	76	93.5	0.9
Kyrgyz Republic					100.0	0.2		100.0	6.7		84.5	0.2
Lao PDR	18	79.9	2.0		34.8	1.0		84.4	2.9	70	100.0	2.0
Latvia		100.0	0.8		100.0	0.1		100.0	1.9	61	96.3	1.6
Lebanon	82	98.7	0.4		100.0	0.7	54	100.0	1.8		100.0	1.4
Lesotho	76				65.7	0.7	63	91.7	1.1	47	95.0	1.8

(continued)

Annex 5.1   Country-level Annual Changes in Key Health Services (Continued)

Country or territory	DPT3 coverage 1990	DPT3 coverage projected 2015	DPT3 annual change	SBA rate 1990	SBA projected 2015	SBA annual change	TB case detection rate 1995	TB case detection projected 2015	TB case detection annual change	TB successful DOTS treatment 1995	TB successful DOTS treatment projected 2015	TB successful DOTS treatment annual change
Liberia					64.8	0.9		64.7	1.8	79	76.0	0.0
Libya	84	100.0	0.5		100.0	0.3		100.0	0.0		65.3	−0.1
Lithuania		100.0	1.1		100.0	0.6		100.0	16.8		69.2	−0.7
Macedonia, FYR		99.7	0.4		100.0	0.4		100.0	4.3		88.0	0.3
Madagascar	46	62.7	0.3		46.3	−0.3	51	98.6	2.1	55	96.3	1.9
Malawi	87				62.0	0.3	38	36.9	−0.2	71	80.6	0.6
Malaysia	90	100.0	0.5		100.0	0.3	64	79.3	0.7	69	84.5	0.5
Maldives	94	100.0	0.2		48.2	−1.8	101	63.8	−1.6	97	90.7	−0.2
Mali	42	84.8	1.9		72.3	2.4	14	25.7	0.5	59	59.2	−0.2
Malta	63	94.4	0.4		100.0	0.2		11.2	−1.6	100	67.5	−1.5
Marshall Islands	92				98.3	0.2		100.0	11.4		100.0	1.5
Mauritania	33	88.7	2.3		78.7	1.6		53.6	0.8		68.0	0.2
Mauritius	85	95.8	0.3	91.1	100.0	0.4	34	23.2	−0.5		92.0	0.2
Mayotte												
Mexico	53	100.0	1.3		93.4	0.4		100.0	8.8		100.0	1.6
Micronesia, Fed. States of	85	81.6	0.0		90.7	0.0	19	100.0	8.5	80	100.0	1.2

Moldova		100.0	1.4		100.0	0.3		93.5	4.2		61.0	-0.7
Mongolia	84	100.0	1.3		100.0	0.7	7	100.0	7.9		96.5	0.8
Morocco	81	100.0	0.8		91.5	2.6	93	66.3	-1.3	90	84.9	-0.2
Mozambique	46	95.7	1.9		56.8	0.7	54	37.8	-0.6	39	100.0	3.5
Myanmar	88	84.9	0.3		65.6	0.5		100.0	7.6	66	94.7	1.0
Namibia	59	86.8	0.8		88.2	0.9	22	100.0	4.3		73.9	0.8
Nepal	43	100.0	2.4		21.3	0.6		100.0	8.3		88.5	0.1
Nicaragua	66	93.7	0.8		77.1	0.7	73	98.7	1.0	80	89.2	0.5
Niger	22	63.6	1.9		25.5	0.5		100.0	4.6		89.4	1.5
Nigeria	56			30.8	45.9	0.6	11	29.8	1.0	49	100.0	2.9
Northern Mariana Islands					100.0	0.5		15.9	-5.3		74.1	-0.2
Oman	98	100.0	0.2		100.0	0.6		100.0	0.0	84	97.8	0.5
Pakistan	54	84.6	1.6		29.6	0.5	1	46.0	2.4	70	91.4	1.2
Palau	99	100.0	0.5	99	100.0	0.1	115	100.0	0.0	67	76.6	0.3
Panama	86	100.0	1.0		100.0	0.6		100.0	18.9		100.0	2.6
Papua New Guinea	67				33.5	-0.8		45.0	2.3		30.2	-2.6
Paraguay	67	80.3	0.6	66.8	83.6	0.8	14	0.0	-1.9	51	100.0	3.6
Peru	72	100.0	0.8		90.5	1.8	101	64.6	-1.6	83	95.2	0.4
Philippines	88				65.1	0.6		100.0	10.2		97.3	0.8
Poland	96	100.0	0.3		100.0	0.6		100.0	10.3		97.5	1.5
Portugal	89	100.0	0.4		100.0	0.0	75	100.0	1.8	69	98.7	1.3
Puerto Rico					100.0	0.7		82.1	1.0	65	78.1	0.5
Romania	96	99.6	0.1		99.3	0.0		22.0	-0.8		85.2	0.5

(continued)

Annex 5.1 Country-level Annual Changes in Key Health Services (Continued)

Country or territory	DPT3 coverage 1990	DPT3 coverage projected 2015	DPT3 annual change	SBA rate 1990	SBA projected 2015	SBA annual change	TB case detection rate 1995	TB case detection projected 2015	TB case detection annual change	TB successful DOTS treatment 1995	TB successful DOTS treatment projected 2015	TB successful DOTS treatment annual change
Russian Federation		100.0	1.7		100.0	0.2		28.1	1.5	65	72.4	0.4
Rwanda	84	96.9	0.9		45.1	0.8	34	22.2	-0.9		69.2	0.2
Samoa	90	92.3	0.0	76	100.0	1.8	47	86.5	2.3	80	78.6	-0.5
São Tomé and Príncipe	92	100.0	1.1		80.7	0.2						
Saudi Arabia	92	99.0	0.3		97.8	0.4		69.3	2.4		100.0	2.6
Senegal	51	79.5	1.0		75.1	1.3	61	41.1	-0.9	44	98.5	2.7
Serbia and Montenegro		100.0	0.8		97.2	0.2		48.4	1.4		100.0	1.0
Seychelles	99	100.0	0.1					68.3	-0.8	89	47.7	-2.3
Sierra Leone		76.3	1.8		56.8	1.0	28	35.4	0.0	69	96.3	1.2
Slovak Rep.		100.0	0.1		100.0	0.6	80	0.0	-4.3	64	100.0	2.2
Slovenia					100.0	0.0		76.6	0.4	90	81.6	-0.2
Solomon Islands	77	83.8	0.5		89.3	0.2		100.0	6.0	65	100.0	1.6
Somalia	19	52.5	1.4		25.1	-0.3		66.6	2.2	86	90.8	0.3
South Africa	72	95.5	0.9		100.0	1.1		100.0	10.9		67.5	-0.1
Sri Lanka	86	100.0	0.9		100.0	0.3	59	79.9	0.9	79	85.6	0.4

Country												
St. Kitts and Nevis	99				100.0	0.3		−20.7	0.0		100.0	3.8
St. Lucia	89				100.0	0.1		−2.0	44.4		50.7	−1.4
St. Vincent and the Grenadines												
Sudan	98	99.2	0.0		100.0	0.3		1.4	53.3		88.3	−0.1
Suriname	62			69.4	85.4	0.5		3.9	83.6		100.0	1.7
Swaziland	83	80.8	0.1		74.4	−0.9		0.7	44.8		55.6	0.6
Syrian Arab Rep.	89	100.0	0.6		98.5	1.9		4.9	100.0		79.8	−0.4
Tajikistan	91	82.1	0.0		63.2	−0.5		−0.9	0.0		95.7	1.1
Tanzania	78	96.3	0.7		63.6	−0.7	56	−1.1	32.4	73	91.6	0.9
Thailand	92	100.0	0.6		45.9	0.3		9.2	100.0		82.6	0.7
Timor-Leste	77	61.3	0.6		100.0	0.5	13	0.1	52.3		93.8	1.2
Togo	94				18.0	−0.4		0.2	15.6	60	71.8	0.4
Tonga	82	98.6	0.2		74.9	1.4	49	5.8	100.0	75	100.0	1.2
Trinidad and Tobago	93	100.0	0.8		94.8	0.1						
Tunisia	84	100.0	0.3		97.2	0.0		−0.4	88.4		93.8	0.3
Turkey		83.4	0.3		100.0	1.3		−3.6	0.0		100.0	1.3
Turkmenistan	45	100.0	0.8		91.7	0.7		3.8	85.4		97.6	1.6
Uganda		94.6	1.9		100.0	0.4		−2.0	19.8		100.0	3.3
Ukraine	97	100.0	0.5		47.6	0.5						
Uruguay					100.0	0.2	77	−0.6	72.6	68	100.0	1.3
Uzbekistan		100.0	1.5		96.8	0.0		4.4	74.4		87.8	0.6

(continued)

Annex 5.1 Country-level Annual Changes in Key Health Services *(Continued)*

Country or territory	DPT3 coverage 1990	DPT3 coverage projected 2015	DPT3 annual change	SBA rate 1990	SBA projected 2015	SBA annual change	TB case detection rate 1995	TB case detection projected 2015	TB case detection annual change	TB successful DOTS treatment 1995	TB successful DOTS treatment projected 2015	TB successful DOTS treatment annual change
Vanuatu	76				89.7	0.1		100.0	10.5		72.1	-0.8
Venezuela	63	80.4	0.8		97.0	0.2	72	70.3	-0.2	74	91.3	0.8
Vietnam	88	97.4	0.3		100.0	1.8	30	100.0	4.5	91	94.9	0.3
West Bank					100.0	0.5		0.0	-2.6		94.4	0.5
Yemen, Rep. of	84	88.7	1.5		40.1	1.0	2	100.0	4.4	66	93.4	1.0
Zambia	91				38.4	-0.5		93.7	3.4		87.7	0.8
Zimbabwe	88				83.6	0.7		34.3	-0.7		70.7	0.0

Source: United Nations, UNICEF, World Bank, World Health Organizations and Demographic and Health Surveys.
SBA = skilled birth attendance.

CHAPTER 6

Institutional Context of Health Services

Gerry Bloom, Hilary Standing, and Anu Joshi

Summary

Objectives: To identify the main institutional factors that influence the delivery of health services in LMICs and to describe the domains of governance that affect the implementation of health policy.

Method: A qualitative review of literature concerning institutional arrangements and health systems was conducted.

Key messages: Implementation of health services is dependent on eight institutional dimensions for planning or assessing strategies to strengthen health services:

- Degree and breadth of commitment to the stated objectives of the strategy or intervention
- Rules about how critical stakeholders are involved, and the incentives to make them work
- Incentives and disincentives for health workers (and ultimately organizations) to perform well
- Capacity of government to be a regulator of the health system

(continued)

- Mechanisms for accountability in health systems
- Co-accountability of national health systems to external bodies providing financial and technical support
- Level of statehood
- Institutional development

Reasons for Conducting the Review

Many LMICs have implemented a wide range of health system development strategies that have included investments in appropriate facilities,
personnel, and complementary inputs; the establishment of financing
mechanisms; and interventions to improve the performance of public and
private providers. Yet the outcomes have varied considerably in terms of
both service delivery and health status. There are many possible explana-
tions for the divergence, and one in particular is the difference in the institutional context within which the strategies were implemented. This
study draws on developments in understanding institutional development
in LMICs to stimulate thinking about the influence of political and institutional factors on health system development.

The *World Development Report* 2004 (World Bank 2003) conceptualized this issue as one of realigning incentives to encourage good performance. This involves the design of financing and management systems that
provide appropriate signals to service providers. It also involves measures
to make these providers more accountable to their clients and the community, particularly the poor. The *World Development Report 2004* identifies two main approaches to improve accountability and performance:
the "short route" entails measures that enable communities to influence
local health facilities; the "long route" concerns political accountability.
Both routes alter the incentives faced by decision makers in health facilities and agencies responsible for policy formulation and implementation.
Given the recognition of the importance of incentives and accountability
in service delivery, what can be learned about the main institutional factors that influence health services delivery in LMICs?

Objectives of the Review

This study sought to identify the key institutional issues that explain how
different strategies to strengthen health services are implemented in

LMICs, and to use this information to describe some of the key institutional dimensions that influence health policy implementation. The study seeks to illuminate the relevant issues for strengthening health systems and services in very different institutional contexts.

Methods Used

This qualitative analysis, based on a literature review of institutional arrangements, highlights the relevant issues surrounding the nexus between institutional arrangements and health systems. It adds to the framework used in the *World Development Report 2004* by incorporating an understanding of the influence of institutional arrangements on development (North 1990; Fukuyama 2004; Centre for the Future State 2005). North (1990) distinguishes between institutions, which are formal and informal "rules of the game" that constrain behavior, and organizations, which operate within these rules. He points out that people must internalize rules as behavioral norms and they must believe that transgressors will be punished, if the rules are to be effective. He argues that the more trust that is necessary for achieving a social end, the more important are the institutional arrangements. For example, the capacity of a society to invest in research and translate new knowledge into widely available goods and services requires a high level of trust among many organizations, implying sophisticated social rules. The same factors are relevant to health systems, whose functions require a high level of trust between various stakeholders and, consequently, effective, predictable, rules-based institutional arrangements.

The institutional arrangements of a successful health system are defined as a series of explicit and implicit "contracts" that accord service providers and other key actors a high social status and an appropriate income in exchange for acting in the interests of the community and patients (Bloom 2004; Bloom et al. 2008). These contracts involve formal rules and informal understandings, and are underpinned by socially accepted norms of behavior.

What Are the Main Limitations, Findings, and Implications?

This study is limited by the scope of its analysis and methods of enquiry, that is, a qualitative literature review that brings in other institutional frameworks. It has identified critical institutional factors that should be considered in developing and implementing strategies to strengthen health services based on past experience and evolving theory, but it cannot predict which factors will be most influential in a particular country. Although it raises questions for consideration, it does not identify how the answers will evolve or what effects they may have. Measurement of governance, institutional capacity, and statehood are not well developed, and continue to be evolving constructs. Moreover, there are as yet no definitive models to classify country characteristics that can predict health service performance.

The study identifies eight key institutional dimensions for planning or assessing strategies to strengthen health services. Findings and propositions are summarized below under each of the eight dimensions.

Degree and Breadth of Commitment to the Stated Objectives of the Strategy or Intervention

Aspiration of policy or intervention, versus cynicism of politicians. It is often difficult to distinguish between those policies or interventions included as a general aspiration or made in response to a particular stakeholder; and those that government leaders believe are important to their legitimacy and political survival. As an example, governments tend to issue large numbers of policy statements, health development plans, and so forth, which often include a plethora of targets and objectives, and therefore delineate the needs of perhaps multiple stakeholders. In terms of legitimacy, it is important to note that, in many countries, the government that came to power in the immediate postcolonial or postrevolutionary period made commitments to provide universal access to health services. These promises were important elements of the legitimacy of these regimes. However, as it became clear that they were unable to meet these promises, governments have been unwilling to alter their original commitments publicly. This was apparent in the Russian government's unwillingness to discuss openly the policy implications of the widespread use of informal payments by health workers (Mackintosh and Kovalev 2006). Such circumstances have created difficulties in formulating realistic policies that make the best use of available resources (Bloom and Standing 2001).

National need versus narrow interest. In many cases, national policies and multiyear plans are largely produced by government officials. Other stakeholders may be consulted, but these moves are often informal and do not commit stakeholders to specific responsibilities. This can become problematic, as in the case of a disruption of a multiyear health development program by a change in government following competitive multiparty elections, where the health sector plan or strategy in question may be dismantled as it is perceived as a product of the previous regime.[1]

Incentives for key actors. Many countries have created regulations and policies but government officials and other actors have made little effort to enforce them (Ensor and Weinzierl 2006). This analysis supports the notion that reviews of country institutional arrangements and health system development should explore the degree to which these regulations were translated into political commitments, the incentives for key actors to translate policies or regulations into changes in health system performance, and whether the public evaluated government performance on the basis of how far such policies were implemented.

Health Sector Stakeholders, Interests, and Common Agreements

The effective functioning of a health system relies on the existence of rules-based arrangements between actors. Therefore, any national plans for strengthening health services should explore the processes for establishing these relationships and the incentives for stakeholders to make them work (table 6.1). Planners should also explore stakeholders' specific interests and the degree to which particular institutional arrangements operate in favor of more powerful stakeholders, and identify countervailing strategies to give voice and influence to the poor.

Influence of Incentives and Disincentives on Performance

A key characteristic of the health sector is the importance of skilled workers, and so the incentives that workers face have an important influence on both an individual's performance and that of the overall health sector. In light of this, approaches to health system strengthening should pay specific attention to the incentives and disincentives that health workers face, including: short-term livelihoods, long-term benefits linked to opportunities for further training and promotion, extent to which poor governance and oversight have produced or encouraged perverse incentives (for example, rewards for poor performance), and norms and moral codes to ensure ethical behavior of health workers.

Strength of Government Capacity to Serve as Regulator and Steward of the Health System

Government officials' regulatory duties. In order for government to play an effective role, the responsibilities of senior officials and those responsible for enforcing regulations and monitoring health system performance need to be clearly defined; this aspect of institutional development should therefore

Table 6.1 Key Health Sector Stakeholders and Interests

Actor	Incentives for making institutions work	Specific stakeholder interests	Strategies to counterbalance stakeholder interests
Central government	• Strong identification with particular policy • Degree to which government officials are answerable for successful implementation of policy	• Possibilities for rent seeking (abuse of power) • Hijacking/appropriation of agendas to serve specific constituencies (for example, urban elites, ethnic groups)	• Involve other stakeholders in planning and monitoring. • Provide public information. • Powerful, charismatic leadership can win public support for an intervention.
Local government	• Degree of political accountability to the population • Monitoring of performance by higher levels of government	Possible partnerships with local power brokers, patron–client relations, favoritism in for example, suppliers, transfers	• Create service delivery and regulatory partnerships. • Provide information on resource use and service delivery. • Establish robust local monitoring arrangements, strengthen governance capacity of political representatives.
Facility owners/ managers	Reputation, trust, attract patients	Pressure to maximize income, prescribe unnecessary treatment	• Report on facility performance. • Ensure direct accountability to the local population. • Improve facilities-level incentives; for example, return revenue for improvements to services.
Pharmaceutical suppliers	Reputational risks from counterfeits, need for reputation for social responsibility, establish stable market	Competitive strategies that deny information or push unnecessarily high use of products	• Implement strong government regulatory systems. • Widely disseminate information on products and prices.

Community-based organizations	Voice of local groups		• Provide transparency in access to resources and use of them. • Strengthen governance arrangements in such organizations.
Professional associations	Reputation, social standing	Possible representation of narrow group • Closure from below and misuse of power for economic gain • Refusal to address gross urban bias in human resources	• Include nonprofessionals in governance. • Negotiate contractual bargains on service delivery for underserved populations.
Trade unions	Pay and promotion	Resistance to public sector reforms and measures to improve efficiency	Test demand-side approaches and competition.
Donor agencies	Success in achieving institutional goals	Short-term career moves and tendency to undervalue long-term institutional development	• Commission systematic studies of long-term impact of interventions feed into internal monitoring arrangements. • Sponsor training/orientation in political and institutional analysis.
International advocacy groups	High motivation to address specific needs	Focus on short-term targets with little interest in other consequences	• Widen governance arrangements. • Improve analysis and forecasting.

Source: Authors.

be further explored when strategies to strengthen health services are planned or evaluated.

Government officials' incentives. Many countries have quite well-developed legal rules in the health sector that are largely not enforced. Moreover, there is often little incentive for local officials to enforce such rules. These issues may be related to levels of pay, political influence over promotion, and widespread corruption. They may also reflect insufficient funding of the regulatory agency itself. In light of these findings, countries would benefit from relating health system performance and general measures of strengthening government performance.

Regulatory partnerships. In many instances, government works in partnership with other stakeholders to design and implement regulations. The stakeholders may include organized professions or pharmaceutical companies. In recent years, a variety of partnerships have emerged that include representatives of health workers, community-based organizations, and so forth. These regulatory partnerships—and their potential to mediate conflicts of interest—should be assessed in more detail when considering strategies to strengthen health services.

Media role. In many cases, scandals or pressure by the media have brought problems to the surface and placed pressure on government to act. In understanding the nexus between institutional arrangements and health system development, the role of the media should be further explored in identifying issues and providing incentives for government action.

Mechanisms for Accountability in Health Systems

Health in the political system. The degree to which health issues play a part in major political statements and electoral politics—evaluating the importance of health in political manifestos—should be considered when developing strategies to strengthen health services. It is important to assess whether there is evidence that health has influenced political decisions, and identify whether there are specific committees to deal with health issues in representative bodies, as well as their level of influence in decision making.

Community-based and nongovernmental organizations. Many countries have used a variety of mechanisms to make service providers more responsive to the local population. These include formal health committees, organizations concerned with specific programs, and organizations that include a local service delivery component. In developing and pursuing health services strengthening strategies, it would be useful to consider the role of these types of organizations in improving health system performance.

Co-accountability of National Health Systems to External Bodies Providing Financial and Technical Support

Management of co-accountable projects. A gradual shift has occurred in the pattern of external transfers so that an increasing proportion of them finances service provision. There have been attempts to design systems to manage co-accountability in this new environment (for example, SWAps), but there are few examples of long-term systematic construction of capacity by all relevant partners.

Specific support programs and wider impact. Program design should take into account the objectives of both meeting current health-related needs and building sustainable health systems that provide appropriate incentives for key actors. In some cases, there has been a disproportionate emphasis on the former, leading to unintended consequences from perverse incentives.

Systems of accountability. Program design needs to take into account the explicit and implicit incentives that specific support programs provide for relevant national actors. Those designing programs should assess the extent to which program managers should be held accountable for their performance, the persons to whom they will be accountable, and the performance criteria on which they are to be judged.

External agencies' relationships. Program design needs to take into account the nature and quality of the relationships that have developed between national actors and external agencies.

Level of Statehood

Level of statehood refers to the extent to which the government has effective control over its territory, is not excessively dependent on external or mineral resources, observes the constitution, and is guided by the rule of law and the degree to which institutions of government, political parties, and civil society organizations are stable, predictable, and routine.

One illustration of the relative weakness of the state in many countries has been the emergence of pluralistic health systems, where a large proportion of health care transactions take place outside the public sector (Bloom and Standing 2001). This may involve private providers operating within well-defined regulations and much larger numbers of practitioners working outside the legal framework (Berman 1998; Harding and Preker 2004). It may also involve government employees charging for services legally or without legal sanction (Ferrinho et al. 2004). A notable feature of many countries with pluralistic health systems is the limited capacity of government to influence the system's performance (see below). A sign of this weakness has been a growing gap between the language of policy and agreements with donor agencies, and the reality on the ground (Bloom and Standing 2001; Mackintosh and Kovalev 2006). To begin bridging this gap, much more attention must be paid to the institutional and political context within which agreements are negotiated. The same policy will play out very differently, even in apparently similar countries.

Institutional Development

The level of institutional development refers to the following three main elements: the extent to which government has the capacity to carry out its programs (for example, in-post staff who are paid regularly) and to provide the resources for supporting initiatives; the degree to which functioning accountability mechanisms exist; and the extent to which corruption is prevalent. Government capacity is particularly relevant to health systems because of its reliance on the existence of functioning rules-based institutional arrangements in the public domain. For example, public sectors in countries with strong states are often categorized as "Weberian bureaucracies," in which employees are expected to act in the public interest in exchange for status and secure employment. In many other countries, public sector jobs deviate considerably from this ideal and it is widely understood that government employees pursue livelihood strategies to secure an adequate income. These strategies include requesting informal payments or working privately. It is often difficult to draw a clear boundary between accepted market practices and corruption (Lewis 2006). Pritchett and Woolcock (2004) argue that arrangements that work quite well in the advanced market economies perform differently in these circumstances, and they suggest that this explains the growing interest in demand-side approaches and community-based development as mechanisms for limiting opportunities for opportunistic behavior. Similarly, Minogue (2005) argues that regulatory systems reflect levels of institutional development and cultural norms. Further, Leonard (2000) suggests that organized professions also function quite differently in many LMICs.

Afterword

It is difficult to measure these eight dimensions of governance, which depend largely on subjective assessments by individuals who know the country context well. However, Kaufmann et al. (2005) have constructed composite indicators of governance that provide rough indicators. Importantly, these indicators should be supplemented with detailed local knowledge about the state of governance, which is particularly relevant to health system performance.

Note

1. The Malawi Social Action Fund, however, provides a positive example of a large intervention that attained national status and received support from all political parties (Bloom et al. 2005). This was achieved through the creation of transparent decision-making rules and through a very active publicity campaign that involved a variety of media.

References

Berman, P. 1998. "Rethinking Health Care Systems: Private Health Care Provision in India." *World Development* 26(8): 1463–79.

Birdsall, N., and R. Hecht. 1997. "Swimming against the Tide: Strategies for Improving Equity in Health." In *Marketizing Education and Health in Developing Countries*, ed. C. Colclough. Oxford: Clarendon Press.

Bloom, G. 2004. "Private Provision in its Institutional Context: Lessons from Health." DFID Health Systems Resource Centre Issues Paper. London.

Bloom, G., W. Chilowa, E. Chirwa, H. Lucas, P. Mvula, A. Schou, and M. Tsoka. 2005. "Poverty Reduction During Democratic Transition: The Malawi Social Action Fund, 1996–2001." Institute of Development Studies Research Report 56, Brighton.

Bloom, G., and H. Standing. 2001. "Pluralism and Marketisation in the Health Sector: Meeting Health Needs in Contexts of Social Change in Low and Middle-Income Countries." Institute of Development Studies Working Paper 136.

Bloom, G., H. Standing, and R. Lloyd. 2008. "Markets, Information Asymmetry and Health Care: Towards New Social Contracts." *Social Sciences & Medicine* 66(10): 2076–2087.

Centre for the Future State. 2005. *Signposts to More Effective States*. Brighton: Institute of Development Studies.

Department for International Development. 2003. Drivers of Change Team. http://www.chronicpoverty.org/toolbox/PolicyInfluence_MediaEngagement/3.1%20Power%20and%20Country%20Level%20Analysis/1-DFID_DoC%20summary%20(DB).pdf.

Duncan, A., I. Sharif, P. Landell-Mills, D. Hulme, and J. Roy. 2002. "Bangladesh: Supporting the Drivers of Pro-poor Change." Report to DFID. http://www.opml.co.uk/economic_policy/development_policy/ei453e_banglades.html

Ensor, T., and S. Weinzierl. 2006. "A Review of Regulation in the Health Sector in Low and Middle Income Countries." Oxford Policy Management Working Paper, Oxford

Ferrinho, P., W. van Lerberghe, I. Fronteira, F. Hipolito, and A. Biscaia. 2004. "Dual Practice in the Health Sector: Review of the Evidence." *Human Resources for Health* 2(1): 14.

Fukuyama, F. 2004. *State Building: Governance and World Order in the Twenty-First Century*. London: Profile Books.

Gilson, L. 2003. "Trust and the Development of Health Care as a Social Institution." *Social Science and Medicine* 56: 1453-68.

Harding, A., and A. Preker, eds. 2001. *Private Participation in Health Services Handbook*. Washington, DC: World Bank.

Kaufmann, D., A. Kray, and M. Mastruzzi. 2005. *Governance Matters IV: Governance Indicators for 1996–2004*, www.worldbank.org/wbi/governance/pubs/govmatters4.html.

Leonard, D. 2000. Lessons from the New Institutional Economics for the Structural Reform of Health Services in Africa, in Leonard, D (ed.) *Africa's Changing Markets for Health and Veterinary Services: The New Institutional Issues*. Basingstoke: Macmillan Press.

Lewis, N. 2006. "Governance and Corruption in Public Health Care Systems." Center for Global Development Working Paper 76.

Mackintosh, M., and S. Kovalev. 2006. "Commercialisation, Inequality and Transition in Health Care: The Policy Challenges in Developing and Transitional Countries." *Journal of International Development* 18: 387–391.

Minogue, M. 2005. *Apples and Oranges: Problems in the Analysis of Comparative Regulatory Governance*. Centre of Regulation and Competition, Institute for Development Policy and Management, University of Manchester Working Paper 94.

North, D.C. 1990. *Institutions, Institutional Change and Economic Performance*. New York: Cambridge University Press.

Ovretveit, J. 2006. Strengthening Health Services in Low Income Countries. Unpublished background document (summarized in chapter 4).

Oxford Policy Management. 2003. *Drivers of Change: Reflections on Experience to Date*. Oxford Policy Management, Oxford.

Pierson, P. 2000. "Increasing Returns, Path Dependency and the Study of Politics." *American Political Science Review* 94: 251–267.

Pritchett, L., and M. Woolcock. 2004. "Solutions When the Solution is the Problem: Arraying the Disarray in Development." *World Development* 32(2): 191–212.

Standing, H. 2000. "Gender: A Missing Dimension in Human Resource Policy and Planning for Health Reforms." *Human Resources for Health Development Journal* 4(2).

Thelen, K. 2003. "How Institutions Evolve." In *Comparative Historical Analysis in the Social Sciences*, ed. J. Mahoney and D. Rueschemeyer. Cambridge: Cambridge University Press.

Tibandebage, P., and M. Mackintosh. 2005. "The Market Shaping of Charges, Trust and Abuse: Health Care Transactions in Tanzania." *Social Science and Medicine* 61: 1385–1395.

World Bank. 1993. World Development Report 1993: Investing in Health. Washington, DC: World Bank.

———. 2004. *World Development Report 2004: Making Services Work for Poor People*. Washington, DC: World Bank.

CHAPTER 7

Evaluation of Changes in Health Results in World Bank-assisted Health Projects

Savitha Subramanian and David H. Peters

Summary

Objective: To identify how World Bank-assisted health projects measure changes in health services, financing, and impact on health status; and to identify project characteristics associated with improvements in health services, financing, and status.

Methods: A review was made of all 118 implementation completion reports of World Bank projects that had a health component and that were completed in the three fiscal years 2003 to 2005.

Key messages:

- Sectorwide approaches may well improve health services or health status more than other programs.
- Among project activities, contracting and logistics support were likely to show improvements in health services and status, respectively.

(continued)

- Projects organized around disease-control programs suggested improvements in health services and outcomes.
- No type of project input was associated with improvements in health services or status.
- More consistent measurement of results is needed, to better assess whether individual country efforts produce the desired changes.

Reasons for Conducting the Review

Despite the wide consensus that health systems and the services they produce are critical factors in the achievement of international and local health and development goals, there are relatively few systematic attempts to evaluate health systems performance across countries. There are also few organizations that have the data that can be used for such analysis. The World Bank is one such body, and provides an opportunity to examine its multiple-country experience related to its financial assistance in the health sector and to examine what can be learned about improving health services.

The most recent in-house evaluation of the entire health, nutrition, and population (HNP) portfolio of World Bank assistance recognized many positive contributions of the World Bank, but noted that "the Bank typically focuses on providing inputs rather than on clearly defining and monitoring progress toward HNP development objectives" (Johnston and Stout 1999). This view was supportive of the World Bank's first HNP Strategy (1997), which identified the need to monitor progress against objectives. The three priorities identified in the strategy to guide the direction of the World Bank's work in the HNP sector were to work with client countries to improve HNP outcomes of the poor; enhance the performance of health care systems; and secure sustainable health care financing. Subsequently, with the World Bank developing a new HNP strategy in 2006, it became timely to examine what had been learned about progress toward the main priorities of the first HNP strategy.[1]

There is considerable debate over which approaches to providing development assistance in health are the most effective. Over the last few decades much of the debate has been between priority programs for specific diseases on the one hand, and other approaches to strengthening health systems on the other. These other approaches include comprehensive area-based projects, community development projects, those designed to develop management support systems (essential drugs, equipment, etc.), sectorwide approaches, and other organizational approaches (Mills 2005). Table 7.1 defines the common organizational approaches as used in the discussion paper of Subramanian et al. (2006). More recently, debate has focused on the relative merits of general budget support compared to assistance given directly to the health sector (Cordella and Dell'Aricca 2007; Koeberle et al. 2006).

In addition to considering broadly how development assistance is organized for health, insights into more specific types of inputs or activities are related to improvements in health services, financing, or health outcomes are also important. For example, are projects that offer technical assistance more likely to have an impact on health services or health

Table 7.1   Definitions of Approaches to Organizing Development Assistance in the Health Sector

Approach	Description
General budget support	Development assistance provided as general support to the government, not targeted at the health sector. It is sometimes considered an extrasectoral approach. Projects rely on government systems to manage the funds, on the basis of policy agreements to achieve broad objectives, which include the health sector. Projects provide general budget support without earmarking of funds to a sector (such as "Poverty Reduction Support Credits," Structural Adjustment Loans").
Health sector	
Disease program	Strengthening a priority program organized around control of a specific disease (HIV/AIDS, tuberculosis, malaria) or a specific set of health services and conditions (immunization, family planning)
Geographic priority	Strengthening management and delivery systems in a particular geographic area of a country, often chosen because of the characteristics of a particular population
Management support system	Focusing on a particular management support system (for example, systems to provide key inputs such as essential drugs, buildings, or equipment)
Sectorwide approach	Investments and actions based on common sectoral policy and objectives, expenditure framework, and systems for implementation and review. In some cases, funding is provided as budget support but with specified allocation to the health sector; in some cases, funding is labeled "adaptable program loans."
Others	Projects organized around other approaches, such as health providers, financing mechanisms, community engagement approaches, and accountability approaches

Source: Subramanian et al. 2006.

status? Do investments in training or pharmaceuticals have an impact on health services or health status? Given the lack of skilled human resources working in the health sector in many LMICs, do projects that focus on systems for human resources have a higher likelihood of demonstrating a change in health services?

Some of the main types of inputs and activities that were assessed across World Bank-assisted projects were as follows:

- *Project inputs:* salaries of health workers; training of health workers; technical assistance; pharmaceuticals (including vaccines and contra-ceptives); purchase, repair, or maintenance of equipment; building or repair and maintenance of buildings; and computer software
- *Project activities:* human resources systems (including increasing the number of health workers, improving health worker capacity, or systems to manage human resources); health services management systems (including quality of care approaches and health management infor-mation systems); logistics systems (such as selection, procurement, and distribution of drugs and other commodities); policies or activities to regulate health providers; contracting of health organizations; and involvement of civil society organizations or the public in planning.

Objectives of the Review

The specific aims of this review were to:

- Identify how World Bank-assisted HNP projects measure changes in health services, health financing, and impact on people's health, the three priority areas of the World Bank's HNP strategy prior to 2006
- Identify project characteristics associated with improvements in health services, health financing, and health status. The main project characteristics of interest are how the project was organized to pro-vide assistance, types of project inputs, and types of project activities.

This type of review was intended to show whether an adequate level of evaluation of health services, financing, and status was being carried out in World Bank-assisted projects, in order to give some assurance to national stakeholders that progress was being made in these relevant areas. By com-paring results across countries and by accounting for different country characteristics, it was hoped that a plausible level of association between certain types of project design features and improvements in health serv-ices, financing, and status could be detected.

For many decision makers, knowing whether a relevant improvement has been made during a project is sufficient to assess whether the particular approach was successful, and perhaps whether it is worth continuing or expanding in that country. In the context of this review, this means that measurements were drawn at a minimum of two points in time for a relevant measure of health services, health financing, or health status for a given project. Information on how often this occurs provides some insight as to whether a minimal level of evaluation is being performed, allowing local decision makers and the public to know whether progress is being made. If certain approaches to project design can be shown to be associated with improvements, that would provide additional information to support particular strategies.

If alternative designs for health assistance are being considered (either by national decision makers or those from international agencies), then it becomes more useful to compare projects from other countries in determining whether there are typical approaches, inputs, or activities that are more likely to show improvements. Countries can serve as comparisons to each other, in which case it becomes useful to try to account for factors within countries that might also explain some of the differences in health services, financing, and health status. These differences would include factors such as the income level of a country, literacy rates, and the types of policies and institutions, although many other factors could also be considered. By accounting for these other factors, there is greater plausibility that the effects of project characteristics can be found that are associated with improved health services, financing, or health status. (However in this review, too few projects evaluated changes in health financing for analysis.)

Methods Used

The review was limited to an inventory and systematic evaluation of results that were measured and reported in the official project evaluation reports of completed World Bank-assisted projects—implementation completion reports (ICRs).

The review examined all World Bank projects that contained a health component and were completed during the three fiscal years 2003 to 2005.[2] Project information was extracted from all 118 ICRs that were completed in this time and that had a health sector component. Each ICR was prepared by the unit of the World Bank responsible for designing and supervising the project, with input from the government to document their achievements. For this review, each project ICR was systematically assessed using a checklist of the assessment criteria to document which indicators were used for measuring health services, financing, and status, and the characteristics of interest: the primary organizational approach, and the types of inputs and activities involved. In order to achieve consistency in the data entry process between the two data collectors, data were double entered. When data were inconsistent between the two entries, the two data collectors investigated the problem and resolved it. Two other reviewers were used to assess the data entered and reconcile any remaining discrepancies.

Table 7.2 defines the outcome variables used in the review: changes in health services, health financing, and health status. The main independent variables were derived from table 7.1 and the project inputs and project activities bullets, above.

Table 7.2   Definitions of Health Services, Financing, and Health Status Used in the Review

Change in outcome variable	Description
Health services	Any measurement of an indicator that measures the utilization, coverage, quality, efficiency, or distribution of health services, including changes in health behaviors of individuals. These types of indicators are usually defined as project outcomes, but may also be defined as health service outputs in the evaluation frameworks.
Health financing	Any measurement of an indicator that describes the financing dimensions of health, whether for individuals, government, or other organizations. Health financing indicators can be impact-level measures (for example, income protection for individuals), or output and outcome levels (for example, enrollment levels in health financing schemes, contributions by government or individuals, cost of services).
Health status	Any measurement of an indicator that describes the long-term effect on the health, nutrition, and population status of the population. Mortality rates, disease incidence and prevalence rates, case fatality rates, cure rates, and rates of malnutrition and fertility are all examples of health status measures. These indicators can be considered as project outcomes, although they tended to be identified as project-impact or project goal-level indicators.

Source: Subramanian et al. 2006.
Note: The review examined any measurement of health services, health financing, and health status in the projects, and focused on those projects demonstrating any change in these indicators taken from at least two measurements at different points in time.

The review used exploratory data analysis to describe each variable, followed by tests of statistical association between the outcome and explanatory variables. Multiple logistic regression analysis was used to control for potentially confounding variables and derive odds ratios for two outcome variables: improvements in health services and improvements in health status (too few projects evaluated changes in health financing). Further details on the methods used are available in the discussion paper (Subramanian et al. 2006).

Main Findings

One of the most striking features of the review is how infrequently World Bank-assisted projects in the field of HNP evaluated changes in health services (42 percent of projects), health financing (17 percent), or health status (33 percent). However, the good news is that those projects that paid attention to measurement were associated with better health services and health status. When at least two measurements were taken of an indicator, they nearly always demonstrated an improvement. Yet given the importance of equity considerations, it is remarkable that none of the projects included measurements of equity of health services, financing, or status.

The analysis also provided further indications about how health projects are designed. The majority of projects were financed from within the health sector (73 percent), rather than outside it. Nearly all projects provided technical assistance (88 percent) or training (75 percent), but salary support was much less common (21 percent). Most projects involved activities to support human resource management (81 percent) or health services management systems (72 percent), but very few involved the public in planning the program (16 percent), contracting with service providers (27 percent), or regulating health providers (39 percent). (Annex table 7.1 provides the details of the project characteristic by global region.)

In examining which type of organizational approach is associated with improvements in health services or health status (health financing had too few cases to assess), both SWAps and disease-control programs did better than others (figure 7.1).

A regression analysis was used to control for other variables. This resulted in identifying only a few project characteristics that were associated with improvements in health services or health status. (Annex table 7.2 has the full models.) In this analysis, this means that the odds ratio for an improvement of health services or health status was greater than 1. Of the different types of project organizational approach, only SWAps achieved an

Figure 7.1   Percentage of Projects Showing Improvements in Health Services, Health Financing, or Health Status, According to Organizational Approach

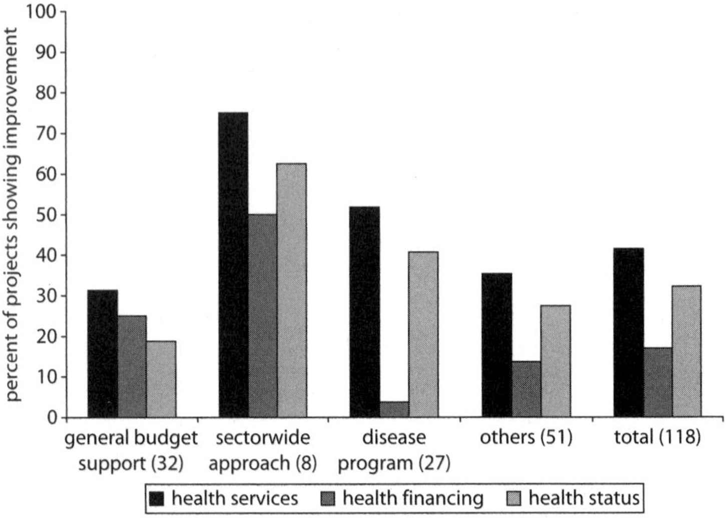

Source: Authors.

odds ratio that was statistical greater than 1 at a level of p value <0.05 for both health services and health status (figure 7.2).

The significantly higher odds of programs that use SWAps making improvements, compared to others, is potentially important, though the sample size was quite small. It is possible that the emphasis on regular review of performance, which forms part of most SWAps, means that they are more likely to measure and report changes. Whether SWAps are actually more effective at achieving improvements is not clear, largely because of poor reporting of performance by most projects, and weak evaluation designs. However, the multivariate analysis reinforced the association of SWAps with measurement of improved outcomes.

No type of project input was associated with improvements in health services or status. Of the project activities, those using contracting were more likely to show improvements in health services, and those providing logistics support showed improvements in health status (figure 7.2). These findings suggest that the use of contracting and support for logistics is likely to be an important element in success.

Main Limitations

The main limitation of this review is that it is unclear if the factors associated with improvements in health services or health status actually

Figure 7.2   Odds Ratios for Improving Health Services and Health Status According to Organizational Approach and Project Activity

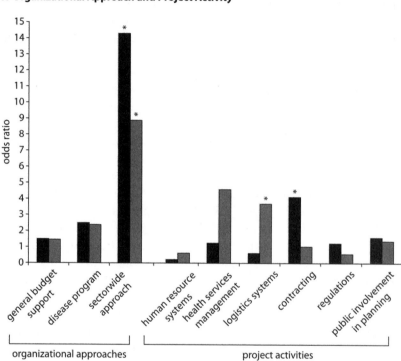

Source: Authors.

Note: Based on multiple logistic regression models (annex table 7.2). Geographic priority, management support system, and other approaches not shown.

An odds ratio > 1 means that improvement is more likely to occur when that variable is present.

* P value <0.05 (the probability of making an error in concluding there is an effect, when in truth there is not, is less than 5%).

caused the differences. To the decision maker, it may be adequate or even plausible to accept these factors as contributing to improvements. Most researchers, though, will remain skeptical about the findings, even if they stimulate further hypotheses to test, concerning which conditions these organizational designs and activities are likely to cause improvements. Equally, the limitations of this study design prevent it from providing probabilistic estimates about how well different types of projects can be expected to improve health services or health status. Since the act of measuring of improvement is likely an endogenous factor to the change itself, these associations could be demonstrating the likelihood of measuring outcomes rather than causing the improvement.

The primary project approaches and other characteristics were not randomly assigned (many of these approaches were not reasonably randomized, such as SWAps or general budget support), and a multitude of factors outside the control of a project are likely to have influenced its outcomes. To help improve the plausibility of the assessment, the review controlled for the influence of country context factors such as income levels, geographic regions, and policy and institutional assessments, but these were unlikely to provide tight "control" of all other factors influencing health services and health status.

Because the review was primarily interested in how projects measured change in the three priority areas of the World Bank's HNP strategy, it did not evaluate each project based on its individual development objectives, nor of the relevance of the indicators used to the project's development objectives. Nor did it consider other important project effects that were not captured by the three main types of strategic outcomes. For example, it did not assess establishing new institutions or improving processes, unless they could be assessed through the type of outcomes measured.

Many other useful activities may not be captured by quantitative measurements. For example, about 48 percent of the projects involved pilot testing of new schemes in a country. However, in most instances, it was not clear what became of the pilot study, and it was not possible in this review of ICRs to fairly assess their status at the end of the project.

Implications for Decision Makers

Despite the limitations of the review, the findings are still useful enough to address its objectives. One major conclusion is that decision makers and the public need to demand more rigorous evaluation of health sector investments made with World Bank funds, and of development projects more generally. When projects can consistently assess changes in health services, health financing, and health status, these constituents will be better informed and better able to assess the adequacy of programs. Stronger evaluation designs will help them decide which strategies are the most effective and efficient in improving health services and health status.

There is plausible evidence from this analysis that SWAps and projects involving contracting and support for logistics have a better chance of being able to demonstrate improvements in health services or health status, at least when receiving assistance from the World Bank. Projects organized around disease-control programs were also suggestive of improvements in health services and outcomes, though the effects were not as strong. More consistent measurement of results would provide a better basis for assessing whether individual country efforts are actually producing the desired changes.

Notes

1. This chapter is based on the discussion paper of Subramanian et al. 2006.
2. The fiscal year ends on June 30.

References

Cordella, T., and G. Dell'Ariccia. 2007. "Budget Support Versus Project Aid: A Theoretical Appraisal." *The Economic Journal* 117 (523): 1260–1279.

Johnston, T., and S. Stout. 1999. *Investing in Health: Development Effectiveness in the Health, Nutrition, and Population Sector*. Washington, DC: World Bank.

Koeberle, S., Z. Stavreski, and J. Walliser, eds. 2006. *Budget Support as More Effective Aid? Recent Experiences and Emerging Lessons*. Washington, DC: World Bank.

Mills, A. 2005. "Mass Campaigns versus General Health Services: What Have We Learnt in 40 Years about Vertical versus Horizontal Approaches." *Bulletin of the World Health Organization* 83(4) 325–30.

Subramanian, S., D.H. Peters, and J. Willis. 2006. "How are Health Services, Financing and Status Evaluated? An Analysis of Implementation Completion Reports of World Bank Assistance in Health." World Bank: Health Nutrition and Population (HNP) Discussion Paper.

World Bank. 1997. *Health, Nutrition, & Population Sector Strategy*. Washington, DC.

Annex Tables

Annex Table 7.1 Characteristics of Project Evaluations Analyzed
(%)

	Africa (n=38)	East Asia and Pacific (n=10)	Europe and Central Asia (n=20)	Latin America and the Caribbean (n=27)	Middle East and North Africa (n=12)	South Asia (n=11)	Total (N=118)
Main outcomes							
Health services indicator—Any measurement	76.3	90.0	60.0	70.4	83.3	90.9	75.4
Health services indicator(s)—Improvement shown	50.0	50.0	20.0	48.2	16.7	54.6	41.5
Health financing indicator—Any measurement	21.1	0.0	20.0	33.3	8.3	45.5	21.2
Health financing indicator(s)—Improvement shown	18.4	0.0	10.0	22.2	0.0	36.4	17.0
Health status indicator—Any measurement	50.0	70.0	30.0	37.0	41.7	63.6	45.8
Health status indicator—Improvement shown	44.7	40.0	20.0	33.3	16.7	18.2	32.2
Type of development assistance							
Budget support (extrasectoral)	42.1	10.0	25.0	25.9	0.0	27.3	27.1
Health sector approach	57.9	90.0	75.0	74.1	100	72.7	72.8
Organizational approach							
Disease program	29.0	30.0	5.0	22.2	25.0	27.3	22.9
Geographic priority	5.3	10.0	20.0	7.4	16.7	36.4	12.7
Management support system	7.9	30.0	20.0	14.8	58.3	0.0	17.8

Sectorwide approach	10.5	10.0	0.0	7.4	9.1	6.8
Other approaches	5.3	10.0	30.0	22.2	0.0	12.7
Project inputs						
Salaries	26.3	20.0	20.0	11.1	45.5	21.2
Training	71.1	90.0	70.0	70.4	90.9	75.4
Technical assistance	84.2	90.0	90.0	81.5	100	88.1
Pharmaceuticals	68.4	80.0	45.0	44.4	81.8	60.2
Equipment	60.5	90.0	60.0	59.3	63.6	66.1
Buildings	60.5	60.0	55.0	40.7	63.6	58.5
Software	36.8	50.0	60.0	59.3	45.5	49.2
Project activities						
Human resources systems	79.0	90.0	75.0	77.8	90.9	80.5
Health services management systems	63.2	90.0	80.0	70.4	90.9	72.0
Logistics systems	76.3	80.0	70.0	59.3	36.4	67.8
Contracting with organizations	34.2	40.0	5.0	25.9	45.5	27.1
Regulation of health providers	31.6	30.0	65.0	44.4	36.4	39.0
Public involvement in planning	15.8	0.0	10.0	22.2	27.3	16.1

Source: Authors.

Note: Improvement is based on a positive change from at least two measurements.

Annex Table 7.2 Logistic Regression Results for Improvements in Health Services and in Health Status

Variable	Health services			Health status		
	Odds ratio	P value	95% CI	Odds ratio	P value	95% CI
Organizational approach						
(other)						
General budget support	1.49	0.69	0.21-10.50	1.45	0.77	0.12-16.93
Disease program	2.49	0.19	0.65-9.61	2.38	0.22	0.60-9.38
Sectorwide approach	**14.30**	**0.02**	**1.57-130.01**	**8.89**	**0.03**	**1.21-65.42**
Project inputs						
Salaries (none)	0.88	0.84	0.24-3.15	2.01	0.25	0.61-6.60
Training (none)	1.60	0.63	0.23-11.21	0.54	0.60	0.05-5.39
Technical assistance (none)	2.45	0.39	0.32-18.92	0.69	0.76	0.07-6.93
Pharmaceuticals (none)	1.39	0.63	0.37-5.18	0.54	0.39	0.14-2.17
Equipment (none)	0.50	0.42	0.09-2.68	1.20	0.86	0.16-9.06
Buildings (none)	1.97	0.34	0.50-7.82	3.69	0.10	0.79-17.29
Software (none)	2.63	0.14	0.73-9.52	1.27	0.71	0.36-4.45
Project activities						
Human resource systems (none)	0.22	0.17	0.02-1.96	0.62	0.69	0.06-6.50
Health services management (none)	1.25	0.76	0.29-5.40	4.59	0.06	0.93-22.69
Logistics systems (none)	0.62	0.42	0.19-2.00	3.69	0.05	1.02-13.41
Contracting (none)	**4.12**	**0.04**	**1.07-15.94**	**1.03**	**0.97**	**0.31-3.42**
Regulations (none)	1.23	0.72	0.39-3.84	0.57	0.34	0.18-1.79
Public involvement in planning (none)	1.59	0.50	0.42-6.08	1.37	0.66	0.34-5.49

Country policy and inst. assessment

(Low: <3)						
Moderate: 3–3.5	0.28	0.17	0.04–1.75	0.92	0.92	0.17–4.99
High: >3.5	2.00	0.39	0.41–9.62	1.76	0.47	0.37–8.25
Region						
(Africa)						
East Asia and Pacific	1.56	0.66	0.22–11.17	1.21	0.84	0.19–7.65
Europe and Central Asia	4.01	0.20	0.47–34.19	0.29	0.32	0.03–3.28
Latin America and the Caribbean	1.98	0.55	0.21–18.46	0.46	0.49	0.05–4.18
Middle East and North Africa	2.37	0.53	0.16–34.31	0.65	0.75	0.05–8.64
South Asia	0.89	0.90	0.15–5.22	3.21	0.20	0.54–19.02
Economy						
(Low-income)						
Lower-middle-income	0.14	0.07	0.02–1.19	1.83	0.56	0.24–14.05
Upper-middle-income	1.17	0.90	0.12–11.58	1.27	0.84	0.12–13.54
N		118			118	
Pseudo R^2		0.274			0.226	

Source: Authors.

Note: Parentheses indicate reference group. Too few projects evaluated changes in health financing to be included in the regression. Statistically significant relationships are in bold.

CHAPTER 8

Seven Country Case Studies

Sameh El-Saharty, Katja Janovsky,
Banafsheh Siadat, and Finn Schleimann

Summary

Objectives: To describe the strategies of significant scale for strengthening health services delivery in the real-life context in which they occurred in seven low-income countries.

Methods: Case studies involved mixed methods of document reviews, key informant interviews, and quantitative analysis of data from the seven countries.

Key messages:

- Each country situation is unique. Hence generalizations and comparisons across countries are limited.
- Success in implementation of the selected health services delivery strategies is driven largely by several factors related to the country-specific macro environment, to the health sector micro environment, or to both.
- As the country context changes, the health system components also evolve in response to the changing environment.

(continued)

- In virtually no country can overall health services improvements be linked to a particular strategy.
- Political stability, security, and economic growth, as well as legislation, regulation, and the capacity to monitor and enforce, are all macro-environment factors—mainly related to the country context—that influence how strategies are implemented. They are usually outside the control of the "strategy implementers."
- Leadership, the status of NGOs and faith-based organizations, the size of donor support, and aid approaches are factors related to the health sector (the micro environment) that are not under the control of the strategy implementers. But these elements should be seriously examined and considered as they directly influence how the strategy is implemented.
- A set of "strategy-related" factors was found to be critical. These factors are directly related to the design, adaptation, and implementation of the strategy, and are usually under the control of the strategy implementers. They include: seizing the "boost" of new beginnings, ensuring capacity building as a central tenet, modulating the pace of implementation, balancing supply- and demand-side interventions, anticipating consequences and resource requirements for going to scale, and recognizing the fragility of reforms and the need for their institutionalization.

Introduction

This chapter reviews the implementation of a range of health services delivery strategies and the factors that influenced the results achieved in seven countries: Afghanistan, Ethiopia, Ghana, Rwanda, Uganda, Vietnam, and Zambia. These country cases were selected on the basis of a grant, which was provided by the Government of the Netherlands to investigate health services in low-income countries, and which was intended to include a range of countries, particularly in Africa, that had undertaken efforts to improve health services through decentralization, public oversight, or community empowerment strategies over the previous 10 years. The initial seven countries were selected after widespread consultations within the World Bank. The rationale for selection is outlined in table 8.1.

The aim of this chapter is to reach a better understanding of how similar strategies were implemented in different contexts. It considers the impetus for adopting a particular strategy, identifies key drivers of change,

Table 8.1   Rationale for Selection of Countries Based on Strategies to Strengthen Health Services

Country	Strategies pursued
Afghanistan	Postconflict innovations involving contracting strategies to improve the performance of state and nonstate providers
Ethiopia	Decentralization of health service responsibilities to local governments, improving access through rehabilitation and expansion of health facilities, health extension package of services, and introduction of a new cadre of health workers
Ghana	Longstanding SWAp with decentralization of funds to subnational levels, but with an entrenched institutional conflict at central level between the Ministry of Health and the health services delivery agency (Ghana Health Service), and initiation of a community planning and monitoring approach (Community-based Health Planning and Services) with a new cadre of health workers and numerous pilot studies in service organization
Rwanda	Numerous policy reforms, including scaling up of contracts to districts and communities for health behaviors, contracts to nonstate providers to improve performance, and micro-insurance approaches
Uganda	Significant decentralization strategies and a large influx of disease-specific funding (HIV/AIDS and malaria) and social marketing approaches
Vietnam	Rapid decentralization across sectors with evolving institutions, and rapid increases in health services delivery coverage across sectors
Zambia	Longstanding SWAp with decentralization of funds to subnational levels

Source: Authors.

examines the enabling and inhibiting factors, and sets out the results achieved. It identifies issues and lessons learned on the basis of the country case studies. These studies show that successes and failures of particular strategies cannot be divorced from the specific context in which they were implemented. Nevertheless, collectively they do highlight a set of systemic issues related to health services strengthening strategies, potentially providing lessons for policy makers and development professionals that are applicable beyond the individual case studies.

Research Questions

Each of the seven country case studies sought to address the following broad questions:

- Which strategies to improve service delivery that were intended to be of significant scale were adopted and implemented?
- Where did the ideas and the impetus for the strategy come from: local, national, or international sources?

- How has the implementation of the strategies under review been organized and managed, including political advocacy and management?
- What were the pace and degree of implementation, including sequencing and relationships to other strategies?
- What factors in the health sector and in the broader macro environment, including enabling and inhibiting conditions, have influenced adoption, implementation, and outcomes?
- What results have been achieved?
- Are there discernable intended or unintended benefits to the poor?
- What lessons have been learned that are likely to be applicable and useful in other countries?

The answers to these questions have been synthesized across the country case studies and are presented in the rest of this chapter.

Methods

The country case studies, using mixed methodologies, identify how these low-income countries have adopted and implemented strategies to improve health services. A detailed and standardized terms of reference was developed for use in each country to identify the key strategies to improve health services, understand their development, and identify the critical stakeholders and factors affecting implementation.

The specific objectives were to:

- describe strategies to strengthen health services in the real-life context in which they occurred;
- illustrate how adoption and implementation of health systems strategies relate to their context across a variety of LIC settings;
- explore a situation in which an intervention being evaluated has no clear, single set of outcomes; and
- investigate the presumed causal links between program components and program effects in real-life interventions that are too complex for survey research or experimental strategies.

Each country case study involved: (i) collection and analysis of documentation of significant health service improvement strategies in the recent past (5–10 years) in the selected country; (ii) central- and periphery-level field interviews of critical stakeholders in-country to identify their role and assessment of health strategy development and implementation processes, examining both the intended health service outcomes and key unintended consequences; and (iii) identification and analysis of enabling and inhibiting factors and conditions at the macro-environment, health sector, and strategy levels that affected the strategy's adoption and implementation.

Limitations

This chapter presents summaries of in-depth country case studies; hence, detailed country-specific findings are not presented here. The following section highlights only the major findings of each strategy pursued, which are extracted from the background case studies for this chapter.

It is also important to highlight the challenges in conducting a comparative analysis across countries. Success in implementation of the selected health services delivery strategies is driven largely by several factors related to the country-specific macro environment and/or to the health sector micro environment. Many of the results observed are highly contextual and hence generalizations and comparisons across countries are limited. Moreover, as the country context changes, the health system components also evolve and adapt in response to the changing environment. This dynamic relationship makes it even more difficult to ascribe some of the enabling and inhibiting factors to a particular health system component that is constantly adapting.

Importantly, there are also limitations in attributing the observed results (for example, health outcomes, health service outputs) to a specific strategy, particularly when there is usually concurrent implementation of multiple strategies in any given country. In addition, the sequencing of the strategies under investigation within a given country, often in a phased manner, or incrementally but not adhering to plans, further limits the tracing of causal linkages. Finally, given that many of the strategies were implemented only recently, it is difficult to ascertain how these strategies have affected health services delivery in both the medium and long term. In many instances, only the immediate or short-term effects were observed during field visits.

Hence, this chapter focuses more on how the strategies were implemented and what factors influenced their results. It also provides some interpretation of the relationship between the strategies under review and observed outcomes, although it cannot establish direct causality or attribution.

Country Findings

This section provides an overview of key health services delivery strategies of significant scale for each of the seven countries.

Afghanistan

Afghanistan is an important example of a country emerging from conflict. It has pursued innovations in service delivery strategies, under four headings.

Capacity building. Between 2002 and 2004, there was a strong focus on institutional capacity building. However, since 2005 capacity building has been more narrowly focused on the training of individuals (health worker capacity building). There has also been a massive influx of expatriate expertise, much of it in the form of technical assistance (TA), amounting to approximately $1.6 billion since 2002.

The key stakeholders driving capacity building were the main international development partners in so far as they provided TA to strengthen capacity—successful or otherwise. On the other hand, the government, specifically the Ministry of Public Health (MOPH), also had a keen interest in seeing capacity further developed. Management Sciences for Health (MSH), a United States-based NGO, has undertaken much of the work in capacity building (i.e. in terms of human resource development) with the ministry, bolstered with funds from the United States Agency for International Development (USAID).

Health worker capacity building specifically, as well as other strategies in Afghanistan, was well resourced and was therefore rapidly implemented. The concurrent and near-simultaneous nature of this and other strategies has been pivotal to their collective success.

Notably, there has been a tremendous degree of variation in the quality of TA received within the MOPH and there is recognition at present of the need to improve coordination of TA among donors and for donors to relinquish much of the control they have over TA. Some have seen capacity building as driving the short-term objectives of donors, rather than meeting local needs.

Public sector reorganization. In mid-2002, the public administration reform program (PAR), a government-wide multi-donor-supported initiative, was established to strengthen the bureaucracy. One aspect of PAR is the priority reform and restructuring program (PRR) which was planned as an interim measure (2002–05) to restore vital administrative capacity.

The PRR was also designed to help ensure consistency across ministries pursuing reforms with the support of different donors.

Generally, reorganization of the public sector through PAR and PRR was supported by the multi-donor trust fund (ARTF)—with strong interest from the MOPH. PAR and PRR were rapid and well-resourced initiatives, particularly between 2002 and 2004. The public reorganization strategies were also implemented concurrently with health worker capacity building, along with public oversight and community empowerment strategies. However, PRR is to be discontinued and supplanted by a more comprehensive pay and grading reform that will include merit-based appointments, vetting procedures, and performance-based reviews.

Contracting out with nonstate providers and contracting in at MOPH. Health services delivery is contracted out to nonstate providers in four-fifths of the country's 34 provinces, with the financial support of three major donors (World Bank, USAID, and European Commission), and with strong buy-in from NGOs that provide health services. All contracting involves the provision of a basic package of health services. The contracts affiliated with each donor are designed differently, reflecting different approaches to aid management and concerns over the capacity of NGOs to deliver services across an entire province.

Three of the 34 provinces deliver health services through the Ministry of Public Health Strengthening Mechanism (MOPH-SM). The MOPH-SM has become a form of contracting in with the recruitment of managers into the MOPH itself, and includes performance incentives based on third-party evaluation. The remaining districts and provinces are supported through routine MOPH support, often with small NGOs.

The impetus for both contracting-out and contracting-in stemmed from international development partners. Contracting out in Afghanistan was an internationally driven strategy, promoted by the World Bank. Although real collaboration was seen among many important stakeholders in initial discussions, NGOs were marked by their absence. The MOPH was to a certain extent on the sidelines, hampered by its lack of exposure to current technical issues, scarcity of interpreters, and the numerous competing demands made on it by the international community.

Early on, one of the major concerns among some health stakeholders was that there was to be a "big bang" approach in the first year post-conflict in Afghanistan, in contrast to Cambodia where, even seven years after the end of the conflict, basic health services had been contracted out to NGOs in only a few districts. Moreover, many personnel also had moral and ethical concerns, as they questioned the assumptions that the public sector was too weak to be strengthened to deliver health services; that NGOs had a better capacity to manage services even on a large scale that included the district hospital level; and that NGOs were too few to ensure a valid competitive process. There was also concern that contracting out was the first step toward the privatization of health services.

The various contracting mechanisms were carried out rapidly, made possible by the substantial donor support. To aim for effective management of the various contracting strategies, World Bank funds were used to establish and provide running costs for the Grants and Contract Management Unit (GCMU) within the MOPH's Policy and Planning Department. The GCMU is a well-functioning unit that employs local staff as consultants. With respect to contracting out, the GCMU manages the contracting processes involved with nonstate providers. The GCMU also manages funds for the MOPH-SM (contracting-in facilities), hiring managers at market rates to help bolster the delivery of basic health services. However, the GCMU's functions have been questioned, since the unit has taken on tasks that could potentially sit in other MOPH departments.

Figure 8.1   Health Services Indicators, Afghanistan

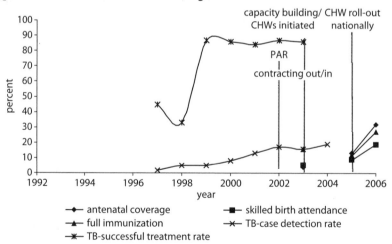

Source: Afghanistan Ministry of Public Health, 2006 Afghanistan Health Survey (AHS); Japanese Institute of Public Health database (TB figures only).

Note: Data on child bednet use and HIV knowledge not available. Antenatal coverage: reflects trends in skilled antenatal coverage use in rural Afghanistan from 2003 Multiple Indicator Cluster Survey (MICS), 2005 National Risk and Vulnerability Assessment (NRVA), and 2006 AHS. Skilled birth attendance: reflects trends in use of skilled birth attendance in rural Afghanistan from 2003 MICS, 2005 NRVA, and 2006 AHS. Full immunization: reflects rural median from 2003 MICS, 2005 NRVA, and 2006 AHS, for children aged 12–23 months fully vaccinated, i.e., BCG, measles, three doses of DPT and polio (excluding polio 0).

Results from a third-party evaluation of the basic package of health services have shown that each of the contracting sites (three types of contracting out and the contracting in) have outperformed the noncontracted facilities in terms of coverage of services, reaching women and the poor, and improving different dimensions of quality. There is no clear leader among the different contracting approaches, as different types of facilities have performed differently according to the various measures of performance. Those facilities with management autonomy tended to have the largest improvements in structural areas, such as the provision of drugs and contraceptives. It is also clear that the government, through the GCMU, has been able to manage contracts effectively. This is a notable achievement given that there was no simultaneous approach to reform elements of central government bureaucracy. In addition, both contracting out and MOPH-SM–supported services have benefited the poor through other means, such as exemptions for user fees.

Expanding access through community health workers. Community health workers were deployed to provide populations in remote and rural areas with access to basic health services. The MOPH has executed several measures through NGOs to train and equip CHWs. CHW homes were expected to serve as community health posts which, consisting of two trained CHWs, were to serve a catchment area of 1,000–1,500 people and provide a limited array of curative services. The use of CHWs was supported by the MOPH, with key financial backing from WHO.

Afghanistan health services delivery trends. This case study found that there have been important improvements in the delivery of health services since 2002, though there is no single strategy that can claim the credit. The various strategies analyzed in this study have been developed concurrently, and are complementary to each other and closely linked. Importantly, their concurrent development, rather than sequencing, appears critical, as they are mutually reinforcing.

Ethiopia

Ethiopia is a country at a crossroads in development. Several reforms have been implemented since the 1990s in different sectors, yet many challenges remain. In the health sector, a 20-year Health Sector Development Program was developed. This program focused primarily on maternal and child health programs such as reproductive health and immunization; communicable diseases such as malaria and HIV/AIDS; and nutritional disorders. It was implemented in the context of a broader government strategy of "decentralization." In this study, we examined the implementation of "government decentralization" as the primary strategy together with other "corollary" strategies at the national level, as well as an assessment of strategies pursued in four (out of nine) regions: Amhara; Oromia; Southern Nations, Nationalities, and People's Region (SNNPR); and Afar.

Government decentralization. Government decentralization in Ethiopia was initiated in 1994 in the form of "devolution of authority and accountability" to manage public services.

Devolution was conceptualized, initiated, and driven by the federal government, with strong support from donor agencies. Implementation occurred in two phases: devolution of authority to the regional level (phase 1) and, subsequently, to the district (*woreda*) level (phase 2). The corollary strategies under devolution were implemented simultaneously in each phase. However, the first phase was extremely delayed (the Constitution was approved in 1994 but implementation of health sector changes really began in 1998). The first phase of implementation was relatively slow, with implementation varying significantly across strategies and regions. The second phase was introduced in 2002, even though many regions still had weak capacity, and were not in a position to manage further devolution to the districts. Whereas it may have been technically sound to modulate the implementation of the second phase to match regional and district capacity, it was seen as politically unfeasible to exclude certain regions from the process.

Under devolution, the federal government retained authority over policy development and strategic planning, while delegating the organization and management of local services to regional authorities. Authority over fund allocation to each region remained centralized, but was dictated by a formula accounting for population size, poverty level, and degree of development, which is approved by the Parliament and which intends to ensure equitable distribution of resources.

Regional health bureaus maintained equal authority and responsibility under decentralized regional governments to manage health services and implement the corollary strategies. These bureaus were mainly accountable to regional government authorities as well as to the federal Ministry of Health. Notably, the organization of health services related to the corollary strategies varied significantly across regions because of a variety of factors, including: the stability of the regional health management team; the capacity of the team to manage health programs in their respective areas; and the ability of the team to mobilize local resources for the implementation of the Health Sector Development Program.

Figure 8.2   Health Services Indicators, Ethiopia

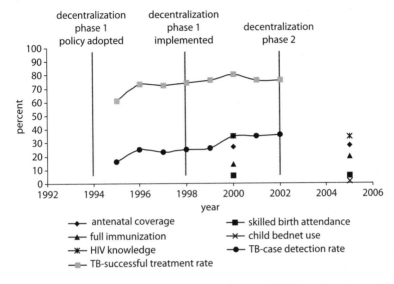

Source: Ethiopia Demographic and Health Survey 2000, 2005. TB Rates from WHO "Making Health Systems Work" working series.

Note: The reference period is five years preceding the survey. Antenatal coverage: % of mothers receiving antenatal care from health professionals (doctor, nurse, midwife) for their most recent birth in the five years preceding the survey. Skilled birth attendance: % of births delivered with the assistance of a trained health professional, that is, a doctor, nurse, or midwife. Full immunization: children aged 12–23 months fully vaccinated, i.e., BCG, measles, three doses of DPT and polio (excluding polio 0). HIV knowledge: % of women who know that HIV/AIDS can be prevented by using condoms and limiting sex to one uninfected partner. Child bednet use: % who slept under an insecticide-treated bednet the previous night.

At the subnational level, these strategies required collaboration between regions and districts. In 2002–03, the Amhara, SNNPR, and Oromia regional governments enacted laws that established district government structures in their localities. In turn, district governments received a budget in the form of block grants from regional governments and distributed these funds among public sector government offices, including those in health, in accordance with district priorities. District governments were, in turn, responsible for all economic development and social services within the district. Implementation, however, varied significantly across districts and was directly linked to the degree of development and management capacity at the regional level.

Corollary strategies. Devolution of authority and accountability in managing health services to subnational levels included the following corollary strategies: improving health services delivery and quality of primary health care, through facility expansion and rehabilitation; expanding access to primary health care; human resource development; improving availability of pharmaceuticals; strengthening information, education, and communication; improving health sector management; and improving health care financing.

The various strategies were implemented with different degrees of success. Decentralization to the regional level had a positive impact on improving health outputs. However, these results started from a very low baseline level. Two corollary strategies were successfully implemented and even exceeded the planned targets: the strategy for improving access through rehabilitation and expansion of facilities, which increased coverage; and the strategy for human resource development through health extension workers, which filled a critical gap in primary health care, particularly in rural and remote areas.

In contrast, the unavailability of essential drugs remained problematic. The implementation of information and communications activities fell short of stimulating greater demand for the available services. Management capacity increased in some areas more than others, and the health management information systems that were needed to support management remained fragile. Finally, the health care financing strategy succeeded in mobilizing some additional resources from the donor community, but did little to increase overall per capita health spending. Public funding to the health sector was reduced due to the conflict with Eritrea, which contributed to stagnation in the performance of health services. Donor funding played a key role in protecting some basic health services, particularly for child health, but also led to an increased dependence on donor financing.

At the subnational level, decentralization was more effective in those regions that increasingly strengthened their management and institutional capacity and where regional governments were able to prioritize their needs and adapt corollary strategies to local needs. However, the effectiveness of decentralization was influenced by limited community voice in the local decision-making process, which made the available resources subject to political influence.

Ethiopia health services delivery trends. This case study found observed improvements in health outcomes, but these could not be attributed to the strategies implemented. At the regional level, the results achieved in the SNNPR were overall better than in the other three regions, mainly due to the stability and management capacity of the regional health management team, and its ability to mobilize local resources.

Ghana

Health sector reform in Ghana has been marked by two distinct changes in recent years. First, the 1997 first Program of Work, as part of a SWAp, involved a large pooled-funding arrangement for external donors, and focused on providing increased and flexible resources to improve health services delivery at the district level. The second major change followed a 2001 government transition, and was characterized by the creation of a National Health Insurance Scheme (NHIS), which was intended to eventually replace the "cash and carry" user-fee system (an election promise), and the full operationalization of the Ghana Health Service (GHS) agency model for service delivery.

Decentralization of budgeting and planning. Due to dynamic leadership in the 1990s within the Ministry of Health, which initially focused on strengthening district health management teams and promoting capable district medical officers, the health sector institutionalized a model of deconcentration through "budget and management centres" under the first Program of Work. While decentralization of budgeting went down to the subdistrict level, the accounting took place at the district level (and above), reflecting a compromise between the desire to provide more autonomy to lower levels while still assuring proper financial management. All district and subdistrict budget and management centres involved in accounting had to be certified in accordance with specific readiness criteria to handle funds and, if they did not qualify, the level above them would manage the finances on their behalf until they had rectified the shortfalls. The budget and management centre system is still functional. In some observers' view, the biggest problem has been that, in many districts, subdistricts have little autonomy due to their lack of direct control over funds, and it seems that some districts use their control to favor district-level expenditures (rather than handing down funds to the subdistricts).

Initially, a key part of the decentralization reform was performance-based service agreements, a type of internal contracting within the public budgeting framework, which was introduced at the subdistrict and district levels in 1997. In regions where there was a serious attempt to introduce such contracts, evidence suggests that they had the promise of both motivating health workers and changing the incentives for their behavior. However, the initiative was short-lived. A major problem was that the promise of timely funding was not kept, which undermined the concept of committing to locally negotiated targets within nationally set indicators on the basis of a known budget ceiling. Another issue may have been the lack of confidence in subdistrict staff by higher managers, or even their reluctance to relinquish control.

Another set of performance contracts was attempted between the Ministry of Health and GHS, and with faith-based NGO providers. But the contracts between the GHS and the Ministry were rendered meaningless by the power struggle between them.

Establishment of the Ghana Health Service agency model. This model was introduced in 1996, but only fully implemented beginning in 2001. It is responsible for service delivery at the regional level and below, while the Ministry of Health retains the main policy-setting role. It has clearly illustrated the problems of strong but conflicting leadership, and the complexities associated with establishing two apex institutions in a country with fairly weak regulation, and with systems characterized by excessive negotiations of power. These problems were thoroughly analyzed by government and with external experts, but have not been acted on in a decisive way. The change of government in 2001 resulted in the placement of new staff perceived loyal to the new government within the Ministry of Health, and many senior staff transferred to the GHS. Personality conflicts and political rivalries were brought to the forefront through structures that seemed to compete with each other for resources and authority. Some observers are of the view that a model based on regional agencies might have been able to combine the advantages of both systems and avoid some of the major drawbacks. This power struggle has likely impaired the sector's performance, particularly at the central level. Recent changes in leadership may bring an opportunity to improve relationships and resolve conflicts between the two organizations.

Introduction of the national health insurance scheme. The NHIS consists of independent district-based mutual health insurance schemes supported by a National Health Insurance Fund. Membership for government employees is compulsory and financed out of their existing Social Security and National Insurance Trust contributions. Other members, apart primarily from indigents, pay a fairly low premium. A 2.5 percent levy using the same mechanism as the existing general value-added tax (VAT) provides most of the NHIS financing.

The introduction of NHIS was driven by an election promise. The initial implementation left much to be desired, but the arrival of competent management has the promise of realizing far-reaching reforms. With enrollment reaching 55 percent and actual cardholders 42 percent of the population (2007), combined with the high overall sector funding and the acceptability of the "health VAT" as a financing source, the NHIS seems fairly consolidated. There remains a risk of financial collapse, ironically because of its success in increasing enrollment. Many nonindigent poor people are excluded from insurance coverage, and face relatively high user charges at government facilities. The government has only recently started to address this problem by looking into modalities for the Ministry of Health to pay premiums for the poor.

The first lesson drawn from the implementation of the NHIS is how the government, faced with strong reluctance from donor partners (based on the judgment that the scheme was financially unsustainable and unlikely to achieve high coverage or promote equity), chooses to rely on domestic advice, partly from Ghanaians living abroad. The second is that the political imperative and individual interests initially led to subpar implementation, but impressive enrollment rates. A third lesson is how the autonomous National Health Insurance Board can change senior NHIS management and introduce a technically capable leadership.

Collaboration with nonstate providers. Ghana, like most other countries, has policies to guide private sector involvement in health, but has seen no major developments for several years. The longstanding tradition of paying staff salaries in faith-based organizations, and the payment of a part of their running costs, have made financing of the private not-for-profit (PNFP) sector in Ghana more robust than in, for example, Uganda. Also, the collaboration and trust between the two systems seem to work better in Ghana. Considering that institutions affiliated with the Christian Health Association of Ghana deliver close to 40 percent of health services, the Association has played too little a role in shaping policies and strategies. Recently, there have been attempts to strengthen the Association's capacity in this respect.

Introduction of community-based health planning and services. The Community-based Health Planning and Services (CHPS) strategy aims at placing a nurse with the necessary resources and support in communities that lack access to health services, particularly in poor areas. This involved a bottom-up process of consultations with communities and the training of CHWs. Output-linked incentives to CHWs were provided.

The CHPS model arose from intervention research (the Community Health and Family Planning Experiment initiated in 1994) conducted by the Navrongo Health Research Center. The experiment had considerable

Figure 8.3   Health Services Indicators, Ghana

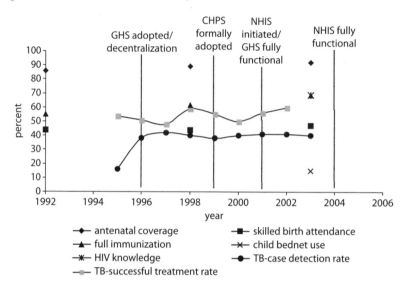

Source: Ghana Demographic and Health Survey 2003; TB rates from WHO "Making Health Systems Work" working series.

Note: The reference period is five years preceding the survey except for 1993, which refers to three years. Antenatal coverage: for women who had a live birth prior to survey. Skilled birth attendance: medically assisted deliveries. Full immunization: children aged 12–23 months fully vaccinated, i.e., BCG, measles, three doses of DPT and polio (excluding polio 0). HIV knowledge: % of women who know that HIV/AIDS can be prevented by using condoms and limiting sex to one uninfected partner. Child bednet use: % who slept under an insecticide-treated bednet the previous night.

buy-in from key decision makers in the health system, and CHPS was formally adopted by the Ministry of Health in 1999. Key elements of the CHPS include a community health nurse retrained to become a community health officer; a community health compound including essential equipment and community health volunteers; and modalities for community participation.

Having been successfully replicated outside a research scenario, the CHPS strategy was included in the second Program of Work (2002–06) and rolled out at a greater pace. The original Program of Work II target was for 1,570 functional CHPS but, in 2005, this was adjusted to only 400. Targets for rolling out the CHPS became part of the PRSP (2005), which many feared would mean too much attention on construction and less on the crucial community and planning components. Insufficient budget allocations have resulted in the lack of infrastructure becoming an important limiting factor, although reports also note that, where construction has actually taken place, community entry activities are also lagging behind.

Whereas all districts have taken the first step and established CHPS zones, the number of fully functional CHPS in 2006 was only around 200. This figure may be an underestimate as it excludes construction by local government authorities. Other constraints have been insufficient personnel and problems in finding appropriate places for CHPS zones. There have thus been considerable problems in scaling up the CHPS strategy. However, the government and its partners still see it as a key strategy.

Ghana health services delivery trends. Although there have been slow and mixed changes in health services in Ghana, the overall results cannot be linked to particular strategies. It is easy to cite the conflict between the Ministry of Health and the GHS as undermining the enabling environment, but attributing the lack of more substantial progress in health services to this is rather speculative. The deconcentration model for reassigning responsibilities and resources within the public health sector seems to have been implemented fairly well. There may have been missed opportunities to further integrate with the local government system, but it is difficult to predict what effect that would have. The level of collaboration between the health sector (GHS) and local government differs from district to district, and has depended on individual managers within both systems. On the other hand, there are similarities between the creation of the NHIS, establishment of the budget and management centres, and implementation of the CHPS strategy in terms of strong buy-in from national decision makers and strong national involvement in the development of the concepts. However, both the latter strategies received considerable external support. In contrast, the attempt to shift to performance-based service agreements in 1997 was less thoroughly prepared and probably had too little support among key stakeholders.

Rwanda

Rwanda has largely emerged from its 1994 genocide. Its health system has settled into a decentralized model of care with a prominent role for faith-based providers. Health strategies have had a high profile in the country, with the president directly involved in their promotion. Within this context, the Rwanda case study has focused on three health services delivery strategies: fiscal decentralization, performance-based financing, and community health insurance *(mutuelles)*.

Fiscal decentralization. Fiscal decentralization (policy adopted 2001, law enacted 2006) served as an essential component of Rwanda's decentralization agenda to devolve authority to the district level. It involved the transfer of fiscal responsibilities and financial resources to facilities directly, across sectors. Fiscal decentralization involved unearmarked funds in the form of block grants to districts through the Local Authority Budget Support Fund to pay the salaries of administrative district level staff; earmarked transfers to districts for—among other things—health worker salaries and health centers; and other transfers to districts.

The objective was to bring services closer to the people and to improve the financial viability of districts. Fiscal decentralization was rolled out rapidly—perhaps too rapidly—without the necessary support structures in place. For example, until June 2007 districts lacked accounting software to manage financial transactions, and currently local capacity remains limited in managing financial and human resources. (In terms of sequencing, fiscal decentralization was implemented 3–5 years after both the performance-based financing and *mutuelle* pilot schemes were initiated.)

Fiscal decentralization was organized by the central government which, from the outset, determined the degree of authority delegated to local levels and delineated relevant policies and standards. In these efforts, the central government received significant technical assistance and guidance from multiple development partners that organized their support in the form of a SWAp. Decentralized units at local levels had the authority to manage the flow of funds (once received) as well as the delivery of health services. In essence, decentralization has transformed health facilities into autonomous entities, with the ability to manage financial and human resources as they deem most appropriate, according to local needs. This includes complete control over the hiring and firing of health personnel.

Performance-based financing. Performance-based financing (PBF)—modeled on the principle of separating purchaser–provider functions—involved the purchase of outputs by the Ministry of Health, rather than the financing of inputs, on the basis of facilities' performance across a range of indicators taken from the basic package of health services. PBF also drew on contracting schemes in Afghanistan and Cambodia.

The motivation for PBF came from the low quality of services and the need to improve quality so as to increase *mutuelle* membership. The government implemented PBF in order to provide additional incentives to health workers to improve efficiency and outcomes. Additional support came from international actors who financed the pilot schemes. Based on the success of these pilot projects, the central government then pushed the expansion of PBF coverage.

The pace of implementation of the PBF strategy, like most reforms in Rwanda, was remarkably fast. PBF was complementary to the *mutuelle* strategy, and was initiated in 2002, soon after *mutuelle* schemes with NGO support. PBF was expanded to 23 districts (out of 30 districts nationwide) in the next phase, using a national PBF model that is a hybrid of the original three pilot schemes. The seven remaining districts are adopting the national PBF model in the last phase.

In terms of the organization of PBF, the Ministry of Health is responsible for the establishment of norms and standards within the national health policy whereas the district, as a decentralized body, is responsible for management and oversight of day-to-day operations. A system to administer PBF payments is based on the collaboration of a pool of technical assistants from 11 Ministry of Health departments and technical agencies.

A steering committee has been established in each district to independently monitor health center performance indicators that, in turn, determine the amount of funding received by each center. This committee includes representatives of local health bodies, the community, and *mutuelles*. PBF at the district hospital level is managed through an informal structure in which three or four district hospitals peer review one another's work. Reports on the peer evaluation are then sent to the central level authority on PBF for final review.

Community health insurance (mutuelles). Community health insurance (prepayment) schemes were designed to spread the financial risk of seeking care across their membership base. The goal was to respond to the low utilization of health services (due in part to user fees) by improving financial access to health services, particularly for underserved populations. The package of services reimbursed by *mutuelles* to health facilities has expanded over time, and currently covers all services delivered within a health center as well as drugs from the national essential drug list. *Mutuelles* also cover the majority of costs for health services and drugs delivered at district and referral hospitals, when *mutuelle* members receive referrals for these higher levels of care.

In essence, the adoption of *mutuelles* in Rwanda reflected a bottom-up strategy, driven largely by local communities, and were particularly motivated by the success of the initial pilot schemes. Subsequently, the strategy was driven and scaled up by the central government. Currently, it is the central government that sets forth national guidelines and policies, including *mutuelles'* management capacities financial sustainability and package of services; their partnerships with health facilities; community

Figure 8.4   Health Services Indicators, Rwanda

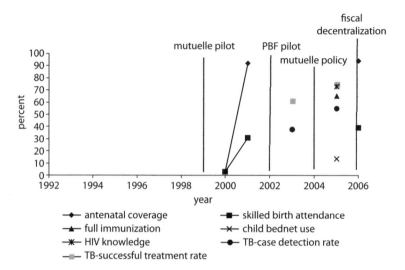

Source: Ministry of Health Annual Reports 2003, 2004, 2005; Rwanda Demographic and Health Survey 2005.

Note: The reference period is five years preceding the survey. Antenatal coverage: % of women receiving antenatal coverage from a skilled provider (at least 1 visit). Skilled birth attendance: % of births delivered with the assistance of a trained health professional, that is, a doctor, nurse, or midwife. Full immunization: children aged 12–23 months fully vaccinated, i.e., BCG, measles, three doses of DPT and polio (excluding polio 0). HIV knowledge: % of women who know that HIV/AIDS can be prevented by using condoms and limiting sex to one uninfected partner. Child bednet use: proportion of children under 5 who slept under an insecticide-treated bednet the previous night.

involvement; and monitoring and evaluation. At the local level however, *mutuelles* are organized and run by community representatives and local health care providers. They also serve as a forum to promote dialogue between the community and providers on the quality and range of health services offered. In this way, community members are better able to hold providers accountable for services delivered.

Rwanda health services delivery trends. Although implementation of fiscal decentralization, PBF, and community health insurance have likely contributed to marked improvements within the health sector, in terms of both health service outputs and health outcomes, these gains should be examined against the backdrop of a doubling in per capita health expenditure, from $17 to $34 between 2003 and 2006.

Uganda
The Uganda health reforms presented in the 2000/01–2004/05 Health Sector Strategic Plan (HSSP), covered all aspects of the health system,

including financing and user fees, the latter of which were abolished (March 2001) within public health facilities (with the exception of private wings in hospitals), leading to a surge in use of primary health care services within the public sector, particularly among the rural poor. The HSSP also highlighted the need to further scale up those disease-specific programs that had proved successful in a given area.

In addition to the three strategies now highlighted, this case study examines supportive supervision as a cross-cutting dimension. The ideas for reform are largely home grown, albeit with considerable inputs from the international community in the context of an emerging SWAp.

Decentralization: Focus on subdistrict and health centers. Decentralization from the district to the subdistrict level was signaled in the 1999 National Health Policy and served as "the big reform" of the HSSP in 2000, and involved two main components: improved referral capacity—each subdistrict was to have an upgraded health center or hospital—and improved day-to-day oversight of all subdistrict health facilities.

Improving the referral capacity took longer than intended. A review of upgraded health center operations in 2006 found that, on average, only half of the expected services were provided and only 22 percent of upgraded health center operating theatres were functional.

Little guidance was provided on implementation in Ministry of Health policy documents for subdistrict oversight functions. Subdistrict management training began nationally four years after the policy was adopted. District health teams were largely excluded, and this is a key reason why there has been little follow-up supervision and mentoring. Several development partners active in subdistrict capacity building reportedly prefer a more harmonized approach, linked to HSSP objectives.

Oversight strategies for nonstate providers. Uganda's Public-Private Partnerships in Health (PPPH) strategy was developed in recognition of the sizable contribution of private providers in the delivery of health services, and of the need to coordinate efforts. A PPPH Unit was established in 2000 and the policy was drafted in 2003. However, the policy was neither formally adopted nor fully implemented. After a short period, resources for the PPPH Unit waned and it has now become largely inactive.

The major nonstate providers are PNFP providers, NGOs, and civil society organizations; and private for-profit providers and drug shops.

Most PNFP providers are faith-based organizations. In 2002 they accounted for 40 percent of hospitals and 34 percent of Uganda's total health workforce. Approximately 86 percent of PNFP providers are located in rural areas. PNFP providers have a long history of collaboration with government. During the 1960s, mission facilities received government subsidies but, during the conflict in the 1970s and 1980s, these ended. However, in 1997, a new and charismatic Minister of Health established a taskforce to work out a new cooperation modality. Subsidies to PNFP providers rose, both as a share of PNFP providers' recurrent budget (from 4 percent in 1997 to 30 percent in 2003/04), and as a share of the total health sector budget (from 0.5 percent to 7 percent in 2002), but they have stagnated since. Salary differentials between PNFP providers and the public sector are a major issue driving the attrition of staff, with losses of key cadres amounting to 20–30 percent in 2006. In terms of results, PNFP provider utilization and productivity increased between 1999 and 2003 as judged by outpatient, inpatient, and delivery statistics. Given that many PNFP facilities are located in poor rural areas, these increases in utilization have been, arguably, pro-poor.

An increasingly large number of NGOs and civil society organizations provide health-related activities. Most service delivery NGOs are international NGOs, such as the African Medical and Research Foundation and Médecins Sans Frontières. The relatively few local NGOs that are directly involved in service delivery tend to have a religious affiliation. Expansion is fairly localized geographically, with both international and local NGOs mushrooming in the post-conflict zone of the north. The creation of many new organizations has been driven by external funds—especially from the U.S. president's Emergency Plan for AIDS Relief and the Global Fund to Fight AIDS, TB, and Malaria. Limited oversight is provided by the Uganda Aids Commission, but international NGOs and donors are the most direct source of contact for many NGOs.

The private for-profit sector is large and diverse, but information on it is scant. Moreover, the current legal framework for the licensing and regulation of health workers and facilities is fragmented. Professional councils regulate and supervise professional standards. Facilities are also recommended for licensing by the Medical Council but in practice, there is rarely any inspection before licenses are granted. There are a small number of full-time private doctors, nurses, and pharmacists but dual practice is widespread. Legally, a health professional may practice anywhere once registered, but the Medical Council acknowledges this is a gray area and private practice is harder to regulate.

Drug shops are known to be a major source of care, and are believed to often provide substandard drugs and incomplete courses of treatment.

Licensing and inspection of private pharmacies and drug shops are the responsibility of the Uganda National Drug Authority. Inspection is a challenge but some prelicensing inspection of pharmacies and drug shops occurs and has increased. Nevertheless, many unlicensed drug shops remain—in towns and along trade routes, often run by nursing assistants working out of hours.

Community engagement: Village health committees and village health teams. Community participation has long been a key element of national policy in many sectors. In health, the many approaches have had multiple objectives: community empowerment for health development, service delivery oversight and accountability, and actual service delivery. In the 1970s and 1980s, several NGOs supported community-based health care through village health committees and CHWs, but this lost momentum in the 1990s as financial support waned and a new approach emerged.

Figure 8.5   Health Services Indicators, Uganda

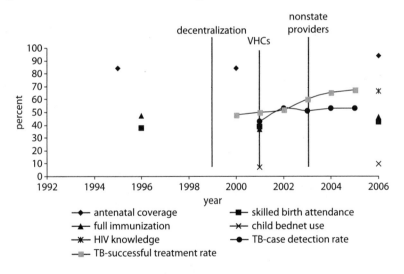

Source: Deliveries, full immunization, and TB rates from Uganda annual Health Sector Performance reports. TB rates from WHO "Making Health Systems Work" working series. Child bednet use and HIV knowledge from Uganda Demographic and Health Survey 2006. Historical data from Demographic and Health Survey 1995.

Note: The reference period is five years preceding the survey. Antenatal coverage: % of women receiving antenatal coverage from a skilled provider. Skilled birth attendance: % of births delivered with the assistance of a trained health professional, that is, a doctor, nurse, or midwife. Full immunization: children aged 12–23 months fully vaccinated, i.e., BCG, measles, three doses of DPT and polio (excluding polio 0). HIV knowledge: % of women who know that HIV/AIDS can be prevented by using condoms and limiting sex to one uninfected partner. Child bednet use: % who slept under an insecticide-treated bednet the previous night.

In 2000, HSSP introduced village health committees in every village as part of the health delivery system. Voluntarism was central to the concept. Although an implementation strategy was approved in 2001, the lack of clear conceptualization and a fragmented process led to delays. The village health team approach—consisting of 5 to 10 volunteers, drawn mainly from existing CHWs—was piloted with external support at 30 sites in 30 districts, largely in northern Uganda. However, the two village health team evaluations that were conducted do not provide information on some key aspects of scaling up: the approximate time dedicated per volunteer, the time spent on supervision, and the costs of scaling up and sustaining these teams. Nationwide rollout has been slow and poorly coordinated as scale-up costs had not been fully worked out beforehand, and the implementation seems costly. Sustained supervision is also an issue. Only 65 of 1,190 villages in Mukono and 4 of 61 parishes in Kabarole have village health teams.

Supportive supervision, monitoring, and mentoring. The Ministry of Health began introducing a quality management process that included district supervision as early as 1984. Today, it provides three main types of supervision: integrated supervision, technical supervision, and ad hoc visits in emergency disease outbreaks. Supervision teams were designed as high-level multidisciplinary teams headed by a commissioner to do quarterly, week-long "integrated support supervision" visits to districts and subdistricts. These teams function fairly well overall but with high variability. Individual category programs have continued to carry out technical supervisory visits. While program visits are uncoordinated and may be too many for district staff to easily cope with, the content is more specific, and visits offer more time for discussion. Several district interviewees in this case study considered these visits to be more useful than the integrated support supervision visits.

Uganda health services delivery trends. Although early successes in implementation of the above strategies were enabled by increases in government funding for health, government allocations to districts, growth in subsidies to PNFP providers, a strong Minister of Health who championed change in the health sector, and more flexible funding by donors, these gains were limited, particularly as the strategies under investigation were only partially implemented.

This case study raises the question as to whether too much emphasis was placed on reporting whether targets had been achieved, and not enough on whether the targets (and the strategies) had been the right ones in the first place, whether they were achievable, what adaptations were necessary, and what were the factors hindering progress. This is seen particularly in the village health team approach: revisiting the feasibility of country-wide implementation would have been more useful than attempting to prove the validity of the concept on the basis of a few pilots and some notable successes in the unique postconflict context of northern Uganda.

Vietnam

Since its adoption of market-friendly economic reforms in 1986, Vietnam has become one of the best-performing developing countries in the world, both in terms of economic and human development. It is also pursuing pro-poor policies, which are reflected in two recent health reforms discussed in this case study. The hospital user fees introduced in 1989 and the hospital autonomization policy launched in 2002 were undertaken to promote cost savings, staff morale, and operational efficiencies in government health facilities. To counter the possible adverse effects of user fees, the poor and other disadvantaged groups were initially exempted from paying them and, from 1991, were also given financial protection through various health insurance programs. Crucially, the approach to most of the health sector reforms in Vietnam (including expansion of disease-specific programs) involved initial piloting within a given province or district, followed by efforts to scale up nationally.

Hospital autonomy and user fees. Hospital user fees were introduced in 1989. This move sought to provide financial incentives to health staff to provide services, with fee exemptions for specific groups. Ultimately, greater financial autonomy was granted to health facilities in the context of a much broader public administration reform (PAR) program. In 2002, the central government, as part of the PAR, granted financial autonomy to all revenue-generating public entities, including hospitals. In effect, these entities were given the authority to manage both revenues and expenditures, subject to financial audits and budget approval of relevant state agencies.

Essentially, hospital autonomy reflected a top-down strategy that was developed and organized by the central government. Although the Ministry of Health does not play a direct managerial role, it supports the strategy's user fee policy. Political advocacy is not a relevant issue, as dissent from the policies articulated by the Communist Party is rarely seen. In addition, management of day-to-day operations has been delegated to facilities (for example, with the hospital director granted managerial autonomy to run the hospital), and oversight of the strategy is provided by the provincial Department of Health and the provincial People's Committee.

The pace of implementation has been slow with, for example, only 46 percent of eligible facilities implementing the strategy by 2005, while hospitals in well-off regions and higher-level facilities (such as central hospitals) more rapidly implemented the strategy. No province has fully implemented the strategy in all health facilities, but all provinces have committed to do this.

The financial status of hospitals has improved due to the revenue generated from user fees, and from the cost savings generated by increased efficiency. Initial evidence suggests a shifting of services toward more lucrative, fee-based services.

Social health insurance for the poor and other groups. In 1992, Vietnam introduced a national health insurance program, comprising a compulsory and a voluntary scheme. The poor and other vulnerable groups were not explicitly targeted in these schemes, although a government ordinance in 1995 stipulated coverage for war veterans, orphans, the disabled, and other groups under the compulsory scheme. In 2002, Health Care Funds for the Poor followed, which mandated all national and local public health facilities to provide preventive and curative care free of charge, under guidelines set forth by the Ministry of Health, for the poor and ethnic minorities.

Social health insurance for the poor, like most policies in Vietnam, was mandated by the central government and supported by the Ministry of Health. Actual management, however, is conducted at the provincial level by the Fund Management Board. Political advocacy from the Ministry of Health is apparent only as it relates to setting premiums. The current arrangement leaves room for conflicts of interest, given the multiple roles of the Fund Management Board as insurance payer, service provider, and purchaser.

Implementation was slow initially. At the outset, provinces had the option of choosing between direct reimbursement and prepaid health insurance card schemes, and most opted for direct reimbursement due to capacity constraints. Direct reimbursement was subsequently phased out in 2005 and the move to insurance card schemes began in 2006. These schemes are now implemented in full and, under these, beneficiaries are entitled to the same benefits as individuals under compulsory health insurance.

Figure 8.6   Health Services Indicators, Vietnam

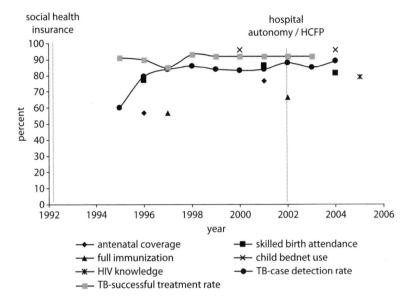

Source: WHO "Making Health Systems Work" working series; Vietnam Demographic and Health Survey 2005; Japanese Institute of Public Health database.

Note: The reference period is five years preceding the survey. Antenatal coverage: % of women receiving antenatal coverage from a skilled provider. Skilled birth attendance: % of births delivered with the assistance of a trained health professional, that is, a doctor, nurse, or midwife. Full immunization: children aged 12–23 months fully vaccinated, i.e., BCG, measles, three doses of DPT and polio (excluding polio 0). HIV knowledge: % of women who know that HIV/AIDS can be prevented by using condoms and limiting sex to one uninfected partner. Child bednet use: % who slept under an insecticide-treated bednet the previous night.

Vietnam health services delivery trends. The World Bank has conducted a preliminary impact evaluation of the health insurance scheme, illustrating that improved targeting (with the poorest quintile accounting for at least 50 percent of the beneficiaries) raised financial protection coverage from 3.3 million to 4.8 million beneficiaries from 2003 to 2005. Utilization of services has also increased, with inpatient admissions rising by 45 percent and outpatient visits by 20 percent.

The financial autonomy policies were part of the government's overall program to modernize state management, though they were not easily applied to the health sector. Although these policies were intended to reduce the fiscal burden of the state and secure additional income for workers, they did not work this way in all places. For example, they did not take into account the weak demand for health services in the poorest regions in the country, where potential hospital revenues are very limited, and where health workers earned little. Outside urban areas or provincial centers, hospital user fees were either not implemented or unsuccessfully implemented because of the reduced demand for health services. These unintended consequences were known early in implementation, yet action was not taken to address them at that time.

The user fee schedules were not based on actual costs of providing the service or on the ability of the buyers to pay, limiting the ability to generate enough user fee revenue to recover recurrent costs or to generate additional resources for capital investments. Whereas income of hospital staff improved in some places, the hospital buildings, medical equipment, and other capital resources remained badly maintained. In some places, a two-tier system resulted, in which nonpaying patients were given less attention than paying patients. With closer monitoring and management, this situation might have been avoided.

Zambia

Zambia faces many challenges in providing an equitable health system for its people. It is a poor nation with one of the highest HIV rates in the world. Infrastructure is not well developed and corruption is significant. Zambia has also been heralded for ambitious plans to decentralize power within the health structure. It has also allowed NGOs to lead service delivery using CHWs, and has encouraged greater community participation.

Decentralization. This process began in the 1990s and marked a significant departure from the previous centralized model. District health management teams received much decision-making power under new district health boards. This provided health districts with a moderate choice over expenditures, user fees, contracting, and governance. Further, actions were taken to create district management capacity and allocate some health financing to districts.

Decentralization involved the sequencing of several reforms initiated between 1992 and 1999, in which new management structures were created, including the development of the Central Board of Health (1995) and the appointment of various district health boards and hospital management boards (1992–93). However, many of them were abolished in 2006, along with user fees in response to a perceived failure of the Central Board of Health to fulfill its mandate by a newly elected government intent on bringing a "new deal" for Zambia that included a focus on health care and a more centralized model of health services delivery.

Impetus for the decentralization strategy had come with a new government in 1991, supported by a core group of health reform champions from the Ministry of Health leaders, academicians, and other prominent government officials. The strategy also had strong popular support. However, opposition emerged at the outset from some Ministry of Health officials, as well as some physicians. The Ministry of Finance and civil service unions would later oppose the strategy, particularly with the transfer of personnel employment contracts from the civil service to district and hospital boards. Frequent changes in the Minister of Health after 1996 also marked the slowing of the reforms and loss of direction and motivation for decentralization at large.

Changes in outputs or health outcomes could not be attributed with any certainty to decentralization, but it is possible that the health of the poor was better as a result of decentralization than it would have been otherwise, given the downward negative trends in most indicators and the impact of HIV/AIDS in the 1990s; these downward trends ultimately leveled off. Such trends must, though, be seen in a context of a marked increase in financing: allocations to the health sector as a proportion of total government expenditures increased from 5.7 percent in 1991 to 13.4 percent in 1994. User fees increased health facility income marginally, although the cost of collection was estimated to exceed the income generated. There also appeared to be substantial declines in utilization of health services, particularly among the poor.

NGO-led services delivery through community health workers. Large-scale actions to mobilize, train, supervise, and motivate volunteer CHWs, most notably for HIV/AIDS activities, have been carried out since the late 1990s with donor financing, and primarily by church health services and HIV/AIDS-centered NGOs. A few central NGOs carried out this work. The strategy involved the formation and training of government community health committees at all levels.

NGO-led services delivery was motivated by the experience of pilot projects providing health worker outreach activities, and a general desire by government to develop the nongovernmental sector in health services delivery, particularly given the limited number of government personnel to provide services. It was developed as a bottom-up strategy initiated by trusted local health care providers rooted in their communities. Subsequently, however, it became top-down, supported by significant resources and effective management, which were needed for scaling up.

These NGO/CHW programs expanded rapidly after 2000 which reflected, in part, the greater speed and cost-effectiveness of donors working with the nongovernmental sector versus the public sector. The rapid pace of implementation was further facilitated by the additional donor financing available between 2002 and 2007 for HIV/AIDS, tuberculosis, and malaria.

Throughout implementation, the government retained a great deal of control in the shape and design of the strategy, so much so that it was difficult to distinguish government from nongovernmental programs.

This strategy has prompted increases in the number of CHWs, who have become the largest health labor force in Zambia. There are significant results, in terms of cost-effectiveness and reaching the poor in difficult-to-serve areas, mainly in those districts where this strengthening strategy has been pursued. There is less evidence of improvements in health outcomes, although some can be gleaned from specific project evaluations. However, no changes in national health indicators could be attributed with certainty to a specific set of NGO or CHW activities.

Community participation. Community participation in health involved the establishment of formal participatory structures at the community and district levels to plan and manage community health. A series of health groups at lower levels was created to foster community health planning and management through the election of community members into various local structures, including neighborhood health committees. However, implementation varied, as did the degree and type of participation of each of the different groups. In 2006, with the resumption of centralized control, these community structures weakened significantly. The remaining neighborhood health committees are not supported by the Ministry of Health, and they have little influence on central government decisions.

The introduction of community participation structures in Zambia were supported by the commitment and will of the newly elected government in 1991, of key government champions of the reform, and of the community. (Popular support for radical change also played a part.) These three sets of actors often viewed community participation structures as a way of enabling individuals to feel more vested in the health system. This aim was largely not achieved though, partly because the communities had no previous experience with this type of participation and because the government did little to communicate the nature of the change and the objectives to the public, or to train community members for their specific roles. The strategy was implemented well where NGOs provided training and supported and used these structures (especially neighborhood health committees) and where government health personnel were not only supportive, but spent time facilitating and encouraging membership of community participation groups.

Figure 8.7   Health Services Indicators, Zambia

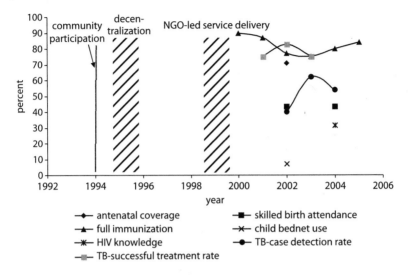

Source: Zambia Demographic and Health Survey 2001/02; Japanese Institute of Public Health database. Immuniza-tion data obtained from presentation at 134th APHA Meeting in Boston, 2006, "RED Strategy Improves Community Participation in Immunization of Children: Zambia's Experience."

Note: The reference period is five years preceding the survey. Antenatal coverage: % of women with at least 4 Antenatal coverage visits. Skilled birth attendance: % of births delivered with the assistance of a trained health professional, that is, a doctor, nurse, or midwife. Full immunization: children aged 12–23 months fully vaccinated, i.e., BCG, measles, three doses of DPT and polio (excluding polio 0). HIV knowledge: % of women who know that HIV/AIDS can be prevented by using condoms and limiting sex to one uninfected partner. Child bednet use: proportion of children under 5 who slept under an insecticide-treated bednet the previous night.

Although district health board members added a local "user" and rep-resentative perspective to district health plans, which sometimes ensured that these were more needs-oriented, at least with respect to the commu-nities represented, district health boards never had real influence over local human resources because they did not gain the authority or funding to manage employment contracts as was originally envisaged.

Zambia health services delivery trends. This study found that a closer examination is needed of NGO capacity to deliver health services, health worker shortages, and community groups, in promoting the rapid scaling up of health services to the poor.

Key Implementation Factors and Lessons Learned

This section aims to depict lessons that have been learned about imple-mentation from some or all of the seven case study countries and that are likely to be applicable and useful in other countries. What drives or impedes change is obviously very context specific (obviously including the political and institutional background), and the effectiveness of the very same implementation strategies can vary considerably according to circumstances. This is partly because "there are no general laws in social science that are consistent over time and independent of the context in which they are embedded" (Rein 1976). Although there are patterns as to what is important in implementation across the case studies, the point bears repeating: each case study has a unique context.

The key implementation factors that emerge from the country case studies may be broadly grouped into three categories. Macro-environment factors that are mostly related to the *country* context and are usually outside the control of the "strategy" implementers; micro-environment factors that are mostly related to the *health* sector; and factors that are related to the *strategy* (figure 1 in the overview). The micro-environment factors are not under the prerogative of the "strategy" implementers but should be seriously examined and considered as they directly influence how the strategy is implemented. The last but most important set of factors are the "strategy" factors. These are directly related to the design, adaptation, and implementation of the strategy and are usually under the control of those implementing it.

Macro-environment or Country Context Factors

Role of political stability, security, and economic growth. The case studies strongly suggest that political stability, security, and economic growth are highly beneficial to continuity in developing and implementing strategies. They also provide an enabling environment. Yet these three factors are preconditions, not guarantees, as seen for example in a comparison of Afghanistan and Zambia. The former country saw considerable gains in a situation of insecurity and uncertain economic growth, while the latter witnessed serious reversals in a relatively stable environment. Uganda is an unusual case where the postconflict environment in the north of the country is embedded within the stable and relatively secure situation found within most other parts of the country. Notably, the Ugandan north has benefited from considerable donor attention and resources, and from greater willingness to experiment and innovate than other areas in the country.

What also appears to be important is how the strategy for improving health services is developed and implemented. In the case of Afghanistan, a relatively high level of transparency and accountability of service providers has made health services improvement possible, despite the fragile security situation.

Legislation, regulation, and the capacity to monitor and enforce. Legal and regulatory frameworks are in place in all the countries studied. In some places, Vietnam for example, there are highly developed laws and decrees. However, even in Vietnam, which is approaching middle-income status, the gap between the framework and the capacity to monitor and enforce compliance is considerable. In decentralized systems it is particularly difficult to ensure the fit between central intentions and local capacity. In some countries, with Vietnam and Ethiopia good examples, the power of the party and the central control that it exercises remain the single most important factor in securing adherence to the aims of the state. However, whereas in Vietnam market orientation has led to the dismantling of some previous structures, Ethiopia has remained essentially statist in its approach.

In Zambia, the framework for decentralization was initially confined to the health sector, while in Ethiopia the devolution of government functions to the regions and subsequently to the districts covered all sectors. The Ethiopian model represents a more fundamental political commitment to decentralization that is less likely to be reversed.

Overall, however, there is insufficient evidence that can be construed from the case studies to answer questions as to which of the different models of decentralization is more effective. In Uganda, government health sector spending initially decreased by one-third when local government first took over allocation of resources. This trend was eventually reversed—at least partly—by introducing earmarked funds for primary health care.

Some case studies (in the Ghana case study, conflict between different groups; and in the Uganda case study, not just dual practice but also drug shops and NGOs) also point to the effect that the vested interests of provider groups may have on applying (or not) regulations, or adopting effective self-regulation. Statutory bodies designed to oversee the work of health professionals and facilities are frequently weak, at best capable of first-time registration, and policies to strengthen them have remained ineffective because of lack of financial and human resource allocated to monitoring, inspection, and quality assurance. In Uganda, although this is an explicit part of its health sector strategy, government has failed to take action, and civil society groups have failed to exert effective pressure for greater attention to these quality of care issues.

Decision makers need to analyze the legal and regulatory frameworks and assess the enforcement capacity before considering new sector strategies. The case studies suggest that robust regulatory frameworks that are commensurate with the enforcement capacity are more likely to support the successful implementation of health sector strategies.

Micro-environment or Health Sector Factors
The critical role of leadership. The quality of political or managerial leadership is an essential ingredient of success in implementing policies. What is less clear is how gains derived from having a charismatic and courageous champion are sustained when changes occur at the top.

In the case studies reviewed, the influence of leadership has been significant. In Rwanda for example, it is the president who has set the tone for reform and is exercising authority both in an inspiring and controlling way, while during Ghana's early successes in the late 1980s and early 1990s it was a farsighted Director of Medical Services who ensured that regions and districts could innovate and thrive. The corollary of course is that deterioration at the political level—for example in Uganda where democratic values have been increasingly neglected; politically expedient decisions, such as increasing the number of districts, have become the norm; and corruption is taking its toll—constitutes a "disabling" environment, as does the kind of patronage prevalent in Afghanistan and Ethiopia, in the latter case largely based on party and regional affiliations.

Status of NGOs and faith-based organizations. The country case studies demonstrate a range of relationship patterns between NGOs and faith-based organizations on one side, and governments on the other. In some cases, government attitudes toward NGOs are at best neutral or even outright discouraging, such as in Ethiopia and Vietnam where local NGOs are virtually absent. It is not clear that a single model emerges as best practice, though it is clear that NGOs are able to contribute more in places where they have been encouraged.

In Uganda, the relationship between faith-based organizations and the government since independence has gone back and forth between regular subsidies and virtually no support at all, between harmonious and acrimonious dialogue. One issue is that ministries of health are concerned that their own financial and staff allocations may be reduced as a result of government subsidies, contracts, and personnel secondments to the churches.

The situation in Rwanda is different: faith-based organizations—running 32 percent of health centers and 46 percent of district hospitals—serve as an integral part of the health system, and are often the first point of contact for the poor. In Afghanistan NGOs provide almost 80 percent of health services, mainly driven and supported by international donors.

There has been a considerable increase in NGOs (not only in the post-conflict countries) due to the huge influx of funds for HIV/AIDS, and the preference of certain development partners to work through NGOs rather than through government. Few effective umbrella NGOs, which can act as interlocutors among government, donors, and smaller NGOs, were found in the countries under review, with the exception of Christian Health Associations acting on behalf of faith-based organizations in Ghana, Uganda, and Zambia. Governments are therefore struggling to ensure that NGOs are following their policies.

Size of donor support and aid approaches. Changes in the aid approaches of the donor community and in the global health architecture in terms of organization and financing have clearly had a profound effect on implementation of health services in LMICs. Determining the precise impact of changes from project funding to SWAps (focusing on the sector as a whole and reducing highly earmarked funding), and from there to global health partnerships (emphasizing specific diseases and interventions, while going back to earmarking contributions), is much more difficult.

Some countries are "donor darlings" and others are "donor orphans." Rwanda is an example of the former, while Uganda has switched to the latter group. Ministries of finance in different countries also take different positions regarding their "fiscal space." In Uganda, for example, the Ministry of Finance has set ceilings for spending on health, which meant reducing government funding when external funds increased, even though many of them were heavily earmarked. As a result, it is only possible to say that the way in which funds are provided makes a difference, and that flexibility, predictability, and reliability are key concerns, but the exact impact of the presence or absence of these conditions is unknown. The International Health Partnership initiative[1] supported by a large number of donors and governments is currently trying to shed further light on this and supports negotiations of the health sector with ministries of finance.

In the case of Rwanda, the size of donor support, which contributed to a doubling of per capita health spending in a few years, and introduction of performance-based contracting, may have played a key role in improving health services and outcomes. Afghanistan is yet another example. Elsewhere, the introduction of SWAps in Ghana in 1991 by donors led to better results. Similarly, the focus on community empowerment (support to NGO/CHW expansion) supported by donors in 2000 improved health services.

Donor support therefore, whether by its size or its approach, provides an enabling environment for successful implementation, but actual success depends heavily on the adaptation and implementation of the strategy.

Strategy-related Factors

Seizing the boost of new beginnings. The studies on Afghanistan and Rwanda offer clear evidence that a fresh start, the absence of bureaucratic "baggage," and an abundance of attention from the international community can enhance innovation, courage, and motivation to go to scale and establish effective implementation structures, even without a full return to stability and security. In Afghanistan, systematic experimentation with contracting out and the rollout of CHWs gained support from different stakeholders and resulted in notable improvements in health services at an early stage. When such a situation is combined with inspired leadership and willingness to learn and adapt, as in Rwanda, huge progress can be made. But reversals are still possible unless successful experiments are implemented at scale and reforms are institutionalized.

Ensuring capacity building as a central tenet. "Capacity building" has been used to mean different interventions ranging from developing individual clinical or managerial skills through training or provision of technical assistance (TA), to institutional capacity of health organizations, or even health systems development. In the country case studies, lack of capacity was invariably cited as a reason for slow or inadequate implementation. However, no clear picture emerges as to why this was the case.

In many instances, what takes place under the heading of capacity building is little more than traditional training for individuals—as in Afghanistan, for example. Yet this type of training alone is not an effective intervention to improve health worker performance or health services, a finding seen elsewhere in this book. Technical assistance of the mentoring and capacity-building type, which supports rather than substitutes national human resources, remains a challenge that is rarely met.

Uganda presents another model in the form of developing the institutional capacity of health organizations. The interventions included the development of a manual for planning and management of subdistrict services coupled by management training and strengthening of different types of supervision at the technical and managerial levels. However, with the change of leadership in the Ministry of Health, the highly promising program featuring supportive supervision and quality assurance was all but abandoned. Similarly, a highly effective quality assurance program in Zambia was also discontinued.

The Afghanistan country study found that capacity building through training drove the short-term objectives of donors, rather meeting the needs of locals. Systems of regular supportive supervision, linked with continuing education and sustained beyond externally funded projects have been developed but have tended to disintegrate when the external funds or inspired leadership (or both) disappeared. Rwanda at present looks promising but, as said earlier, the key will be for systems to be fully institutionalized.

Recent studies on capacity, change, and performance, such as those from the European Center for Development Policy and Management (ECDPM) in Maastricht, offer a broad-based analytical framework that demonstrates how stakeholders, the external context, the intervention, and internal resources all need to combine to create capacity and performance. However, the case studies do not shed much light on the reasons why capacity building can be done well in some countries (Rwanda) and some regions (SNNPR in Ethiopia), and less so in others.

Modulating the pace of implementation. The pace of implementation is an issue in some countries. It is often driven by ideology and political need without sufficient attention to creating capacity for implementation and ensuring a reliable flow of resources. The tension between the need for demonstrable short-term gains and long-term sustainability is well documented, and the case studies show that it can be hard for countries to get the balance right.

In Ethiopia, it has been argued that the pace of decentralizing to the district level was too fast for limited institutional and managerial capacity, and gains in delegating authority to the provincial level should have been consolidated before further decentralization to the next level. However, where decentralization is driven by overriding political concerns, it is usually difficult for the leading health politician to suggest a different pace that would more likely ensure gains in the effectiveness and quality of service delivery.

The pace of implementation is also influenced by resistance to change among stakeholders. In most cases, resistance by the health sector to political decentralization has been counterproductive. In the case of Rwanda, there were pockets of opposition to decentralization reform, particularly at the center, as this was feared to disempower existing central level staff.

Decentralization required a "mindset change" of central officials to accept and embrace reforms. By contrast, the pace of decentralization has worked relatively well in Ghana, where a deconcentrated model was introduced at a moderate pace, dictated by the application of sector-specific readiness criteria for districts to act as budget and management centres. When districts did not yet meet these criteria, the region would perform this function until district capacity had been achieved.

Balancing supply- and demand-side interventions. All case studies show demand-side interventions and demand creation to be largely neglected—an omission bound to influence implementation. Health services delivery issues have been addressed mostly from the supply side with insufficient attention to the way in which ministries of health can engage civil society to create demand.

Most countries built up a cadre of health workers intended to provide a link between health facilities and the community, and to stimulate demand for health services. Many also involved rather vague communications strategies to increase demand for health services. The creation of CHWs in Afghanistan, Ghana, and Zambia and the use of health extension workers in Ethiopia were adopted mostly after it became apparent that supply-side interventions were failing to increase use of available health services. There is clearly a need for greater attention to innovative demand-side interventions from the beginning, rather than as an underfunded afterthought.

Anticipating consequences and resource requirements for going to scale. Key findings in most countries are that plans and strategies are often not implemented at scale, and that institutional structures and resources for scaling up pilots, however successful, are rarely adequate.

The early Zambia reforms aimed at delinking part of the health sector from the civil service suffered detrimentally from a lack of foresight about the implications of this step for health workers' pensions and other benefits. This could arguably have been avoided if the donor community had not only pointed out the problem, but provided one-off funding. Similarly, the creation of and support to village health teams in Uganda was based on an insightful problem analysis and proposed an attractive model for government and United Nations agencies. However, no realistic costing had been undertaken, and requirements for long-term motivation and supervision of community-based workers were underestimated, with the result that the approach has only been fully implemented in one pilot district and in the postconflict north of the country, where external donor resources are abundant.

In Ethiopia, the decrease of government financing to the health sector due to the conflict with Eritrea led to a stagnation of health services. In Ghana, though government financing increased, this was dedicated primarily to salaries and health insurance. With donor funding directed more to general budget support and earmarked programs, flexible funds for health managers were reduced and resulted in lower allocations for critical supplies and outreach activities.

By contrast, the scaling up of the successful performance-based financing pilot projects in Rwanda was pushed by the government and supported by donors, which led to fast and successful implementation. Moreover, large-scale performance-based financing was complementary to the *mutuelle* strategy. This reflects three key factors: political will to support the scaling up of a strategy, the need to mobilize adequate resources for implementation, and the need to ensure that other strategies are complementary or mutually reinforcing.

Recognizing the fragility of reforms and the need for their institutionalization. Several case studies document early successes and then serious reversals. The relationship and potential time lag between policy and management downturns, and deteriorating service outputs, are not, however, straightforward.

In Uganda and Zambia it was the exit of a champion minister that set the process of reversal in motion. In Ghana it was the adoption of a politically motivated policy to create a national health service that proved disastrous, with consequences that are still felt. Even in case studies that have notable successes to report, such as Rwanda, researchers suggest that reversal would be possible if there was a change in political leadership or if external resources decreased prematurely.

In Uganda, the health sector deteriorated also because of multiple issues around resources and financing. Declining allocations by the Ministry of Finance, partly in response to vast amounts of external funds for the health sector (albeit for specific diseases), and a marked retreat from unearmarked funding by the donor community, all combined to create an increasingly unfavorable environment, which also affected the morale of health officials.

The questions that need to be asked are: At which point are reforms sufficiently institutionalized to survive these types of shocks and threats? What is known about institutional sustainability thresholds? What conditions need to be in place in terms of stakeholder buy-in and state capacity beyond government administration, in order to ensure continuity? In Afghanistan and Rwanda, it is probably too early to tell whether institutional reforms are sufficiently robust. In Uganda and Zambia, it is clear that the adopted reforms were insufficiently institutionalized to survive the demise of their champions. Decentralization in Ethiopia is driven by the federal government and is likely to survive at least as long as the present government power structure remains.

A critical mass of human resources for health is clearly important. Ghana is instructive here. The systematic training of large numbers of young medical officers in public health and economics over an entire decade created a critical mass of highly qualified and motivated doctors that set the tone for lasting reforms of regional and district health systems and services delivery, despite reversals at the national level.

The donor community still has a potentially more important role to play (as seen, for example, in the fact that it has already backed champions and innovations), in safeguarding promising policy directions, nurturing leadership, and providing consistent advice and stable support to key institutions during times of political change.

Concluding Thoughts

The case studies of how countries have developed and implemented their strategies demonstrate how each situation is unique. The interpretation of the core meaning of the strategies selected for review is not consistent. Changes in health services or outcomes could seldom be plausibly linked to a package of strategies, much less attributed to a single strategy. This raises the question whether a better specification of how strategies are actually implemented is required not only in order to compare strategies and results, but also to facilitate learning on which factors are likely to influence the adoption and implementation of any particular strategy, and what effects they will have.

The country case studies also shed some light on the diversity in implementing the common strategies identified at the outset in the *Overview* and the factors that influenced the course taken.

Decentralization is perhaps the most diverse subject. The term covers a multitude of aims, directions, and strategies. The messages as to what works and what does not do not point to a single direction. Some case study countries, although formally decentralized, are actually examples of strong central control. Ethiopia is a case in point. However, what does emerge is a sort of checklist of points that need to be monitored. This would include the changes in the role and responsibility of the center, which are often neglected; the importance of finding a locus for continuing "intermediate-level functions," such as monitoring, mentoring, and supervising when the regional or provincial level is abolished; and general and sector-specific approaches to capacity building and to assessing performance.

Community engagement or empowerment, too, covers a wide range of approaches and issues: paid versus unpaid workers, local versus national focus, voice versus service delivery, accountability to community versus accountability to health facility, and so forth. Without greater specificity, it is difficult to say what enhances and what inhibits community engagement. Certainly, there is a political dimension to the issue of voice, which goes far beyond creating the post of village health workers who provides services within their community.

Oversight strategies feature a wide variety of approaches. They do, however, point almost universally to the neglected issue of government capacity to perform stewardship functions in mixed systems of public and private providers. Contracting has great promise and receives a great deal of attention, but is clearly insufficient to address the much broader issue of government capacity for oversight and regulation. In some countries, for example Afghanistan, development partners have established quasi-independent mechanisms for effectively monitoring performance and for managing contracts. This appears to work well. However, it is less clear whether these arrangements are effective in building the required state capacity for oversight. Equally in Rwanda, the international community has played a key role in the initial experimentation and, more recently, in coordinating and managing contracts on a wide scale.

Despite the limitations of these studies, they do underline how different countries have evolved in different ways to both develop and implement health strategies. In fact, as the country context changes, the health system components also evolve in response to the changing environment. In the final chapter, we examine in further detail how some of these processes, such as identifying key stakeholders and gaining their commitment, or using information to hold actors accountable, can be used in the implementation of health strategies.

Note

1. Launched in September 2007, the International Health Partnership is a coalition of international health agencies, governments, and donors committed to improving health and development outcomes in developing countries and getting back on track to reach the health-related MDGs.

References

Agyepong, I., and S. Adjei. 2008. "Public Social Policy Development and Implementation: A Case Study of the Ghana National Health Insurance Scheme." *Health Policy and Planning* 23(2): 150–160.

Asante, F., and M. Aikins. 2008. "Does the NIHS Cover the Poor?" Institute of Statistical, Social and Economic Research and School of Public Health, Legon University, Ghana.

Baser, H., and P. Morgan. 2008. "Capacity, Change, and Performance: Study Report." http://www.ecdpm.org/Web_ECDPM/Web/Content/Download.nsf/0/AE807798DF344457C1257442004750D6/$FILE/Morgan_Baser__2008_Study-Report_Capacity_Performance_Change_06052008.pdf, accessed May 8, 2008.

Capuno, J., and K. Ohiri. 2007. "A Case Study of Vietnam's Recent Health Reform Strategies." Washington, DC, World Bank.

El-Saharty, S., P. Dubusho, S. Kebede, and B. Siadat. 2007. "Ethiopia: Improving Health Service Delivery." Washington, DC, World Bank.

External Review Team. 2007. "Report of the External Review Team on the Ministry of Health Programme of Work 2006." Accra, Ghana.

International Labour Organization. 2006. "Technical Note: Financial Assessment of the National Health Insurance Fund." http://www.ilo.org/public/libdoc/ilo/2006/106B09_342_engl.pdf, accessed May 12, 2008.

Janovsky, K., and P. Travis. 2007. "Uganda Health Services Delivery Case Study." Washington, DC, World Bank.

Lannes, L., B. Siadat, M. Kabera, J. Mathonnat, and A. Soucat. 2008. "Rwanda Health Services Delivery Case Study." Washington, DC, World Bank.

Ministry of Health, Ghana. 2001. "The Health of the Nation: Reflections on the First 50-year Health Sector Programme of Work 1997–2001." Accra: Ministry of Health.

———. 2002, 2003, 2004, 2005, 2006, 2007. "The Ghana Health Sector Programme of Work." Accra.

Nyonator, F. K., J. K. Awoonor-Williams, J. F. Phillips, T. C. Jones, and R.A. Miller. 2005. "The Ghana Community-based Health Planning and Services Initiative for Scaling Up Service Delivery Innovation." *Health Policy and Planning* 20(1): 25–34.

Ovretveit, J., and N. Segaren. 2007. "Strategies to Strengthen Health Services in Zambia: A Case Study." Washington, DC, World Bank.

Peters, D. H., and J. St. John. 2007. "Implementation and Completion Results Report. Republic of Ghana Health Sector Program Support Project II." Washington, DC, World Bank.

Rein, M. 1976. *Social Science and Public Policy*. Middlesex, United Kingdom: Penguin Education.

Schleimann, F. 1999. "Performance Contracting in the Ghanaian Health Sector: Will it Actually improve Efficiency?" Master of Public Administration Dissertation, Copenhagen Business School, Denmark.

Simmonds, S., F. Feroz, and B. Siadat. 2007. "Improving Health Service Delivery in Low Income Countries. Country Case Study: Afghanistan." Washington, DC, World Bank.

World Bank. 2007. "Project Performance Assessment Report: Second Health and Population Project & Health Sector Support Project." Washington, DC: World Bank.

———. 2008. *World Development Indicators*. http://ddp-ext.worldbank.org/ext/ DDPQQ/member.do?method=getMembers&userid=1&queryId=135, accessed May 6, 2008.

———. 2008. HNP Stats, http://web.worldbank.org/WBSITE/EXTERNAL/ TOPICS/EXTHEALTHNUTRITIONANDPOPULATION/EXTDATASTA TISTICSHNP/EXTHNPSTATS/0,,menuPK:3237172~pagePK:64168427~pi PK:64168435~theSitePK:3237118,00.html, accessed May 6, 2008.

CHAPTER 9

From Evidence to Learning and Action

David H. Peters, Sameh El-Saharty, and Katja Janovsky

Findings

Failing to learn from experience is the common dynamic in international development, even though there is a large literature that identifies lessons.[1] In this chapter, we nonetheless identify some key lessons that have emerged from systematic analysis of strategies and case studies to strengthen the delivery of health services in LMICs.[2] We look at what has worked, what has not worked, and offer some insights on how to improve implementation. We finish by turning attention to ways to be better at "learning and doing."

What Has Worked

An important lesson from the studies carried out for this book is that many strategies can be used to improve implementation of health services in LMICs. Yet although many things can work well, there are no "magic bullets" or clear strategies that can be replicated and expected to work well in any country setting. In part this is because the country contexts differ and each strategy takes on a life of its own, so that even having the same label does not mean that the same strategy is being pursued.

Although strategies may not be reproducible to any large degree and can have a wide range of effects, some broad strategies have repeatedly improved the delivery of health services in several LMICs. These are:

- Expanding disease-specific programs that are effective in small areas to a larger area of the country (this was identified as a strategy with having some success across countries in chapter 1, and was described in the Uganda and Vietnam country case studies).
- Developing and using systems for locally adaptive learning, involving frequent reviews of results and testing of approaches by local implementers and other stakeholders. (This was demonstrated as a significant implementation success factor in chapter 1, table 1.4, and specifically among successful approaches for community empowerment in chapter 4, as well as in the country case studies of Afghanistan and Rwanda.) Other dimensions of adaptive learning involve making plans aimed at overcoming locally identified constraints, and encouraging flexibility and modification through stakeholder feedback (as identified in chapter 1, table 1.4).
- Careful consultation and involvement of stakeholders, particularly those involved in implementation and local oversight, as well as beneficiaries. When the community is actively engaged in managing interventions, such as serving on community boards, running revolving drug funds, and deciding on provider bonuses, or where local resources are used as part of program support, improved outcomes have been found (as shown in the analysis of community empowerment strategies in chapter 4, table 4.4 and figure 4.2, and the case of *mutuelles* in Rwanda).
- Training of CHWs can improve outcomes, but no training model was found to be clearly superior. More broadly, training in combination with other interventions, such as supportive supervision, can be effective in improving health worker behaviors (as was described in chapter 3, figure 3.3, the country case study of Afghanistan, and to some degree the case studies of Ethiopia and Ghana).
- Providing incentives to health workers or health organizations for good performance, often in the form of explicit contracts (as highlighted in chapter 7, figure 7.2, and described in the country case studies of Afghanistan and Rwanda), or through supportive supervision of health workers (as identified in chapter 3, figure 3.3), or mechanisms to increase accountability to the public or other institutions (as shown in the country case studies of Afghanistan and Rwanda). In Vietnam, the increased hospital autonomy through Decree 43 has led to increased revenue for some implementing hospitals. Part of this revenue was used

to top up salaries and create an incentive for increased efficiency (but there is also some evidence that hospitals are shifting services to more lucrative fee-based services).

- Ensuring that adequate resources are available is clearly associated with successful implementation, but the implementation challenges have often been how to obtain adequate resources, or how to proceed when resources are not sufficiently available for distribution to units that need the funds. (This was apparent in all the country case studies, even though significant international funding for health became available, often earmarked for specific purposes.) Using community resources can also be an important source of support for programs, but local resources are unlikely to be forthcoming or effectively used without attention to local accountability and involvement.

What Has Not Worked

The other good news from these studies is that no strategy has been tried and obviously fails in a consistent way. Our research strategies depended on the documentation of results, and there were relatively few published studies that had negative results. There were, however, some conditions under which strategies to strengthen implementation were more likely to fail. These include:

- Implementing strategies where there is no strong and consistent leadership usually fail. Strong leadership includes: providing a clearly communicated mandate from the top management that gives authority, resources, and accountability to key leaders and teams throughout an organization (as identified in the review in chapter 1, as well as in chapter 4, figure 4.1; the Ghana case study involved strong but conflicting leadership; Uganda and Zambia had significant leadership changes and subsequent changes in priorities and implementation).
- Overly simplistic strategies, such as providing ad hoc health worker training by itself, or making simplistic policy changes such as introducing clinical guidelines or user fee guidelines without adequate attention to their effects and ability to change course, tend to fail (as shown in chapter 3, figure 3.3). Simply training health workers in Afghanistan, Ethiopia, Uganda, or Zambia had its limitations, but building capacity for supervision systems and other institutional dimensions seems to offer more promise.
- Implementing overly complex strategies that outstrip the management capacity of organizations that provide health services can lead to poor results. This may explain why multiple-component strategies

have higher rates of failure, but also a higher average effect when they succeed. An important task of planning and implementation is to diagnose when a strategy is outstripping the management capacity of service delivery organizations.

- Failing to assure that resources are made available to those responsible for implementing programs or providing services is an obvious but regrettably common condition (identified in chapter 1 and found to some degree in each of the country case studies, particularly concerning resources reaching the most peripheral management units). Resources that are displaced due to corruption have an additional demoralizing effect (identified in chapter 1 and described in the Uganda country case study).

There are also ways to implement the strategies identified that reduce the chances of success. Many of these involve doing the opposite of those factors that are identified above as contributing to success.

Another common trap is to focus almost exclusively on technical aspects of interventions, or on the securing of a particular policy statement at the expense of addressing the key actors or contextual factors that affect implementation.[3] However, badly managed or superficial consultation organized to gain support can also backfire (for example, in the Zambia country case study). Although using resources from within a community can improve the prospects for community empowerment strategies (as identified in chapter 4), not obtaining resources for the additional costs of support and supervision at village level is also problematic (for example, for the village health teams in the Uganda country case, or neighborhood health committees in Zambia).

If community involvement is a key strategy to successful implementation, it should be recognized that there is also a long history of poorly managed community development programs intended to foster community involvement. Community development programs reached a prominence in the 1950s, modeled after India's national rural development schemes and its multi-purpose village worker (Mayer et al. 1958). However, the rapid expansion of community development programs throughout Asia, Africa, and Latin America was nearly finished by the mid-1960s, largely because the expected gains did not materialize. Some important lessons from the implementation failure of these schemes are relevant today (Holdcroft 1978; Korten 1980):

- Excessive pressures for results, usually through delivery of goods and services, drove out the necessary attention to institution building.

- Implementation was frequently done through conventional bureaucratic structures and centrally mandated targets, rather than being responsive to capabilities or needs of local communities.
- Parallel and competing government agencies were often responsible for implementation and coordination, leading to bureaucratic conflict that contributed to the demise of the movement.
- More emphasis was given to expanding social services than in raising incomes of rural residents, and often for services of questionable value. This seems to be a result of pursuing bureaucratic interests rather than those of beneficiaries.
- Existing power structures of villages were accepted as given without any attempts to change them, frequently resulting in the capture of benefits by local elites. Local organizations were kept separate from each other rather than being linked into larger and more powerful bodies.

One factor that is noticeably absent in the set of determinants of successful implementation is the development and use of comprehensive planning. While only a few people would suggest that all planning and budgeting is nugatory, it is also evident that the emphasis of international agencies on comprehensive, costed plans or well-written proposals has little relationship with the successful implementation of those plans and proposals. The review of the literature conducted in chapters 1, 2, and 4 could not identify any evidence that such planning was a determinant of successful implementation. This is not a total indictment of any type of planning, as locally adaptive learning processes, identifying and overcoming constraints, and using local community resources for program support were all identified as factors that improve implementation, as is strong management. The problem appears to be with blueprint planning approaches that ignore or obstruct the need for constant reappraisal and replanning by beneficiaries and those involved in implementation, and the way that it contradicts the managerial flexibility that is required to take advantage of these processes (Brinkerhoff and Ingle 1989; Bond and Hulme 1999).

How to Improve Implementation

The approaches above represent a number of strategies (or components of strategies) that have been shown to either work well or not work well. Many of these lessons should seem self-evident, yet it remains remarkable how often they are ignored. This "knowing-doing gap" is well known in the management field (see for example Pfeffer and Sutton, 2000), yet it is little addressed in the literature on health services in developing countries. Rather than simply produce a list of lessons, another reason for identifying them is to lead decision makers and those facilitating the development of health services toward more important questions about the delivery of health services. What can be learned about *how* implementation of health services can be improved? What can we learn about *why* some strategies succeed or fail? Box 9.1 takes the process further, representing a synthesis of not only the evidence-based approach of what we have seen in this book, but a consideration of an alternative approach grounded in the authors' own experience of many years' work in the field—a "learning-doing" strategy.

Box 9.1

A Learning-doing Strategy

Successful implementation of strategies to improve health services involves knowing what to do, how to do it, and why you are doing it. We already know a lot about what interventions to pursue in the health sector, as there are many interventions known to prevent disease and death at relatively low cost. In this book we have highlighted that there are many strategies that can result in successful implementation, but also that these strategies require local knowledge and learning processes to find ways to implement them successfully in each setting. This box describes some of the learning processes that can be used to improve the prospects for successful implementation.

A word of caution: even knowing what to do or understanding the techniques of how to do it does not guarantee good implementation. Getting good data helps, but does not ensure that good decisions are made. To address some of these difficulties requires moving beyond the questions of what to do and how to improve implementation. It demands a more difficult discussion about why knowledge does not get acted on, and involves an appreciation of the values of leaders and influential groups, and knowing why things should be done.

Although there is no blueprint for improving implementation of health services, we offer some guidance for decision makers to ask the right questions, based on potentially good practices found in the various studies.

(continued)

Box 9.1 *(Continued)*

Use strategies to improve implementation problem solving

Some of these strategies involve some disciplined steps, including:

- Look for leaders and laggards, that is, positive and negative performance outliers across units (for example, states within a country, communities within a district, or neighborhoods within a community). Differences may exist in terms of high and low performance, or where there are differences in the presence of poor and vulnerable groups or of exposure to different risks.
- Use multiple sources of information such as routine health information systems, or other informal mechanisms such as communications with key informants or the media.
- Consider the way in which analysis is related to actions taken by decision makers, be they on the front lines of service delivery, immediate supervisors and middle managers, or policy makers.
- Look for unintended consequences of strategies. When implementing health projects or programs, most people tend only to look at the intended results in the narrow area of the program. But since health systems are linked, it is important to look at the unintended consequences of a strategy.
- Identify sources of information for unintended consequences. Places to look include a range of health services, or the range of health systems actors, inputs, and functions. The factors identified in figure 1 (in the *Overview*) specify some key areas to examine within a health system. Key actors include provider organizations and the professions, community groups, and groups within the state. Key functions include human resources management, information systems, financial management, and how the health system is financed.
- Ask whether any strategy has created the right incentives for critical organizations and people to work toward a common purpose of the strategy.
- Consider factors outside the health system, particularly those related to broader reforms in the public sector, the economy, or social systems. Changes in laws, regulations, leadership, macro organization, or economic/political shocks can radically affect the way in which health services are implemented. Trying to anticipate many of these shocks may be very difficult, but it may be more important to be able to recognize when they are occurring as soon as possible, and to take corrective steps. This again involves good information gathering and feedback mechanisms, not rigid planning requirements.

(continued)

Box 9.1 *(Continued)*

Understand the effects of institutions on health services delivery

As pointed out in chapter 6, understanding the institutional context is critical. Eight key questions to consider include:

- To what degree does the policy or intervention respond to strongly expressed needs and to what degree do politicians or political leaders believe that a response to these needs is important to their legitimacy with the population or political future?
- To what degree was the policy or intervention understood to represent a national need as opposed to a narrow political or financial interest?
- What are the incentives for key actors to translate policies or regulations into changes in health system performance?
- What is the government capacity to serve as regulator and steward of the health system?
- What are effective mechanisms for accountability in health systems?
- What is the degree to which governments and other actors are co-accountable to external bodies?
- What is the level of statehood?
- What is the level of institutional development?

Match capacity with implementation

A common problem for LMICs is weak implementation capacity. Trying to find the right fit between program expectations, beneficiary expectations, and capabilities of implementers, governments, and communities is an ongoing challenge and involves the following:

- Continually ask the question about what types of capacity problems exist. Is it institutions or rules of the game that are impeding progress, or is it the specific human skills or support systems that organizations need to perform their work?
- Assess whether the pace of change is outstripping the ability of organizations to deliver services. This requires intelligence gathering from service beneficiaries and implementers. Asking the problems about high and low performers, as discussed above, may give early warning signs.
- Consider whether reorganization is needed, or whether ongoing reorganization is likely to be a part of the problem or the solution. Decentralization or restructuring the hierarchies within an organization is often part of a change needed to build capacity.

(continued)

Box 9.1 *(Continued)*

- Try to minimize the costs of organizational change, and ensure that the responsibilities, authority, resources, and accountabilities are aligned. Expecting district health units to plan and be held accountable for results, but then not giving them the ability to flexibly use financial and human resources (in short, power without responsibility) is a common recipe for implementation failure.

Use processes that encourage learning and good decision making

A recurring theme throughout this book is that processes that encourage learning and decision making, and action, based on learning have been shown to be particularly effective in improving implementation. A learning-based approach focused on the implementation of policy could involve some of the following steps (and see box 9.2):

- Seeking out local innovations and local innovators (among, for example, communities and health service providers). People can also be encouraged to test new approaches (through incentives or by exposure to new ideas and others' experiences), and not be limited to ideas generated within the health sector.
- Identifying and documenting the depth and variation in which new and existing strategies for strengthening health services are being implemented, and the roles played by key stakeholders over time.
- Making agreements that the results of innovations and other strengthening strategies will be monitored, and that there will be formal evaluations of their results and that lessons learned will be incorporated as part of the process of further developing strategies. Mechanisms to facilitate learning from both successes and failures should be structured into any strategy.
- Finding ways to understand local institutional arrangements and markets, and to involve key actors in the innovation and learning process.
- Engaging government, civil society, and professionals in the learning process, since all these groups will likely need to alter their roles.
- Developing more systematic ways to understand and anticipate the outcome of different strategies and innovations, so as to provide better frameworks within which the learning process can be structured.

Get the Data—Ask the Questions

Even though there is a willingness to test different strategies to strengthen health services in many countries, there is a repeated failure to learn from experience. This begins with a failure to get data and ask the types of questions needed to learn. The four systematic reviews found many articles on strategies to strengthen health services, strengthen health organization performance, improve health worker performance, and empower communities, but relatively few well-designed studies and evaluations (chapters 1, 2, 3, and 4). The study on the changes in health services delivery across countries over time was also marked by the limitations in the basic data that are available for analysis (chapter 5). Among health services, only childhood immunization coverage, tuberculosis coverage and treatment data, and skilled birth attendance were recorded with close to annual frequency at a national level. Other data on health services, and more importantly, assessments of health status, were not available with sufficient regularity. At least for World Bank-assisted projects, changes in health services, financing, and health outcomes are rarely measured (chapter 7). Most of these projects do not achieve a minimum level of measurement to be able to assess change.

In addition to the expense and technical difficulties in obtaining data on health services and health outcomes, other barriers have been the lack of effective demand for data that can be used for accountability to the public and to national and international funding agencies. This also reflects a lack of use of the data for learning and meaningful evaluation and planning (chapters 7 and 8).

Among the country case studies, it was clear that there is relatively little comparable data across countries, and that in many countries, the strategies used do not involve close tracking of changes in implementation or results, particularly at subnational levels or among vulnerable populations (chapter 8). Afghanistan is a notable exception in its extensive use of disaggregated data in decision making, though extensive external assistance has been used to collect and analyze the data. It is also one of the few countries where substantial progress is being made across a wide range of health services parameters, though other factors such as the improvement in security, strong leadership, and a return of talented health professionals, committed NGOs, and large investments in the health sector have also played a substantial role (Hansen et al. 2008).

When data are used well to assess progress of strategies to improve health services, the results tend to be positive. This was seen in some evaluations of World Bank-supported projects, the systematic reviews of different strategies, and the country case studies. In part, this may be due to a bias to publish those studies and evaluations that have positive findings (and the fact that the act of measuring may change the outcome), though there were also suspicions of such bias among World Bank project evaluation documents and country case studies, where the incentive to demonstrate positive results may not be as strong.

But if organizations and decision makers are unwilling to accept error as a means of learning, mistakes are likely to be unmeasured and repeated. It is quite likely that the measurement of key outcomes is a proxy indicator for more successfully managed strategies, and that the use of data contributes to the success of strengthening strategies in health services. Use of data is an important part of a strategy that uses feedback to adapt and change course during implementation, so the availability of data identifies those strategies or contexts where these learning and acting processes take place.

Promoting organizational learning has been identified elsewhere as an important approach to be able to scale up strategies in LMICs (Uvin 1995; Simmons et al. 2002; Cooley and Kohl 2005). This is consistent with the findings of the review of community empowerment strategies and health services strengthening strategies, which found that continuous feedback about needs, constraints, implementation progress, and results is associated with effectiveness of implementation. However, it may not be easy to build in strong feedback and learning processes.

Data are frequently used to set targets for health services and health status. By itself, having targets set does not appear to affect implementation. The targets for health services set by international consensus, such as MDGs, tend to be unrealistic. High aspirations may be helpful for raising attention and funds, but can also be used to place blame. The practice of setting international targets ends up being arbitrarily applied, even when there is a good rationale for them. For example, some immunization targets may be set because of theoretical considerations of reaching herd immunity once certain levels of coverage can be reached. However, the international targets that have been set frequently do not match a country's experience, as is described in chapter 5. These targets also tend to discount the local nature of health services delivery, as they do not take local conditions into account, or the relationships between the targeted health service and other health services. Chapter 5 also shows that different types of health services can change in different rates and directions, meaning that different health services cannot be assumed to be either synergistic (they help each other positively) or antagonistic (gains in one health service take away from gains in another). This reinforces the need to use data in each country setting to see how a broad set of health services are changing, and whether they are behaving synergistically or antagonistically.

The practice of setting international health service targets is flawed in a more fundamental way, representing a simplistic "black box" notion of implementation and deterministic sets of results (figure 9.1). The problem lies in insufficient attention to context, the role of key actors and institutions, and the way in which specific implementation factors emerge in different settings and evolve differently over time. International agencies have a tradition of demanding detailed plans in exchange for development funding, despite the questionable relationships between such plans and results.

The recent interest in results (for example, MDGs, results-based financing) appropriately changes the focus, but largely neglects the most important challenges in development: the challenges of implementation. Detailed planning is most useful when the nature of the problem is well known and predictable (Senge 1994), a situation that does not apply to questions of how to implement health services in diverse communities. To address the issues of implementation, it is important to better understand the factors influencing implementation, most notably those related to capacity, accountability, and the importance of key actors and incentives. Better plans and clear expectations of results will not be enough to produce results, even if more money is made available.

Find the Right Scale

Decision makers and managers rarely learn from experience when they attempt to find the right scale of operations. One manifestation is the frequency with which pilot studies are undertaken and subsequently neglected. For example, nearly half of all the projects assisted by the World Bank in the health sector involved pilot testing of new schemes in a country, but it was usually unclear what became of the pilot study at the end of the project. The literature on strengthening strategies suggest that pilot studies are more likely to be effectively expanded when there are several phases of testing, feedback, and modification by decision makers and those responsible for design and implementation of the strategy. On the other hand, simply replicating strategies tested on a small scale in many sites without scope for local adaptation and learning appears to have little impact.

Figure 9.1   Simplistic Causal Chain from Health Intervention to Health Outcomes

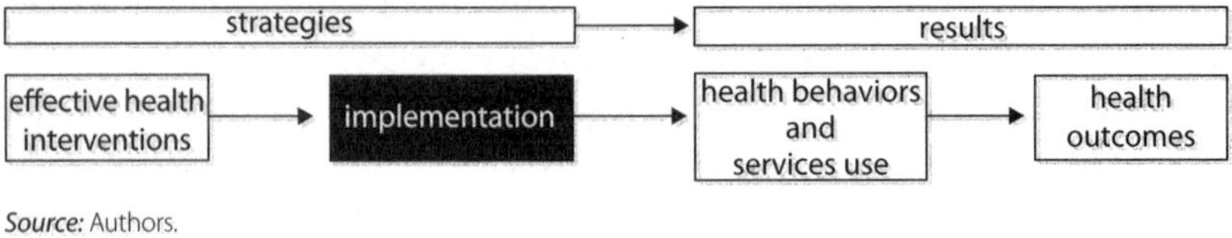

Source: Authors.

Much of the published literature concerns small-scale and short- to medium-term outcomes. It is much more difficult to see if these strategies are able to cover larger populations and have more sustainable effects. As discussed in chapter 1, an unfortunate habit of the health economics and public health literature is to simply assume that implementation can occur on a large scale by either following a correct theory or by replicating what can be demonstrated in a small, relatively controlled environment. In the community empowerment literature review, there were more assessments of larger scale strategies than in the other literature reviews: 25 studies (18 percent of the total) were implemented on a provincial or national scale. But it was not clear whether the scale of strategy is related to the results. Results may be smaller as the scale of implementation increases because of diseconomies of scale due to reduced ability to manage personnel and other resources, or to build relationships and communicate effectively with beneficiaries. If continuous adaptation to local circumstances is a critical element of successful implementation, it appears that adaptation will also be easier on a smaller scale.

Strategies to strengthen specific disease-control programs can be replicated from smaller to larger scale. Although having sufficient resources and political support for these types of programs can more frequently serve as enabling factors, they are also likely to have fewer components in a strategy and be simpler to coordinate as scale increases. Disease-specific programs are also less likely to examine their effects on other parts of a health system, and therefore have benchmarks for successful implementation that are more closely aligned with a narrower set of activities.

Find the Right Scope

In contrast to many specific disease-control programs, multiple strategies (or strategies with multiple components) were shown to have greater average effects, but also to have greater variation and risk of failure. This may be because strategies with multiple actions reinforce each other. When examining community empowerment approaches, it was found that when multiple interventions are built into a foundation of a successful existing program, with a supportive sociopolitical environment, the chances of implementing health services on a larger scale and for the longer term were enhanced.

One way to build reinforcing strategies to strengthen health services is to combine supply- and demand-side approaches (for example, training of health workers and public education), accountability measures (for example, disclosure of health facility performance) and aligning incentives (for example, rewards for good performance). From a supply side perspective, incrementally adding sets of interventions (through training, recruitment, supplies, supervision, and materials) can help improve the quality and range of health services provided.

In either case, as the strategy becomes increasingly complex, implementers run the risk of outstretching their capacity, through difficulties in obtaining consensus and support from communities and the professions, increasing the need for greater management oversight, securing adequate resources, and ensuring that no unintended consequences from each strategy component undermine other components. Learning when a strategy is becoming too complex, unmanageable, or creating perverse consequences is an important part of a learning approach to implementation.

Given that most people's health needs are not restricted to a single condition, and that health organizations and programs need to address more than one set of services, it is important to reorient the measurement of health services across a wider range of dimensions that match what is expected to be implemented. Yet many programs are concerned with success in more narrowly defined dimensions of health services, and few examine other services or dimensions of the performance of an organization. For example, in the systematic review of health organizations, over 127,000 citations were screened because the articles included terms related to the performance of health organizations in LMICs, but only 88 studies ended up with an adequate study design with sufficiently defined outcomes across a minimum of three areas of organizational performance. In the review of project evaluations at the World Bank, SWAps tended to measure a wider range of indicators of health services, and were found to be more likely to measure and demonstrate improvements in health services and health outcomes than World Bank-supported health projects organized around disease control, general budget support, or other project designs.

Recognize That the Same Name May Be a Different Strategy with Different Effects

Many of the strategies described in the systematic reviews and the country case studies are given the same name, yet are clearly very different strategies. Decentralization has a different meaning in each of the country case studies. Both design features and how the strategies are implemented in a given context appear to matter. This is the case even where many different strategies with the same label are said to have positive effects. For example, contracting approaches were found to be associated with measurement of improved health services and health outcomes. The systematic reviews of strengthening strategies and performance of health organizations showed that contracting approaches can be successful in different ways in many different environments. Yet knowing that contracting strategies can work does not mean that they will always work and have the same effects, regardless of where or how they are implemented. Studies that compare different types of contracting in the same environment demonstrate that their effects are not uniform, and that differences in the nature of the contracts, the management autonomy, and the type of evaluation of contractors, and the types of incentives in the contracts result in differential effects in terms of technical quality of health services, productivity, equity of provision, and responsiveness to patients (Arur 2008). Most of the experience on contracting in health in LMICs examines short-term outcomes and a limited range of effects, so it is not clear how long the same set of contracts will work. It is likely that contracting approaches will have variable effects, and that there will be a need to change them over time. The implication is that simply relying on past experience and evidence from elsewhere is not sufficient, and that attention to implementation is an ongoing challenge that requires attention.

What Next?

For decision makers, implementation cannot be seen as a separate process that occurs in isolation of political debate and the interactions among politicians, bureaucrats, managers, front-line workers, and the public. Given the complex way in which agendas are set, policies are formulated, and decisions are made in different countries, a single body of knowledge or experience is unlikely to determine what an appropriate policy is in a given context. Yet if implementation is understood in the most flexible terms, as "what happens between policy expectations and (perceived) policy results" (Furman 1990), then even those most skeptical of rational policy making or rational management will recognize the relevance of demonstrating the linkages between policy expectations and results. Although many models of implementation research have failed to live up to their theoretical or predictive intentions, in part because of the complexities involved, this does not negate the need for careful evaluation and feedback as an integral aspect of implementation (Pressman and Widalvsky 1984). Considering how frequently faulty implementation occurs, there is good justification for using stronger evaluations of implementation experience (DeLeon 1999).

Yet many organizations, managers, and politicians are not interested in producing information that may make them "look bad." Organizational

culture and the attitudes of leaders may be averse to error, experimentation, and disclosure of results. This may help maintain a status quo, but
also ensures that mistakes remain hidden and are likely to be repeated
(Korten 1980; Rondinelli 1993). Several approaches have been developed
to overcome the inadequate use of information, ranging from participatory processes designed to empower those most likely to suffer from the
status quo (Chambers 1997), to the creation of "learning organizations"
(Senge 1994) and flexible and adaptive management systems (Brinkerhoff
and Ingle 1989), to focusing on overcoming information asymmetries
through an emphasis on institutions and the development of new social
contracts (Bloom et al. 2008). Box 9.2 describes a framework for using a
structured learning strategy.

Box 9.2

A Structured Learning Strategy

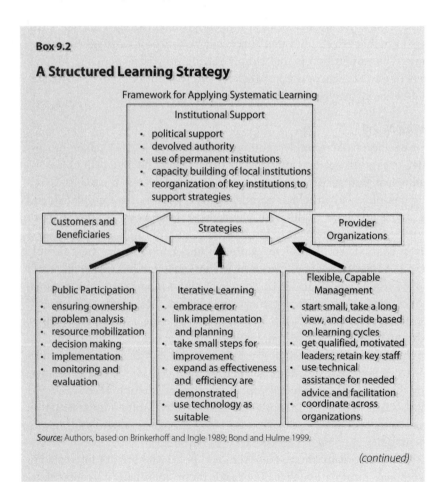

Framework for Applying Systematic Learning

Institutional Support
- political support
- devolved authority
- use of permanent institutions
- capacity building of local institutions
- reorganization of key institutions to support strategies

Customers and Beneficiaries

Strategies

Provider Organizations

Public Participation
- ensuring ownership
- problem analysis
- resource mobilization
- decision making
- implementation
- monitoring and evaluation

Iterative Learning
- embrace error
- link implementation and planning
- take small steps for improvement
- expand as effectiveness and efficiency are demonstrated
- use technology as suitable

Flexible, Capable Management
- start small, take a long view, and decide based on learning cycles
- get qualified, motivated leaders; retain key staff
- use technical assistance for needed advice and facilitation
- coordinate across organizations

Source: Authors, based on Brinkerhoff and Ingle 1989; Bond and Hulme 1999.

(continued)

Box 9.2 *(Continued)*

Building on the work of learning approaches in development (Brinkerhoff and Ingle 1989; Bond and Hulme 1999), the box figure outlines a conceptual framework that recognizes the key institutions and organizations and focuses on the concrete activities they can undertake. This framework is not a reflection of how public institutions may have been designed, or how they currently operate, nor is it restricted to the context of learning processes within private organizations or civil society organizations. Rather, it is an action-oriented framework that builds on all these experiences.

The framework is intended to be a flexible guide to different types of learning process; its application is expected to vary considerably based on local market conditions. At different stages in the design and implementation of strategies to improve the provision of health services, important roles will be played by a variety of actors. Consumer organizations may be directly involved in problem solving, resource mobilization, and monitoring. Service provider organizations will work best if they are able to identify and retain qualified and motivated staff, communicate effectively across organizations, and use professional facilitation and advice in targeted ways (as distinct from the tendency in the many development agencies that see technical assistance as a driving force for change). Critical institutional support includes government policies that encourage local participation and innovation by service providers, using permanent and local organizations for administration and regulatory functions, and a willingness and ability to reorganize and refocus these institutions as needs are identified. Notwithstanding the potential benefits of collaboration and mutual learning, the interests of different stakeholders, such as consumer and service provider organizations, may be in conflict with each other. Resolving such conflicts may require intermediating bodies or other, local solutions.

Even with structured participation, learning, and flexible management and institutional support, there is no guarantee that simply following these practices will lead to better implementation and better outcomes. There is also a substantial literature in the management field that points to the need to move beyond the straightforward replication of processes used successfully elsewhere, and that provides important cautionary tales (Pfeffer and Sutton 2000; Senge 1994):

- There are knowledge practices that can get in the way of implementation. These include:
  - An emphasis on technology and transfer of codified information and specific practices (such as best practices and what works)

(continued)

Box 9.2 *(Continued)*

- Formal systems that do not store or transfer tacit knowledge
- People responsible for data and knowledge do not understand the actual work being done
- There is a need to get beyond processes. Many people have been able to see successful business processes and copy them, yet not replicate their results. They focus on what to do and the procedures for how they do it, but miss the philosophy about why things are done.
- It is important to understand values and philosophy as a reason for why things are done. Values and motivations vary in different countries, different ministries of health, different NGOs, and different development partners. Yet a strong sense of values in an organization, usually demonstrated by the senior leadership and encouraged at different levels, is needed to bridge the gap between knowing what should be done and actually doing it.
- Improving health services usually means taking action. Whereas planning and assessing results is important, the focus should be on using judgment to ensure that action is actually taken to improve services.

The studies in this book point to a clear need to create demand among decision makers and the public for more rigorous evaluation of health sector investments, including those supported by the World Bank. When projects are able to consistently assess changes in health services, financing, and status, decision makers and the public will be better informed, and better able to assess the adequacy of programs. The primary motivation for better assessment of implementation and other results of health services is to be able to learn from experience. This is needed for successful adaptation of strategies, for ensuring accountability and ownership by key actors, for identifying unintended consequences, and for stimulating and rewarding good performance. Stronger evaluation designs will also help indicate which strategies are most effective and efficient in improving health services.

Notes

1. Bond and Hulme (1999) and Holdcroft (1978), for example, outline key lessons that should have been learned but have been ignored.

2. In table 2 in the *Overview*, the "Main lessons and implications" for decision makers are listed for each chapter.

3. Ignoring the interests and incentives for health workers, how a strategy influences the private sector, or whether powerful interest groups will be affected adversely is likely to reduce the chances of success (as shown in chapters 1, 6, and 8). Ignoring the role of civil society organizations and community involvement in the design, adaptation, and accountability of health services also reduces the effectiveness of service delivery and prospects for scaling up (identified in chapters 1 and 4).

References

Arur, A. 2008. "Contracting for Health Services in Afghanistan: An Analysis of the Changes in Outpatient Services Utilization and Quality between 2004 and 2005." PhD dissertation, Baltimore: Johns Hopkins University.

Bloom, G., H. Standing, and R. Lloyd. 2008. "Markets, Information Asymmetry and Health Care: Towards New Social Contracts." *Social Science and Medicine* 66(10): 2076–2087.

Bond, R., and D. Hulme. 1999. "Process Approaches to Development: Theory and Sri Lankan Practice." *World Development* 27(8): 1339–1358.

Brinkerhoff, D., and M.D. Ingle. 1989. "Integrating Blueprint and Process: A Structured Flexibility Approach to Development Management." *Public Administration and Development* 9(5): 487–503.

Chambers, R. 1997. *Whose Reality Counts? Putting the First Last.* London: Intermediate Technology Publications.

Cooley, L., and R. Kohl. 2005. *Scaling-Up: From Vision to Large Scale Change—A Management Framework for Practitioners.* Washington, DC: Management Systems International.

DeLeon, P. 1999. "The Missing Link Revisited: Contemporary Implementation Research." *Policy Studies Review* 16: 311–338.

Furman, B. 1990. "When Failure is Success: Implementation and Madisonian Government." In *Implementation and the Policy Process: Opening Up the Black Box*, ed. D.J. Palumbo and D.J. Calista. Westport: Greenwood Press.

Hansen, P.M., D.H. Peters, N. Niayesh, et al. 2008. "Measuring and Managing Progress in the Establishment of Basic Health Services: The Afghanistan Health Sector Balanced Scorecard." *The International Journal of Health Planning and Management* 23: 1–11.

Holdcroft, L.E. 1978. "The Rise and Fall of Community Development in Developing Countries, 1950–65: A Critical Analysis and an Annotated Bibliography." MSU Rural Development Paper No. 2, 1978.

Korten, D. 1980. "Community Organization and Rural Development: A Learning Process Approach." *Public Administration Review* 40(5) 480–511.

Mayer, A.C., M. McKim, and R.L. Par. 1958. *Pilot Project, India: The Story of Rural Development of Etawah, Uttar Pradesh*. Berkeley: University of California Press.

Pfeffer, J., and R. I. Sutton. 2000. *The Knowing-Doing Gap*. Boston: Harvard Business School Press.

Pressman, J.L., and A. Wildavsky. 1984. *Implementation*. (3rd edition.) Berkeley: University of California Press.

Rondinelli, D.A. 1993. *Development Projects as Policy Experiments: An Adaptive Approach to Development Administration*. (2nd ed.) London: Routledge.

Senge, P.M. 1994. *The Fifth Discipline: The Art & Practice of the Learning Organization*. New York: Bantam Doubleday Dell Publishing Group, Inc.

Simmons, R., J. Brown, and M. Diaz. 2002. "Facilitating Large-Scale Transitions to Quality of Care: An Idea Whose Time Has Come." *Studies in Family Planning* 33(1): 61–75.

Uvin, P. 1995 "Paths to Scaling-up: Alternative Strategies for Local Nongovernmental Organizations." *World Development* 23(6): 927–940.

Glossary

The following glossary gives common definitions and usages of terms.

Accreditation: In international practice, accreditation is a system of external expert examination of correspondence to a set of standards; it is based on the principal of voluntary participation of the examined. Daily compliance to practice and conduct standards by the entire staff ensures that they do everything according to expectations. To obtain an indication of "good practice" (which is an indicator of the level of success) during accreditation, a facility under examination is motivated to demonstrate its actions toward both patient and staff advocacy (AHRQ 1999).

Accountability: Processes through which individuals, organizations, and states determine their decisions and actions, processes by which individuals, organizations, and states report on and explain their decisions and actions, and processes through which individuals, organizations, and states may safely report concerns arising from the decisions and actions of others, and gain redress as and where appropriate. Accountability therefore requires responsible behavior within all three of these domains (HAP n.d.) or the responsibility for actions or decisions (Shortell and Kaluzny 2006).

Adequacy inference: Inferences about the adequacy of program outcomes depend on the comparison of performance or impact of the project with previously established adequacy criteria. These criteria may be absolute—e.g. distributing 10 million packets of oral rehydration salts to children with diarrhea or achieving 80 percent oral rehydration therapy use rate—or may refer to a change—e.g. a 20 percent decline in reported diarrheal deaths in the program area. Even when specific goals have not been established, performance or impact may still be assessed by measuring general time trends, such as an increase in coverage or a reduction in mortality. There are two main types of adequacy evaluations: (a) adequacy performance evaluations assess how well the program activities have met the stated objectives; and (b) adequacy impact evaluations assess whether or health or behavioral indicators have improved among program recipients or among the target population as a whole (Habicht et al. 1999, pp. 2–3).

Agency theory: Agency theory refers to the variety of ways in which agents, linked by contractual arrangements with a firm, influence its behavior. These may include organizational and capital structure, remuneration policies, accounting techniques, and attitudes toward risk taking (Economy Professor n.d.) or in the context of changing views on the roles of the state, how divergent interests are reconciled in a principal–agent relationship between the government owner and hospital management (Preker and Harding 2003, p. 30).

Agenda setting: The ongoing process within organizations through which organizational members identify important problems and search for innovations to address these problems (Shortell and Kaluzny 2006).

Allocative efficiency: This requires that an economy provide its members with the amounts and types of goods and services that they most prefer. In standard economic theory it occurs when resources are allocated in such a way that any change to the amounts or types of outputs currently being produced (which might make someone better off) would make someone worse off. This is sometimes also called "Pareto efficiency" (World Bank 1998).

Autonomization: Reforms that give public provider organizations greater autonomy and rely on market or "market-like" incentives to generate pressures to improve performance. Autonomization and corporatization both change the degrees of decision rights, residual claim, and market exposure. These reforms also create more indirect accountability arrangements, such as oversight boards, which give managers more day-to-day freedom. Obligations related to money-losing services and other social functions are usually made more explicit, and are often funded to ensure continued delivery. However, corporatization offers a greater degree of change of the above five elements than autonomization. Under corporatization, provisions for managerial autonomy are stronger than under autonomization, giving managers virtually complete control over all inputs and issues related to service delivery. The organization is often legally established as an independent entity, making the transfer of control more durable than under autonomization. A corporatized entity's status includes a hard budget constraint or financial bottom line, which often makes the organization fully accountable for its financial performance (World Bank n.d. a).

Balanced scorecard: A management instrument that translates an organization's mission and strategy into a comprehensive set of performance measures to provide a framework for strategic measures and management. The scorecard measures organizational performance across several perspectives: financial, customers, internal business processes, and learning and growth (World Bank n.d. b).

Benchmarking: The process of continuously comparing and measuring an organization against business leaders and best practices anywhere in the world to gain information that will help the organization take action to improve its performance (World Bank n.d. b).

Bilateral monopoly: A market characterized by a single seller and a single buyer, otherwise known as monopoly and monopsony, respectively. Examples of a bilateral monopoly frequently occur in the public sector where a government education employee negotiates with a single teachers' union on pay and conditions (Economy Professor n.d.).

Capital expenditure: The expenditure required for financing permanent or semi-permanent facilities or equipment, such as buildings. Capital expenditure is also called investment or nonrecurrent expenditure (EOHSP n.d.).

Capitation: A fixed payment to a provider for each listed or enrolled person served per period of time, or a payment mechanism whereby an organization receives a fixed, prespecified amount of money per time period (e.g. month, year) for each individual for which it is responsible for meeting defined health needs (e.g. primary care, primary and secondary care), regardless of the volume of services rendered (WBI n.d.). Good and bad sides of capitation: prevents overuse of services, but could limit necessary services (EOHSP n.d.).

Certificate of need: A certificate issued by a government body, such as a state health planning and development agency, to an individual or a health care organization, proposing to construct or modify a facility, incur a capital expenditure, or offer a new or different health service. This method of health planning is designed to prevent excessive or duplicate development of organizations and services (AHRQ 1999).

Clinical care system/management roles: Business process within the health care organization designed to assure appropriate, safe, effective, and efficient patient care to clinically similar patient populations. Management roles involve managing clinical care system-oriented business processes (Shortell and Kaluzny 2006).

Clinical outcomes: See "Health outcomes."

Clinical practice guidelines: Recommendations for medical care based on current research (QAP n.d.).

Coalitions: A temporary alliance of distinct parties, persons, or states for joint action (MWOD n.d.) or informal, voluntary agreements among individuals or groups of similar or complementary interests for purposes of achieving objectives (Shortell and Kaluzny 2006).

Code of ethics: A formal set of principles and guidelines that are used in an organization as the basis for defining the boundaries between good and unethical (not always illegal) business practice. These principles and guidelines are visible and made known to all within the organization, as well as external stakeholders (Shortell and Kaluzny 2006).

Cohort: (a) The component of the population born during a particular period and identified by period of birth so that its characteristics (e.g. causes of death and numbers still living) can be ascertained as it enters successive time and age periods. (b) The term "cohort" has broadened to describe any designated group of persons who are followed or traced over a period of time, as in *cohort study* (Last 2001, p. 32).

Community-based care: The blend of health and social services provided to an individual or family in their place of residence for the purpose of promoting, maintaining or restoring health or minimizing the effects of illness and disability (AcademyHealth 2004).

Community-based organization: A private nonprofit organization which is representative of the . . . community or significant segments of the community and which provides employment and training services or activities (U.S. Department of Labor n.d.).

Community-based services: Bringing services as close as possible to where people live and work (Health Canada 2006).

Community care network: An integrated system of medical care, public health, and human service organizations that is formed to: (a) serve a common population defined at the community level; (b) provide consistent and coordinated access to services across care settings and along the continuum of care; (c) implement mechanisms for ensuring accountability to patients and to the general public; (d) manage the delivery of services within the context of fixed financial resources, such as through risk-adjusted capitation payments or global budgets; and (e) pursue the objective of improving community health status as well as the health status of enrolled populations (Shortell and Kaluzny 2006).

Community-driven development: An approach that gives control over planning decisions and investment resources to community groups and local governments. Such programs operate on the principles of local empowerment, participatory governance, demand-responsiveness, administrative autonomy, greater downward accountability, and enhanced local capacity (World Bank n.d. c).

Community engagement: The process of working collaboratively with groups of people who are affiliated by geographic proximity, special interests, or similar situations with respect to issues affecting their well-being (CDC Committee for Community Engagement 1995).

Community empowerment: Empowering communities means that communities should have voice, decision-making powers, and access to resources. Three key facets of community empowerment are: organizing and improving community participation, financing communities through matching grants, and targeting interventions to ensure the participation of socially excluded sections (World Bank n.d. d). In essence, community empowerment is the process of enhancing the capacity of individuals or groups to make choices and to transform those choices into desired actions and outcomes. Empowerment encompasses the autonomy to mobilize resources, having sufficient education to be able to make informed decisions, and having sufficient power to transform those decisions into desired outcomes (World Bank forthcoming).

Community financing: A resource mobilization mechanism that permits a cluster of individuals or households (a community) to contribute resources (money or in-kind services) collectively (World Bank n.d. c)

Community insurance: See "Community financing."

Community management: See "Community empowerment."

Community mobilization: A process through which action is stimulated by a community itself, or by others, which is planned, carried out, and evaluated by a community's individuals, groups, and organizations on a participatory and sustained basis to improve health. Community mobilization relates to building the capacity of community groups to be able to work together coherently toward achieving sustainable use of natural resources. The objective of community mobilization is therefore to mobilize and enhance communities to adopt appropriate resource management practices and skills (Social Enterprise Development Center 2006).

Community scorecards: A more local and rural hybrid of the citizen report card. Instead of surveys, these scorecards rely on focus group discussions with communities and providers to monitor performance of local public facilities (Citizen Report Cards 2003).

Compact: An agreement or covenant between two or more parties.

Competence: Knowledge, skills, and attitudes, which an individual possesses. Competencies are accumulated and developed through education, training, and experience (World Bank n.d. e).

Conditional cash transfers: Conditional cash transfer programs aim at reducing poverty in the short term through cash transfers while at the same time trying to encourage investments into the human capital of the next generation by making these transfers conditional on regular school attendance or the regular use of preventive health care services (World Bank n.d. f).

Confounding variable/confounder: A variable that can cause or prevent the outcome of interest is not an intermediate variable, and is associated with the factor under investigation. Unless it is possible to adjust for confounding variables, their effects cannot be distinguished from those of the factor(s) being studied. Bias can occur when adjustment is made for any factor that is caused in part by the exposure and is also correlated with the outcome (Last 2001, p. 38).

Consumer groups: These represent users or purchasers of the products or services of producers. They are considered a segment of the public (Health Canada 2006).

Consumer protection: Encompasses all the means necessary to safeguard the interests of consumers and empower them to know their rights and make wise, educated decisions (Porteous and Helms 2005).

Contestability: In this context (see next sentence), the term is used to indicate the lowering of barriers to entry for other providers, which opens up the possibility of switching providers if necessary. The context is: "Going beyond these assessments, I have suggested that the management of the NHS should be guided by the following principles." A commitment to contestability rather than competition is a way of stimulating improvements in performance and providing incentives for efficiency (Preker and Harding 2003, p. 292).

Continuous improvement: Commitment to quality is a hallmark of successful organizations. Recognizing the centrality of quality not only internally but also in terms of the perceptions and expectations of key external constituencies and stakeholders is leading health care organizations toward the principles of continuous quality improvement and total quality management (Shortell and Kaluzny 2006).

Continuous quality improvement (CQI): A management approach to the continuous study and improvement of the processes of providing health care services to meet the needs of patients and other persons. CQI focuses on making an entire system's outcomes better by constantly adjusting and approving the system itself instead of searching for and getting rid of persons or processes whose practices or results are outside established norms. CQI is often considered to be synonymous with "total quality management" (AHRQ 1999).

Contracting: A purchasing mechanism used to acquire a specified service, of a defined quantity and quality, at an agreed-on price, from a specific provider, for a specified period. In contrast to a one-off exchange, "contracting" implies an ongoing relationship, supported by a contractual agreement (Preker and Harding 2003).

Contracting reforms: Organizational reform emphasized on the funding side of moving from budgeting to contracting (Preker and Harding 2003).

Control group approach: In the context of methodological approaches to assessing a reform's effects on hospital performance, the control group approach compares behavior and performance among reforming hospitals to behavior among hospitals presumed to be unaffected by the reform, assuming that any observed differences are due to the reform (Preker and Harding 2003, pp. 137–138).

Copayment: In health insurance, a form of cost sharing whereby the insured person pays a specified amount for each health care product or service obtained (e.g. $10 per prescription drug) (AHRQ 1999).

COPE: A process and a set of simple and practical tools to assess and improve the quality of reproductive health care services. The COPE process encourages self-assessment and joint problem solving by service staff and supervisors. It empowers staff to undertake improvement activities (MSH 2003).

Coproduction: An act in which citizens and governments act together to produce results (Krishna 2004).

Corporatization: See "Autonomization."

Cost-benefit analysis: A technique for deciding whether to make a change. As its name suggests, it compares the values of all benefits from the action under consideration and the costs associated with it (United Nations et al. 2005).

Cost-effectiveness: A type of analysis that compares interventions or programs having a common health outcome (e.g. reduction of blood pressure, life-years saved) in a situation where, for a given level of resources, the decision maker wishes to maximize the health benefits conferred on the population of concern (World Bank 1998).

Counterfactual: Contrary to fact (MWOD n.d.) or, in the context of methodological approaches to assessing a reform's effects on hospital performance, the story of what would have happened without a reform (Preker and Harding 2003, p. 137).

Cream-skimming: A process whereby an insurer tries to select the most favorable individuals with expected losses below the premium charged (or the capitation payment received) in order to increase profits (EOHSP n.d.); or choosing to provide only the most profitable services, or to insure only the healthiest patients, so as to avoid subsidizing public goods and thus obtaining extra profits (Getzen 1997). Cream-skimming can make it difficult or impossible for individuals with high expected losses to purchase private insurance (WBI n.d.).

Decentralization: The transfer of authority and responsibility to lower levels from the central government to peripheral levels or lower levels of government (World Bank n.d. g). The dispersion or distribution of functions and powers, specifically: the delegation of power from a central authority to regional and local authorities (MWOD n.d.).

Decision making: A process by which teams attempt to apply all available information to the problem at hand so as to make correct decisions. Some of the problems that prevent good decision making are free riders, polarization, and groupthink (Shortell and Kaluzny 2006).

Decision rights: Rights to make decisions. Critical decision rights that are transferred to management may include control over inputs, labor, scope of activities, financial management, clinical management and non-clinical administration, strategic management (formulation of institutional objectives), market strategy, sales, and the production process (Preker and Harding 2003, pp. 43–47).

Deconcentration: A form of decentralization (sometimes referred to as "administrator" or "administrative" decentralization) that transfers authority and responsibility from a central Ministry of Health to field offices of the ministry at a variety of levels (regional, provincial, and/or local) (World Bank n.d. g).

Delegation (delegation of authority): Passing of some authority and decision-making powers to local officials. The central government retains the right to overturn local decisions and can, at any time, take these powers back (Meinzen-Dick et al. 2001).

Demand-side financing: Includes a range of interventions that channel public funds for public and/or private (health care) to the individual or family. The focus is on putting the resources into the hands of those who demand (health care) and not those who supply it (Patrinos 2001).

Devolution: The transfer of power and responsibility for the performance of specified functions from the national to the local governments without reference back to central government. The nature of transfer is political (by legislation), in contrast to the administrative nature of deconcentration; and the approach is territorial or geographic, in contrast to sectoral (Meinzen-Dick et al. 2001).

Diagnostic-related group: A way of categorizing patients according to diagnosis and intensity of resources required, usually for the period of one hospital stay (EOHSP n.d.).

District team problem solving: This methodology provides a structured learning-by-doing process with procedural guidelines for use by health administrations to facilitate teams of health services staff from facilities and district level in the analysis and solution design of one high-priority health problem in their geographic responsibility area, and to implement their solution within a year (MSH 2003).

Economics of organization: Deals with considerations of information, motivation, innovation, and the implications for how productive activity can best be organized (Shortell and Kaluzny 2006) and is often used in reference to principal-agent theory, transaction cost economics, property rights, and public choice theory.

Effect: The result of a cause. In epidemiology, this is often a synonym for "effect measure," which is defined as a quantity that measures the effect of a factor on the frequency or risk of a health outcome (Last 2001, p. 57).

Effect modifier: A factor that modifies the effect of a putative causal factor under study. For example, age is an effect modifier for many conditions, and immunization status is an effect modifier for the consequences of exposure to pathogenic organisms. Effect modification is detected by varying the selected effect measure for the factor under study across levels of another factor (Last 2001, p. 57).

Effectiveness: In organizations, the degree to which organizational goals and objectives are effectively met (Shortell and Kaluzny 2006).

Efficacy: In clinical epidemiology, the extent to which a specific intervention, procedure, regimen, or service produces a beneficial result under ideal conditions; the benefit or utility to the individual or the population of the service, treatment regiment, or intervention. Ideally, the determination of efficacy is based on the results of a randomized control trial (Last 2001, p. 58).

Efficiency: Defined as the cost per unit output—organizational, managerial, production, allocative (Shortell and Kaluzny 2006).

Enabling factor: Factors that support efforts or interventions (e.g. financial resources, government management and capacity) (Ovretveit et al. 2006).

Endogenous variables: Those in an economic/econometric model that are explained, or predicted, by that model (OECD n.d.).

Equity: Principle of being fair to all, with reference to a defined and recognized set of values. Equity in health implies that, ideally, everyone should have a fair opportunity to attain their full health potential; and more pragmatically, that no one should be disadvantaged from achieving this potential, i.e. everyone should have geographic and financial access to available resources in health care (WHO 2000a; Witter and Ensor 1997; EOHSP n.d.).

Evaluation: The systematic and objective assessment of an ongoing or completed project, program, or policy, including its design, implementation, and results. The aim is to determine the relevance and fulfillment of objectives, development efficiency, effectiveness, impact, and sustainability. An evaluation should provide information that is credible and useful, enabling the incorporation of lessons learned into the decision-making process of both recipients and donors. Evaluation also refers to the process of determining the worth or significance of an activity, policy, or program. This involves an assessment, as systematic and objective as possible, of a planned, ongoing, or completed development intervention. Note: Evaluation in some instances involves the definition of appropriate standards, the examination of performance against those standards, an assessment of actual and expected results, and the identification of relevant lessons (OECD n.d.).

Evidence-based management: The continual identification and application of available scientific knowledge to improve administrative decision making in health care or other industries. Scientific knowledge may include information about optimal clinical staffing levels, compensation and incentive structures, organization and team design, health care financing arrangements, health care demand and supply projections, consumer preferences, cost-effectiveness information regarding health technologies and services, and information regarding the adoption and diffusion of clinical practices and technologies (Preker and Harding 2003).

Evidence-based medicine: The conscientious, explicit, and judicious use of current best evidence in making decisions about the care of individual patients. The practice of evidence-based medicine means integrating individual clinical expertise with the best available external clinical evidence from systematic research (Centre for Evidence-Based Medicine n.d.).

Fee exemption: The ability to identify specific individuals or households and protect them from having to pay out of pocket for a service or good.

Fee for service: A payment mechanism whereby a provider or health care organization receives a payment each time a reimbursable service is provided (e.g. office visit, surgical procedure, diagnostic test) (World Bank 1998).

Financial incentives: See "Incentives."

Franchising: A franchise is a type of business model in which a firm (the franchiser) licenses independent businesses (franchisees) to operate under its brand name. A firm might choose to expand business through franchising because the arrangement invests capital investment and day-to-day managerial responsibilities in independent businesses, overcoming two major constraints to rapid growth. Franchisers in the health sector, often supported by international donors and nongovernmental organizations, establish protocols, provide training for health franchisees, certify those who quality, monitor the performance of franchises, and provide bulk procurement and brand marketing (Ruster, Yamamoto, and Rogo 2003).

Generalizability: See "Validity, Study."

Governance: The exercise of political, economic, and administrative authority in the management of a country's affairs at all levels. Since the advent of the term "stewardship," the term "governance" is sometimes restricted to the relationship between the owners(s) and the management of an organization, i.e. governance of a private hospital would be exercised by its owners (interested, for example, in making profit) while the government's stewardship role would aim at ensuring, for example, access and socially acceptable costs (EOHSP n.d.) or the relationship between the organization and its owners (Preker and Harding 2003, p. 25).

Governance function: The traditions and institutions by which authority in a country is exercised. This definition encompasses the process by which governments are selected, monitored, and replaced; the capacity of governments to effectively formulate and implement sound policies; and the respect of citizens and the state for the institutions that govern economic and social interactions among them (Kaufmann et al. 2008; Bloom et al. 2006). Governance has been given increasing attention due to the important public trust and social accountability responsibilities of health service organizations (Shortell and Kaluzny 2006).

Health insurance: A system that provides benefits related exclusively to health care. It could be a for-profit or not-for-profit, public or private sector organization (AHRQ 1999).

Health outcomes: The effect on health status from performance (or nonperformance) of one or more processes or activities carried out by health care providers. Health outcomes include morbidity and mortality; physical, social, and mental functioning; nutritional status; and quality of life (QAP n.d.).

Health system: All the organizations, institutions, and resources that are devoted to producing health actions which are defined as any effort, whether in personal care, public health services, or through intersectoral initiatives, whose purpose is to improve health. A health system includes all actors, organizations, institutions, and resources whose primary purpose is to improve health. In most countries a health system has public, private, traditional, and informal sectors. Although the defining goal of a health system is to improve health, other goals are to be responsive to the population it serves. This responsiveness is determined by the environment in which people are treated, and should ensure that the financial burden of paying for health is fairly distributed. Four key functions determine the way in which inputs are transformed into outcomes that people value: resource generation, financing, service provision, and stewardship. The effectiveness, efficiency, and equity of national health systems are critical determinants of population health status (WHO 2004).

Health services research: The multidisciplinary field of scientific investigation that studies how social factors, financing systems, organizational structures and processes, health technologies, and personal behaviors affect access to health care, and ultimately health and well-being. Its research domains are individuals, families, organizations, institutions, communities, and populations (AcademyHealth 2004).

Health systems research: The people, institutions, and activities whose primary purpose is to generate and apply high-quality knowledge that can be used to promote, restore, or maintain the health status of populations. It should also include mechanisms to encourage the utilization of research. The main goals of health systems research are the production of scientifically validated research and the promotion of the use of research results, ultimately to improve health (WHO 2004).

Incentives: Systems that reward and therefore tend to encourage certain types of activity (EOHSP n.d.); or rewards, generally monetary, that are used to compensate staff for good performance and achievement of objectives and/or to motivate employees to improve program quality. Incentives, in addition to salary and benefits, can be a planned part of total compensation (MSH 2003).

Inference: The process of passing from observations and axioms to generalizations. In statistics, the development of generalization from sample data, usually with calculated degrees of certainty (Last 2001, p. 94).

Influence systems: Political activity and informal systems of power that often arise in attempts to influence decisions and activities outside the formal system of authority (Shortell and Kaluzny 2006).

Inhibiting factors: Factors that inhibit or limit actions or interventions (e.g. absence of financial resources, poor government management and capacity) (Ovretveit et al. 2006).

Implementation: What happens between policy expectations and (perceived) policy results (Furman 1990).

Institutions: The rules (formal and informal customs) of the game or activities—the humanly devised and socially shared constraints that shape human interaction and the mechanisms by which these rules are enforced (Preker and Harding 2003, p. 25).

Institutional development: The extent to which an institution (e.g. government) has the capacity to carry out its programs and to provide resources that support initiatives; the degree to which functioning accountability mechanisms exist; and the extent to which corruption is prevalent (Bloom et al. 2006).

Integrated model: Compulsory or voluntary health insurance or third-party funding in which both the insurance and provision of health care are supplied by the same organization in a vertically integrated system (EOHSP n.d.). The term used for the systems of health service finance and management in which both the financing and provision of health services are supplied by the same organization with no separation between purchasers and providers, i.e. the health care providers are directly employed (or "owned") by the third-party payers and managerially accountable to a series of governing bodies. This is commonly found in national health services under the Beveridge and Semashko systems (WHO 1998; EOHCS 2000).

Integration, backward: In relation to the market environment and asymmetry of information, hospitals may "backward integrate" by creating strong links with doctors, thereby insulating themselves from competition for patients (Preker and Harding 2003, p. 56).

Integration, forward: In relation to the market environment and asymmetry of information, in hospitals, doctors may "forward integrate" into diagnostic laboratories or pharmacies and steer their patients toward consumption (Preker and Harding 2003, p. 56).

Integration, horizontal: A strategy in which different types of businesses that are not vertically related are combined to achieve competitive advantage (e.g. the merger of two or more hospitals) (Shortell and Kaluzny 2006).

Integration of services: Often a result in the shift from vertical health programming (e.g. disease-specific programs) to an integrated approach, where functions common to different programs may be integrated or delivered through the same channels. Integrated services at the point of delivery will usually benefit the client so that he or she does not need to go to different sessions for curative, promotive, and preventive care, for example (WHO 2003).

Integration, vertical: A power strategy in which businesses that share input-output relationships are combined to achieve competitive advantage (e.g. integrating hospital and managed care companies) (Shortell and Kaluzny 2006).

Intervention: Intentional change in some aspect of status of the subjects—e.g. introduction of a preventive or therapeutic regimen—or designed to test a hypothesized relationship (Last 2001, p. 99). In the context of this research, interventions refer to relatively simple changes that tend to occur at one level (usually for an individual) and are relatively reproducible. In contrast, strategies are more complex, tend to have multiple components, and operate at the levels of clusters of people or populations.

Job aids: Repositories for information, processes, or perspectives that are external to the individual and that support work and activity by directing, guiding, and enlightening performance (Rossett and Gautier-Downs 1991).

Licensing: A written confirmation provided to a faculty (unit), of a right to carry out certain types of activities; issued by an executive body (AHRQ 1999).

Low- and middle-income country: Those in which 2006 gross national income per capita was $11,115 or less (World Bank HNPStats n.d.).

Management: The measures taken to plan, organize, operate, and evaluate all the many elements of a system and the personnel involved (EOHSP n.d.).

Management information system: An information system consisting of a group of computer programs designed to collect, store, and transmit data to support management in planning and directing organizational operations (AHRQ 1999).

Managerial competencies: Specific skills or abilities such as financial, marketing, change management, and performance assessment (Shortell and Kaluzny 2006).

Market exposure: The extent to which hospitals earn their revenue in the market instead of relying on direct budget allocation; or how much of its services a hospital delivers or sells to earn its own revenue. Hospital services identified as largely private goods may be deregulated, reducing barriers to entry that might prevent private firms from competing in these markets. Organizational reform can further be characterized by the degree to which it exposes the corporatized hospital to market forces in the input (factor) and equity markets. Entry barriers to the medical or nursing professions, other than professional school tuition or professional qualifications, may be reduced, as might any advantages to employment by the corporatized hospital relative to employment by its private sector competitors. Some reforms (e.g. New Zealand) have compelled reformed hospitals to obtain investment funds on the same terms as private hospitals (Preker and Harding 2003).

Marketizing reform: Organizational reforms that shift decision-making control to provider organizations and attempt to expose them to market or market-like pressures to improve performance. These reforms also attempt to create new incentives and accountability mechanisms to encourage management to use its autonomy to improve the facility's performance. These reforms may be categorized under three headings: autonomization, corporatization, and privatization (Preker and Harding 2003, pp. 40–41).

Medical audit: A cyclical evaluation and measurement by health professionals of the clinical standards that they achieve (Merry 1998). A medical audit is a detailed retrospective review and evaluation of patient records along specified dimensions of care, usually conducted by physicians and other medical staff (EOHSP n.d.).

Moral hazard: The possibility of consumers or providers exploiting a benefit system unduly to the detriment or disadvantage of other consumers, providers, or the financing community as a whole, without them having to bear the financial consequences of their behavior in part or in full (EOHSP n.d.).

Motivation: Using influence techniques that appeal to emotion, values, or logic to generate enthusiasm for the work, commitment to task objectives, and compliance with requests for cooperation, assistance, support, or resources; also, setting an example of proper behavior (Shriberg et al. 2005).

Natural monopoly: A market structure with only one firm selling a given good or service and no other firms selling closely related goods or services (World Bank n.d. b).

Neoclassical economics: The neoclassical paradigm lays out the potential sources of market failure. The rationale for public ownership has been its effectiveness as a tool for pursuing social objectives in the presence of market failures. This belief is based on a simple view of the relation between ownership and control. Privately owned companies are generally conceived of as profit maximizers—since by maximizing profits, they maximize benefits to their shareholders (or owners). Sometimes maximizing shareholder benefits is not seen as maximizing benefits to society as a whole (Preker and Harding 2003, p. 28).

New public management: A set of principles for structuring public sector activities that has gained great currency in the industrial world, especially in the Anglophone countries. It has strongly influenced the structure of health sector reforms being discussed and implemented. These reforms are also influenced by similar reforms in government-run infrastructure companies and other public enterprises (Preker and Harding 2003, p. 41).

Nondistribution constraint: A critical component of nonprofit organizational rules—blocking residuals to any individuals (Preker and Harding 2003, p. 77).

Nongovernmental organization (NGO): NGOs are defined as private organizations that pursue activities to promote the interests of the poor, protect the environment, provide basic social services, relieve suffering, or undertake community development. NGOs often differ from other organizations in the sense that they tend to operate independently from government, are values-based, and are generally guided by principles of community and cooperation. There are two major categories of NGOs: (a) operational NGOs, whose primary purpose is the design and implementation of development-related projects; and (b) advocacy NGOs, whose primary purpose is to defend or promote a specific cause and who seek to influence policies and practices (World Bank n.d. h).

Odds ratio: The ratio of two odds. The term *odds* is defined differently according to the situation under discussion.

	Exposed	*Unexposed*
Disease	*a*	*b*
No disease	*c*	*d*

The odds ratio (cross-product ratio) is *ad/bc*. The *exposure-odds ratio* for a set of case control data is the ratio of the odds in favor or exposure among the cases *(a/b)* to the odds in favor of exposure among non-cases *(c/d)*. The *disease-odds ratio* for a cohort or cross sectional study is the ratio of the odds in favor of disease among the exposed *(a/c)* to the odds in favor of disease among the unexposed *(b/d)*. The *prevalence-odds ratio* refers to an odds ratio derived cross-sectionally as, for example, an odds ratio derived from studies of prevalent (rather than incident) cases. The *risk-odds ratio* is the ratio of the odds in favor of getting disease, if exposed, to the odds in favor of getting disease if not exposed (Last 2001, p. 128).

Organizations: The players—the way in which people are structured or organized (e.g. hospitals, clinics, pharmacies, and public health programs) (Preker and Harding 2003, p. 25).

Organizational behavior: The set of formal and informal administrative rules and procedures for selecting, deploying, and supervising resources in the most effective way to achieve institutional objectives (Preker and Harding 2003, pp. 114–144).

Organizational reform: A focus on changing the mapping of functions across agencies, for instance, creating health insurance agencies that collect premiums and purchase health services, and on endowing providers with service provision. Decentralization is another common organizational reform in the health sector (Preker and Harding 2003, p. 40). See also "Marketizing reform."

Organizational reform modalities: See "Autonomization," "Corporatization," "Marketizing reform," and "Organizational reform."

Oversight, government: Refers to external government regulatory structure (Preker and Harding 2003, p. 114).

Patient bill of rights: A set of rights, responsibilities, and duties under which individuals seek and receive health care services (EOHSP n.d.).

Patient-centered care: A multidisciplinary approach to patient care that centers the design of work around patients' needs (Shortell and Kaluzny 2006).

Patient safety: A patient's freedom from accidental injury during treatment. Ensuring patient safety involves the establishment of operational systems and processes that minimize the likelihood of errors and maximize the likelihood of intercepting them when they occur (AcademyHealth 2004).

Patient satisfaction: A measurement that obtains reports or ratings from patients about services received from an organization (health plan), hospital, physician, or health provider (AHRQ 1999).

Peer review: The evaluation by practicing physicians or other professionals of the effectiveness and efficiency of services ordered or performed by other members of the profession (peers). Frequently, peer review refers to the review of research by other researchers (AHRQ 1999).

Performance-based pay (pay for performance): A program of financial incentives given to providers (hospitals and physicians) to improve quality and reduce cost, based on measured performance of selected indicators (Shortell and Kaluzny 2006).

Performance budgeting: A general agreement for funding in exchange for delivering certain services or products—where the funding level is tied to explicit performance results and quality indicators (such as utilization, average length of stay, staffing ratios, and infection rates) (Preker and Harding 2003, p. 50).

Performance gaps: Perceived discrepancies between expected and actual organizational performance. Performance gaps often trigger the innovation processes as organizational members look for new ideas or technologies to bridge the gap (Shortell and Kaluzny 2006).

Performance improvement: Encourages the use of evidence-based "best practices." In place of trial and error, it offers a systematic approach, and managers can use analytical techniques (Lande 2002) or the continuous study and adaptation of a health care organization's functions and processes to increase the probability of achieving desired outcomes and to better meet the needs of individuals and other users of services (Joint Commission 2006).

Performance management: The system, policies, and procedures used by an organization to define and monitor the work that people do, and to ensure that the tasks and priorities of employees support the mission and goals of the organization (MSH 2003).

Performance measures: Methods or instruments to estimate or monitor the extent to which the actions of a health care practitioner or provider conform to practice guidelines, medical review criteria, or standards of quality (AHRQ 1999).

Plausibility inference: Plausibility assessments go beyond adequacy assessments by trying to rule out external factors—confounding factors—which may have caused the observed effects. Plausibility assessments attempt to control for confounding factors by choosing control groups before an evaluation is begun, or afterward during the analysis of data (Habicht et al. 1999, p. 13).

Policy: A definite course or method of action selected from among alternatives and in light of given conditions to guide and determine present and future decisions; a high-level overall plan embracing the general goals and acceptable procedures especially of a government body (MWOD n.d.).

Prepayment: Usually refers to any payment to a provider for anticipated services (such as an expectant mother paying in advance for maternity care). Sometimes prepayment is distinguished from insurance as referring to payment to organizations which, unlike an insurance company, take responsibility for arranging for, and providing, needed services as well as paying for them (such as health maintenance organizations, prepaid group practices, and medical foundations) (AHRQ 1999).

Private health accounts (medical savings account): Allows or mandates people to place money in (tax-free) savings accounts to be used only for medical expenses, usually in conjunction with the purchase of a catastrophic stop-loss health insurance plan (EOHSP n.d.).

Private voluntary organization: See NGO.

Privatization: Involves the transfer of ownership and government functions from public to private bodies, which may consist of voluntary organizations and for-profit and not-for-profit private organizations. The degree of government regulation is variable (EOHSP n.d.).

Probability inference: Probability evaluations aim at ensuring that there is only a small known probability that the difference between program and control areas were due to confounding, bias, or to chance. These evaluations require randomization of treatment and control activities to the comparison groups. While randomization does not guarantee that all confounding is eliminated, it does ensure that the probability of confounding is measurable, being part of the error associated with the significance level used. Thus randomization assures that the statistical statement of association is directly related to the intervention. This means that the statement of statistical probability of such a "probability" evaluation relates directly to the causality of the intervention, and is not simply a statement that the comparison groups are different, as is the case for all other study designs (Habicht et al. 1999, p. 14).

Process improvement: Taking corrective action if results do not meet expectations; documenting processes, the way work should be done in the organization; measuring the results of that work, as seen by customers (WHO n.d. a).

Productivity: The volume of output per unit of input. Productivity is often conceived of as labor productivity: the volume of output per unit of labor input, other input factors assumed to be held constant (EOHSP n.d.).

Program: A (formal) set of procedures to conduct an activity, e.g. control of malaria (Last 2001, p. 144).

Project: A planned undertaking, such as a definitely formulated piece of research or a large, usually government-supported, undertaking (MWOD n.d.).

Property rights theory: In the context of changing views on the role of the state in the health sector, this theory is based on the assumption that private ownership appears to have strong positive incentives for efficiency. It has focused mainly on two issues: the possession of residual decision rights and the allocation of residual returns (Preker and Harding 2003, p. 35).

Public choice theory: In the context of changing views on the role of the state in the health sector, this theory is based on the assumption that all human behavior is dominated by self-interest. Individuals are viewed as rational utility maximizers (Preker and Harding 2003, p. 37).

Public-private partnerships: These are based on medium- to long-term contracts between a public sector contracting authority and a private sector provider for the delivery of specified public services, such as power, transport, water and sanitation, solid waste management, as well as education and health services (Dutz 2003).

Quality assurance: The activities and programs intended to provide adequate confidence that the quality of patient care will satisfy stated or implied requirements or needs (AHRQ 1999).

Quality circle: A volunteer group composed of workers who meet to discuss workplace improvement, and make presentations to management with their ideas. Typical topics are improving safety, product design, and manufacturing processes. Quality circles have the advantage of continuity; the circle remains intact from project to project.

Quality collaboratives: A collaborative brings together groups of practitioners from different health care organizations to work in a structured way to improve one aspect of the quality of service. It involves them in a series of meetings to learn about best practice in the area chosen, quality methods, and change ideas, and to share their experiences of making changes in their own setting (Ovretveit et al. 2002).

Quality control: The use of operational techniques and statistical methods to measure and predict quality (AHRQ 1999).

Quality improvement: The attainment or process of attaining a new level of performance or quality that is superior to any previous level of quality (AHRQ 1999). Also, an approach to the continuous study and improvement of the processes of providing health care services to meet the needs of individuals and others. Synonyms include continuous quality improvement, continuous improvement, organization-wide performance improvement, and total quality management (Joint Commission 2006).

Quality management system: See "Total quality management."

Quality planning: Intentional design of systems aimed at producing high quality (AHRQ 1999).

Quality design: A systematic approach to service design that identifies the key features needed or desired by both external and internal clients, creates design options for the desired features, and then selects the combination of options that will maximize satisfaction within available resources (QAP n.d.).

Randomized controlled trial: An epidemiological experiment in which subjects in a population are randomly allocated into groups, usually called study and control groups, to receive or not to receive an experimental preventive or therapeutic procedure, maneuver, or intervention. The results are assessed by rigorous comparison of rates of disease, death, recovery, or other appropriate outcome in the study and control groups (Last 2001, p. 150).

Redesign: The act of transforming processes of care in a health institution or, at the health systems level, a system transformation (AHRQ 1999).

Reengineering: The term is applied to many process and/or organizational development and process simplification methodologies. Business process reengineering is said to produce organizations that are better suited to the modern speed of communications and a better informed and educated public and work force. Business process reengineering is an organization and management philosophy (World Bank n.d. i).

Reflexive comparison: In the context of methodological approaches to assessing a reform's effects on hospital performance, this approach adopts the implicit assumption that the health organization's behavior and performance prior to the intervention would have continued unchanged, so that any differences are due to the reform (Preker and Harding 2003, p. 137).

Reform, funding, and payment: Payment reforms usually alter the structure of payments to tighten the link between resource allocation and delivery of specific outputs. Retrospective fee-for-service, per diem, or case-based payments are examples of such changes. Some reforms try to encourage efficiency by shifting expenditure risk onto providers via capitated payments or prospective global budgets. Different structural changes are made in funding and payment systems to address concerns about clinical or consumer quality or responsiveness to users. These payment reforms usually also tighten the link between resource allocation and user or payer selection. Examples include limited or fully competitive contracting with providers, fund holding with patient selection, and demand subsidies (health vouchers to be used with providers or insurers). None of these instruments is perfect (Preker and Harding 2003, p. 39).

Reform, management: These reforms have included efforts to strengthen the managerial expertise of health sector managers—both through staff training and through changes in recruitment policies to attract managerial skills. Commonly, these efforts are accompanied by improvements to information systems to facilitate effective decision making. Clinical directorates have been created in some systems, and benchmarking of departmental performance has been introduced (Preker and Harding 2003, p. 38). In the public sector, attempts are frequently made to introduce business-process reengineering, patient-focused care, or quality-improvement techniques. Private organizations have introduced recruitment and compensation policies, based on the best personnel management techniques for finding and motivating high performers (pp. 38–39).

Reforms, technological: Such reforms usually consist of targeted investment in medical equipment, or the computers, databases, and software needed to operate an effective management information system. The skills required to operate the equipment or systems are often lacking. Therefore, technological reforms often include a capacity development component, which supports training for relevant staff (Preker and Harding 2003, p. 37).

Regulation: Intervention by government, by means of rules, in health care markets or systems. Regarded as a stipulation of various standards and their enforcement (EOHCS 2000). Regulation, in the context of health services, is the range of factors exterior to the practice or administration of medical care that influences the behavior in delivering or using health services (World Bank n.d. j).

Relative risk: (a) The ratio of the risk of disease or death among the exposed to the risk among the unexposed; this usage is synonymous with *risk ratio*; (b) alternatively, the ratio of the cumulative incidence rate in the exposed to the cumulative incidence rate in the unexposed, i.e. the rate ratio; and (c) this term has also been used synonymously with *odds ratio*. The use of the term "relative risk" for several different quantities arises from the fact that for "rare" diseases (e.g. most cancers), all the quantities approximate one another. For common occurrences, the approximations do not hold (Last 2001, p. 156).

Report cards: Another reform toward improving public hospital services is the application of "report cards," which use citizen feedback to assess the performance of services (World Bank n.d. k).

Research: A class of activities designed to develop or contribute to generalizable knowledge. Such knowledge consists of theories, principles, or relationships, or the accumulation of information on which these are based, which can be corroborated by acceptable scientific methods of observation, inference, and/or experiment (Last 2001, pp. 157–8).

Residual revenue rights: In the context of residual rights of control, the owner has the right to whatever revenue remains after all funds have been collected and all debts, expenses, and other contractual obligations have been paid (Preker and Harding 2003, p. 34).

Residual claimant status: The organization's residual claimant status reflects its degree of financial responsibility—both its ability to keep savings and its responsibility for financial losses (debt). A hospital's residual claimant status is a key to incentive to generate savings and efficiency gains (Preker and Harding 2003, p. 225).

Residual rights of control: The rights to make any decisions regarding an asset's use that are not explicitly contracted by law or assigned to another by contract (Preker and Harding 2003, p. 34).

Risk: The probability that an event will occur—e.g. that an individual will become ill or die within a stated period of time or by a certain age. Also, a nontechnical term encompassing a variety of measures of the probability of a (generally) unfavorable outcome (Last 2001, p. 159).

Risk pooling: Forming a group so that individual risks can be shared among many people. Also, actors each facing possible large losses agree to contribute a small premium payment to a common pool, to be used to compensate whichever of them actually suffers the loss. Contributions must cover losses plus administration costs (WBI n.d.).

Scaling-up: A multidimensional process through which the impact of a program is broadened and deepened. Dimensions of scaling-up that have been identified include quantitative (physical replication); programmatic (new activities and programs); social (increasing the capacity of the community to engage in development activities, and mobilization of increasing numbers of local residents, including the vulnerable and marginalized); organizational (increasingly effective internal management and financial viability; and political (incorporation of the community-driven development approach by higher levels of government, and the direct entry of grassroots organizations into politics) (World Bank 2004).

Sectorwide approach (SWAp): A SWAp is an approach to organizing and financing a sector based on a comprehensive policy framework and program of work. Through negotiated process, the government works together with donors, NGOs, and other key stakeholders to plan and monitor progress. A SWAp implies a coordinated policy and national strategy with planning, implementation, and regular evaluation under the leadership of national government (Cassels 1997).

Separation of provider–payer reforms: In the context of reforming health care delivery systems, separation of provider–payer reforms include: technological reforms, which focus on enhancing the technological capacity of hospitals; management reforms, which include efforts to strengthen the managerial expertise of health sector managers; and funding and payment reforms, which serve to alter the structure of payments to tighten the link between resource allocation and delivery of specific outputs (Preker and Harding 2003, pp. 38–39).

Service agreement: Agreements that are not legally binding contracts, partly because networks, as public statutory bodies, have limited ability to decline or negotiate terms (Preker and Harding 2003, p. 384).

Service-profit chain: In the context of hospital human resource management, in this service-profit chain of causation, the service value is created by employee productivity, which is derived from employee loyalty. Loyalty is in turn the product of employee satisfaction, which results from the internal quality of work life. The service-profit chain grows in importance as a business becomes more service oriented since, by nature, hospital services require direct interaction between care providers and their patients (Preker and Harding 2003, p. 125).

Skill mix (skill mix and new workers): Determining the most effective mix of skills and workers to deliver care is a key requirement for cost-effective health care services. Skill mix has to be addressed as an issue of long-term change management, rather than a one-off "quick fix" (Buchan et al. 2000). New types of worker are being introduced into country health systems in response to consumer need and efficiency/effectiveness requirements. Many of these "new" workers are cadres developed from within current health professions with advanced and enhanced skills, such as family health doctors and nurse practitioners. Others are generic or "multiskilled" workers, as witnessed in Zambia (Chirwa 1996) and Ghana (Dovlo 1997).

Social functions: "Social functions" delivered by the hospital shift from being implicit and unfunded to specified and directly funded. As reforms motivate the hospital to focus more closely on financial viability, management will move to decrease output of services that do not at least pay for themselves. There are different views on how to define "social function." Reasonable people can disagree regarding the degree to which an individual hospital service can be considered a social function. Some would argue that all care for noninfectious disease is a "private good," because it benefits primarily the recipient, and anyone who does not pay for it can be inexpensively barred from consuming it. Others would counter that treatment of chronic disease among the poor fills the social function of providing a safety net for the most destitute. Still others argue that access to all health care services is a human right, which the government cannot morally deny any citizen. Despite these differences of view, a working consensus may be possible regarding a ranking of hospital services from least to most private. Organizational reform designers may use such a ranking to transfer services agreed to be primarily social functions to government health care services, regulate their production, or compartmentalize them within an administratively separate part of the hospital (thus insulating the rest of the hospital from their production costs). Useful indicators for characterizing this dimension of the intervention are whether or not the issue of protecting social functions has been addressed and, for each identified social function, the nature and degree of protection implemented (Preker and Harding 2003, pp. 120–122).

Social health insurance (or social insurance): Social health insurance (SHI) is a means of mobilizing resources for health care that many high- , middle-, and low-income countries use. The common term in use is "sickness fund." Although SHI has no uniform definition because of the variations that exist among the different countries that have adopted it, there are key characteristics that define such a system. One of them is that the compulsory nature of SHI in the countries that use it. In other words, SHI is usually a legally mandated means of health care financing. Another characteristic is its basis on employment or on individual contributions from payroll taxes (World Bank n.d. l).

Social marketing: A discipline that addresses an issue with a particular regard to those affected by it (the target audience), considering their perspective and perceived wants and needs to develop strategies toward change (CDC n.d.).

Span of control: A term originating in military organization theory, but used more commonly in business management, particularly human resource management, it describes the number of subordinates that report to each manager.

Statehood: The extent to which a government has effective control over its territory, is not excessively dependent on external or mineral resources, observes the constitution, is guided by the rule of law, and has stable and predictable institutions of government (Bloom et al. 2006).

Standard operating procedures: Management processes that describe chronological steps to follow and decisions to make in carrying out a task or function (QAP n.d.).

Statistical approach: In the context of approaches to assessing a reform's effects on hospital performance, when the detailed nature of the reform differs from hospital to hospital, this variation can be statistically analyzed to estimate the effect of each dimension of reform on measures of behavior and performance (Preker and Harding 2003, p. 138).

Strategy: A set of essential measures (preventive, therapeutic) believed to be sufficient to control health problems (Last 2001, p. 173). In the context of this research, a strategy involves greater complexity, number of components, levels of operation, or stakeholders than an intervention, and is less likely to be standardizable or replicable in detail.

Strategic management: Those aspects of management within a firm that link strategy analysis and planning to operational management (Shortell and Kaluzny 2006).

Strategic planning: A way to identify long-term goals and to direct the company (or organization) to fulfilling these goals. Strategic planning involves: assessing the current business environment; defining the company's mission; deciding what the business should look like in five years; recognizing the company's strengths, weaknesses, opportunities, and threats; and mapping out a course to take the company from its current to its desired position.

Stewardship: A function of government responsible for the welfare of the population, and concerned with the trust and legitimacy with which its activities are viewed by the citizenry (WHO 2000b). Stewardship, sometimes more narrowly defined as governance, refers to the wide range of functions carried out by governments as they seek to achieve national health policy objectives. In addition to improving overall levels of population health, objectives are likely to be framed in terms of equity, coverage, access, quality, and patients' rights. National policy may also define the relative roles and responsibilities of the public, private, and voluntary sectors—as well as civil society—in the provision and financing of health care (WHO n.d. b).

Supply chain management: The integrated management of business flows and information flows to manufacture, assemble, and distribute to the end customers a specific product, starting from raw materials, considering the international, and in particular, trade facilitation dimension of such transactions (Global Facilitation Partnership for Transportation and Trade n.d.).

Support supervision: Ensures high-quality health care delivery to patients and clients, enabling and supporting staff to practice robust evidence in an integrated way. It demonstrates how skills development occurs and helps practitioners demonstrate their competencies under the requirements.

Technical efficiency: Production of the maximum level of output given a specified level of input (AHRQ 1999).

Technological capacity: Defined by the following indicators: (a) globalization and information technology: how can the globalization and convergence of information and communications technologies work for everyone? (b) energy: how can growing energy demand be met safely and efficiently? and (c) science and technology: how can scientific and technological breakthroughs be accelerated to improve the human condition? (Glenn and Gordon 2001).

Total quality management: A continuous quality improvement management system directed from the top but empowering employees and focusing on systematic, not individual, employee problems (AHRQ 1999).

Transaction cost economics (TCE): Focuses on the distinctive features of activities organized within an organization, versus those organized through market interactions. TCE looks at questions such as: Why does a company buy some inputs, rather than producing them in-house? TCE analysis sheds the most light on firm boundaries and the conditions under which activities are best arranged within a hierarchy instead of through interactions in a market with suppliers or other contractors (Preker and Harding 2003, p. 131).

User fees: Charges for goods or services that the user, or patient, is required to pay (EOHSP n.d.).

Out-of-pocket payments: These payments include cost sharing as well as private expenditure for services not covered by the respective health plan (EOHSP n.d.).

Unintended consequences: The results of the actions of people, including that of government, that have unanticipated or unintended effects (Concise Encyclopedia of Economics Online n.d.).

Validity, measurement: An expression of the degree to which a measurement measures what it purports to measure (Last 2001, p. 184).

Validity, study: The degree to which the inference drawn from a study is warranted, when account is taken of the study methods, the representativeness of the study sample, and the nature of the population from which it is drawn (Last 2001, p. 184).

Vouchers: Voucher schemes enable donors to purchase outputs rather than inputs while offering beneficiaries a choice of provider, a feature that sets them apart from other output-based approaches, such as supply-side subsidies to providers operating under performance-based contracts. Choice creates incentives to lower prices or raise quality (or both) (Sandiford et al. 2002).

References

AcademyHealth. *Glossary of Terms Commonly Used in Health Care*. 2004. http://www.academyhealth.org/publications/glossary.pdf, accessed August 3, 2006.

Agency for Healthcare Research and Quality (AHRQ). *Health Care Quality Glossary*. 1999. http://www.ahrq.gov/qual/hcqgloss.pdf, accessed August 3, 2006.

Bloom, Gerry, Hilary Standing, and Anu Joshi. 2006. "Institutional Arrangements and Health Service Delivery in Low Income Countries," World Bank, Washington, DC. (Background paper for chapter 6 of this book.)

Buchan, James, J. Ball, and F. O'May. 2000. "Skill Mix in the Health Workforce." Issues in Health Services Delivery, Discussion Paper No. 3. Department of Organisation of Health Services Delivery, WHO, Geneva.

Cassels, A. 1997. *A Guide to Sector-wide Approaches for Health Development: Concepts, Issues and Working Arrangements*. Geneva: WHO.

Centre for Evidence-Based Medicine. n.d. "Glossary of EBM Terms." http://www.cebm.utoronto.ca/glossary/index.htm#e, accessed January 10, 2009.

Centers for Disease Control and Prevention (CDC). n.d. "Glossary." http://www.cdc.gov/od/ocphp/nphpsp/documents/glossary.pdf, accessed August 3, 2006.

CDC Committee for Community Engagement. "Executive Summary." 1995. http://www.cdc.gov/phppo/pce/exec.htm, accessed August 3, 2006.

Concise Encyclopedia of Economics Online. n.d. http://www.econlib.org/library/Enc/UnintendedConsequences.html, accessed August 3, 2006.

Chirwa, B. 1996. "HRD and Health Reforms: The Zambian Experience." In *Workshop on Human Resources and Health Sector Reforms*, ed. J. Martinez and T. Martineau. Liverpool, United Kingdom: Liverpool School of Tropical Medicine.

Citizen Report Cards: A Presentation on Methodology. 2003. http://info. worldbank.org/etools/docs/library/94360/Tanz_0603/Ta_0603/CitizenRe portCardPresentation.pdf, accessed August 3, 2006.

Dovlo, D. 1997. "Health Sector Reform and Deployment, Training and Motivation of Human Resources towards Equity in Health Care: Issues and Concerns in Ghana." *Human Resources for Health Development Journal* 1(3).

Dutz, M. 2003. "PPP Systems for Good Governance of Public Service Provision: A Menu of Support Options for Contract Design, Bidding and Monitoring." http://info.worldbank.org/etools/docs/library/86466/ses2.1_ pppsystemsgoodgov.pdf, accessed August 2, 2006.

Economy Professor. n.d. http://www.economyprofessor.com/economictheories/ aa-theory.php, accessed August 16, 2006.

European Observatory on Health Systems and Policies (EOHSP). n.d. "Glossary." http://www.euro.who.int/observatory/Glossary/TopPage?term=1, accessed August 3, 2006.

European Observatory on Health Care Systems (EOHCS). 2000. "Care Systems in Transition (HiT): Template." WHO Regional Office for Europe, Copenhagen.

Furman, B. 1990. "When Failure is Success: Implementation and Madisonian Government." In *Implementation and the Policy Process: Opening Up the Black Box*, ed. D.J. Palumbo and D.J. Calista. Westport: Greenwood Press.

Getzen, T.E. 1997. *"Health Economics": Fundamentals & Flow of Funds.* Chichester, United Kingdom: John Wiley & Sons.

Global Facilitation Partnership for Transportation and Trade. n.d. *Facilitation and Supply Chain Management.* http://www.gfptt.org/Entities/TopicProfile. aspx?tid=d584aa74-efdb-4b04-b463-3c5ab6416c68, accessed August 3, 2006.

Glenn, Jerome C., and Theodore J. Gordon. 2001. *2001 State of the Future.* Washington, DC: American Council for the United Nations University.

Habicht, J.P., C.G. Victora, and J.P. Vaughan. 1999. "Evaluation Designs for Adequacy, Plausibility, and Probability of Public Health Programme Performance and Impact." *International Journal of Epidemiology* 28: 10–18.

Humanitarian Accountability Partnership (HAP). 2006. http://www.hapinterna tional.org, accessed August 3, 2006.

Joint Commission. *Glossary of Terms for Health Care Staffing.* 2006. http://www. jointcommission.org/CertificationPrograms/HealthCareStaffingServices/ glossary.htm, accessed August 3, 2006.

Kaufmann, D., A. Kray, and M. Mastruzzi. 2008. "Governance Matters VII: Aggregate and Individual Governance Indicators, 1996–2007." World Bank Policy Research Working Paper 4654, World Bank, Washington, DC.

Krishna, A. 2004. "Partnerships between Elected Local Governments and Community-based Organizations: Exploring the Scope for Synergy." Social Development Paper No. 52, World Bank, Washington, DC, accessed August 3, 2006.

Lande, R. E. 2002. "Performance Improvement: Population Reports." Series J, No. 52. The Johns Hopkins Bloomberg School of Public Health, Population Information Program, Baltimore, accessed August 3, 2006,

Last, J.M. 2001. *A Dictionary of Epidemiology*. (4th ed.) New York: Oxford University Press.

Management Sciences for Health (MSH). 2003. *Human Resource Management: Rapid Assessment Tool for HIV/AIDS Environments: Toolkit. A Guide for Strengthening HRM Systems*. Boston. http://erc.msh.org/toolkit/, accessed August 3, 2006, October 30, 2006, and January 10, 2009.

Meinzen-Dick, R., A. Knox, and M. Di Gregorio, eds. 2001. "Collective Action, Property Rights and Devolution of Natural Resource Management: Exchange of Knowledge and Implications for Policy." Feldafing, Germany: Zentralstelle fur Ernaehrung und Landwirtschaft (ZEL), Food and Agriculture Development Centre (DSE).

Merriam-Webster Online Dictionary (MWOD). n.d. http://www.m-w.com/dictionary/, accessed August 3, 2006.

Merry, P. 1998. "Pocket Guide to the NHS." The National Health Service (NHS) Confederation, Birmingham, United Kingdom.

Organisation for Economic Co-operation and Development (OECD). n.d. "Glossary of Statistical Terms." http://stats.oecd.org/glossary/, accessed January 10, 2009.

Ovretveit, J., et al. 2002 "Quality Collaboratives: Lessons from Research." *Quality and Safety in Health Care* 11: 345–351.

Ovretveit, J., D. Peters, B. Siadat, and A. Thota. 2006. "Strengthening Health Services in Low Income Countries: Lessons from a Review of Research," World Bank, Washington, DC. (Background paper for chapter 1 of this book.)

Patrinos, H. A. 2001. "Mechanisms for enhanced equity: Demand-side financing." http://ifcln1.ifc.org/ifcext/CHEPublication.nsf/6d82f1255172104a%208525 6bdd006631e8/b8d97e830bb3bad185256c0f0071fa4a/$FILE/CIES%20demand.pdf, accessed August 3, 2006.

Porteous, D., and B. Helms. 2005. "Focus Note: Protecting Micro Finance Borrowers." Consultative Group to Assist the Poor. http://www.cgap.org/portal/binary/com.epicentric.contentmanagement.servlet.ContentDeliverySe rvlet/Documents/FocusNote_27.pdf, accessed August 3, 2006.

Preker, A. S., and A. Harding, eds. 2003. *Innovations in Health Service Delivery: The Corporatization of Public Hospitals*. New York: World Bank.

Quality Assurance Project (QAP). n.d. "Methods & Tools, QA Resources, A Glossary of Useful Terms." http://qaproject.org/methods/resglossary.html, accessed August 3, 2006.

Rossett, A., and J. Gautier-Downs. 1991. *A Handbook of Job Aids*. San Diego, CA: Pfeiffer.

Ruster, J., C. Yamamoto, and K. Rogo. 2003. "Franchising in Health: Emerging Models, Experiences, and Challenges in Primary Care." *Public Policy for the Private Sector*, No. 263. World Bank, Washington, DC. http://rru.world bank.org/Documents/PublicPolicyJournal/263Ruste-063003.pdf, accessed 2006.

Sandiford, P., A. Gorter, and M. Salvetto. 2002. "Vouchers for Health: Using Voucher Schemes for Output-based AID." *Public Policy for the Private Sector*, 243, World Bank, Washington, DC, accessed August 3, 2006.

Shortell, S.M., and A.D. Kaluzny, eds. 2006. *Health Care Management: Organizational Design and Behavior* (5th ed.). New York: Thompson Delmar Learning.

Shriberg, A., L., D. Shriberg, and R. Kumari. 2005. *Practicing Leadership: Principals and Applications* (3rd ed.). New Jersey: John Wiley & Sons, Inc.

Social Enterprise Development Center, Inc. "Community Mobilization." http://www.sedc.org.pk/portal/general/theme_desc.php?themeid=44, accessed August 3, 2006.

United Nations, European Commission, International Monetary Fund, Organisation for Economic Co-operation and Development, and World Bank. 2005. "Handbook of National Accounting: Integrated Environmental and Economic Accounting." Studies in Methods, Series F, No.61, Rev.1, Glossary, United Nations, New York, para. 1.87.

United States Department of Labor. n.d. http://www.dol.gov/dol/allcfr/Title_ 20/Part_632/20CFR632.4.htm, accessed August 3, 2006.

Wanke, M.I., L.D. Saunders, R.W. Pong, and W.J.B. Church. 1995. *Building a Stronger Foundation: A Framework for Planning and Evaluating Community-based Services in Canada*. Ottawa: Health Promotion and Programs Branch, Health Canada. Available at: http://www.hc-sc.gc.ca/hcs-sss/pubs/hhrhs/ 1995-build-plan-commun/index-eng.php.

Witter, S., and T. Ensor, eds. 1997. *An Introduction to Health Economics for Eastern Europe and the Former Soviet Union*. Chichester, United Kingdom: John Wiley & Sons.

World Bank. 1998. "Health Reform Online: Glossary." http://www.worldbank. org/hsr/class/module1/index.htm.

———. 2004. *Zambia: Issues of Scaling up in Peri-urban Areas*. Social Development Notes 97, World Bank, Washington, DC, accessed August 3, 2006.

————. Forthcoming. "A Systematic Review of Community Empowerment Strategies for Health in Low- and Middle-income Countries." Washington, DC.

————. n.d. a. "Health Systems & Financing: Autonomization/Corporatization." http://go.worldbank.org/1A0ANK1UF0, accessed January 18, 2009.

————. n.d. b. "Labor Toolkit Glossary." http://rru.worldbank.org/documents/toolkits/labor/toolkit/glossary.html, accessed August 3, 2006.

————. n.d. c. "Community Driven Development." http://go.worldbank.org/24K8IHVVS0, accessed January 18, 2009.

————. n.d. d. "Community Driven Development: Community Mobilization and Capacity Building." http://go.worldbank.org/39USEU8W91, accessed January 18, 2009.

————. n.d. e. "Competence." http://go.worldbank.org/1A0ANK1UF0, accessed January 18, 2009.

————. n.d. f. "Health Systems & Financing: Decentralization." http://go.worldbank.org/1A0ANK1UF0, accessed January 18, 2009.

————. n.d. g. "Health Systems & Financing: Decentralization." http://go.worldbank.org/1A0ANK1UF0, accessed January 18, 2009.

————. n.d. h. "Social Analysis: Glossary of Key Terms." http://go.worldbank.org/HSXB13LCA0, accessed January 18, 2009.

————. n.d. i. "Administrative & Civil Service Reform: Functional Reviews & Reengineering." http://go.worldbank.org/LCFM2RV5E0, accessed January 18, 2009.

————. n.d. j. "Health Systems & Financing: Regulation." http://go.worldbank.org/1A0ANK1UF0, accessed January 10, 2009.

————. n.d. k. "Health Systems & Financing: Hospitals." http://go.worldbank.org/1A0ANK1UF0, accessed January 18, 2009.

————. n.d. l. "Health Systems & Financing: Social Insurance." http://go.worldbank.org/1A0ANK1UF0, accessed January 18, 2009.

World Bank HNPStats. n.d. http://go.worldbank.org/N2N84RDV00, accessed 2007.

World Bank Institute (WBI). n.d. "The Flagship Program on Health Sector Reform and Sustainable Financing." http://www.worldbank.org/wbi/healthflagship/about.html.

World Health Organization (WHO). n.d. a. Management Effectiveness Program. http://www.emro.who.int/mei/mep/Process.htm, accessed August 3, 2006.

————. n.d. b. "Stewardship." http://www.who.int/healthsystems/topics/stewardship/en/index.html, accessed August 3, 2006.

————. 1998. "Terminology: A Glossary of Technical Terms on the Economics and Finance of Health Services." Regional Office for Europe (document EUR/ICP/CARE0401/CN01).

————. 2000a. "Health Futures: Glossary." http://www.who.int/terminology/ter/ Health_futures.html. Geneva.

————. 2000b. *The World Health Report 2000. Health Systems: Improving Performance.* http://www.who.int/health-systems-performance/whr2000.htm.

————. 2003. *Vaccines and Biologicals.* "Health Sector Reform (HSR): The Impact of Health Sector Development on Immunization Services." http://whqlibdoc. who.int/hq/2003/WHO_V&B_03.21.pdf, accessed August 3, 2006.

————. 2004. "World Report on Knowledge for Better Health: Strengthening Health Systems," pp. 14–15, Geneva.

Index

Boxes, figures, notes, and tables are indicated by b, f, n, and t following the page number.

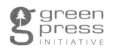